Jonas Salk

JONAS SALK

A Life

Charlotte DeCroes Jacobs

OXFORD
UNIVERSITY PRESS

OXFORD
UNIVERSITY PRESS

Oxford University Press is a department of the
University of Oxford. It furthers the University's objective
of excellence in research, scholarship, and education
by publishing worldwide.

Oxford   New York
Auckland   Cape Town   Dar es Salaam   Hong Kong   Karachi
Kuala Lumpur   Madrid   Melbourne   Mexico City   Nairobi
New Delhi   Shanghai   Taipei   Toronto

With offices in
Argentina   Austria   Brazil   Chile   Czech Republic   France   Greece
Guatemala   Hungary   Italy   Japan   Poland   Portugal   Singapore
South Korea   Switzerland   Thailand   Turkey   Ukraine   Vietnam

Oxford is a registered trade mark of Oxford University Press
in the UK and certain other countries.

Published in the United States of America by
Oxford University Press
198 Madison Avenue, New York, NY 10016

© Charlotte DeCroes Jacobs 2015

Library of Congress Cataloging-in-Publication Data
Jacobs, Charlotte.
Jonas Salk : a life / Charlotte DeCroes Jacobs.
pages   cm
Includes bibliographical references and index.
ISBN 978-0-19-933441-4 (hardback)
1. Salk, Jonas, 1914–1995.   2. Virologists–United States–Biography.
3. Poliomyelitis—United States—History.   4. Poliomyelitis—Vaccination—
United States—History.   5. Poliomyelitis vaccine—History.
6. Influenza vaccines—History.   7. AIDS vaccines.   I. Title.
QR31.S25J33   2015
579.2092—dc23
[B]
2014040267

1 3 5 7 9 8 6 4 2

Printed in the United States of America
on acid-free paper

To my husband, Rod

Unless otherwise indicated, all quotations are taken from interviews conducted by the author between June 2004 and May 2013.

Contents

Jonas Salk

Two Plagues

IN THE SUMMER of 1916, New York's playgrounds stood empty. No children splashed in public swimming pools; none sold lemonade on the sidewalks. No cats roamed the alleys, peering into garbage cans. Troops of sanitary workers in white uniforms hosed down the city streets. Fathers hurried home from work, fear imprinted on their faces, averting their glances from the tiny wooden caskets lined up outside the tenements. Policemen patrolled the streets. New York was a city under siege.[1]

Poliomyelitis had crept into Brooklyn while the public was busy watching the war unfold in Europe. It smoldered for a while between Henry Street and Seventh Avenue. Health officials barely paid attention, assuming it would soon die out. But it didn't. When the press began to attach names and faces to the disease, the community became alarmed. Helen Downing, paralyzed just before graduation from Public School no. 134, received her diploma in bed.[2] After five-year-old Frederick Chaplin made his kindergarten's honor roll, his brother took him to Coney Island. Five days later, he was dead.[3]

Before long, the names and faces gave way to numbers, and they kept escalating. On June 28, Health Commissioner Haven Emerson announced that Brooklyn might be experiencing an epidemic. Although a scientist had identified the poliovirus eight years earlier, no one knew how it spread. Assuming it behaved like other contagious diseases, the commissioner ordered every family bearing a case quarantined. A placard was placed in the window; bed linens and clothing were disinfected; windows were screened to prevent flies from disseminating the disease. Street cleaners worked overtime to collect garbage and cleanse tenement halls and stairwells. Stray cats, suspected of harboring the virus, were rounded up and exterminated—seventy-two thousand by summer's end. The commissioner closed playgrounds and banned children from theaters. He instructed parents to keep food covered and to wash their youngsters' noses and throats with saltwater daily. But filth and flies and cats had nothing to do with the spread of poliomyelitis, and even with these precautions, more children contracted the disease.

The illness started innocently enough—a sore throat, a runny nose.[4] At the end of the day, the child spiked a fever, became restless. Then the pains began—electric shocks that darted through the back, legs, neck, and shoulders. Muscles twitched, and spasms twisted him into a peculiar posture, the shoulders pulled forward, hips rotated, toes pointing downward. All night, the child thrashed about in his bed, drenched in sweat; his face became pallid. When the fever broke, he appeared to be recovering—a deceitful interlude as poliovirus left the bloodstream and invaded the nervous system.

Within a day or two, paralysis struck as abruptly as the fever had, and no one could predict the nature of its onslaught—a weak leg which improved in a few days or an arm dangling useless forever. Poliomyelitis impaired motor control of either one muscle or a group of muscles, yet it left sensation intact. The puzzled child could feel his feet but not move them. Three-quarters of those afflicted survived, many condemned to life in a wheelchair, on crutches, or in bed. They joined a generation of cripples.

If the poliovirus attacked the nervous system higher up, in the base of the brain, death soon followed. Paralyzed throat muscles impeded swallowing. A sip of water streamed out the youngster's nose or drained into his windpipe, causing him to sputter and cough. Unable to swallow saliva, he foamed at the mouth. Breathing gave way to gurgling. As his mother wiped the blood-tinged froth from his lips, he gasped for air, drowning in his own secretions. The struggle over, his eyes rolled back, followed by a few muscle jerks, and the mother held her lifeless child.

Poliomyelitis seemed to have a predilection for striking infants and toddlers. During the second week of July, 412 new cases were reported in New York; the next week, 712. Terrorized parents watched the figures more closely than the stock market. The disease erupted in Staten Island, Manhattan, the Bronx; it didn't distinguish between immigrants and the upper class. Those who could fled. Mothers swarmed into Grand Central Station and the ferry docks, dragging their children into the crowds they should have avoided. The exodus of almost 1,200 children a day halted when towns began to bar them. In Hoboken, New Jersey, guards patrolled city entrances. Policemen blocked 150 families trying to enter Hastings-on-Hudson. Distraught, they returned to New York, where the death toll continued to rise.

Families unable to afford medical assistance at home were ordered to deliver their infected children to Brooklyn's Kingston Avenue Hospital for Contagious Diseases, where they were held in isolation for eight weeks. Prohibited from visiting, parents heard stories of hallways lined with metal cribs, children crying out in pain or pleading for water with no one to hold them. A knock at the door and a telegram notified parents to come retrieve their child's body. When parents looked up at the dark, looming fortress of Kingston Avenue Hospital, many turned away, hiding their youngsters at home. But once a public health nurse discovered a poliomyelitis case in a neighborhood, the Sanitary Squad conducted a house-to-house search for others. Watching a policeman snatch a child from her mother's arms reminded some of the pogroms that they had fled.

By August, every isolation bed in New York was occupied; many held three children. A baby died approximately every two and a half hours. Fear, bordering on hysteria, permeated the city. Then, when the weather turned cool, poliomyelitis disappeared just as unexpectedly as it had come. In America's first major poliomyelitis epidemic, the poliovirus had infected approximately 8,900 in New York, leaving 2,400 dead and many of the remainder paralyzed. Nationwide it had afflicted twenty-seven thousand, mostly children under five years of age. For the next forty years, the carefree spirit of summertime was marred by the specter of this disease, now known simply as polio.

❖

TWO YEARS LATER, another disease ravaged New York—influenza.[5] In 1917, with the country preparing to join the war in Europe, reports of a few cases sounded no alarm. Outbreaks occurred every winter. Characterized by fever, muscle aches, and intense exhaustion, the disease usually ebbed in a week, posing a threat mainly to the elderly and infirm. But in the fall of 1918, influenza metamorphosed into a vicious monster. With no warning, a previously healthy person complained of an excruciating headache, like a demon pounding his temples with a hammer, stabbing his eyes. A temperature spike up to 105 degrees ushered in agonizing muscle pains, profuse sweating, and shaking chills. When the fever broke and relief seemed at hand, the coughing began. Mild at first, the cough deepened; the sputum turned bloody. A viscous fluid filled the lungs, and the patient gasped for breath, suffocating. No longer did it prey on the elderly; they seemed to be immune. Instead, this virulent form of influenza picked young, healthy adults as its victims.

No one was prepared for its fury. Initially the military was the hardest hit as overcrowded camps and close quarters aboard ships favored its rapid transmission. In September, more than twelve thousand soldiers at Camp Devens, outside Boston, contracted influenza. Before long, it spread to civilian populations. As the point of embarkation for troops, New York felt the brunt of the disease early on. The city came to a standstill as taxi drivers, telephone operators, and teachers lay ill. Garbage went uncollected, mail undelivered. When news got out that Franklin D. Roosevelt lay near death, it became clear that this disease ignored socioeconomic boundaries. Trying to allay the growing panic, the New York health commissioner, Royal Copeland, issued positive reports—"no reason for alarm" and "disease on wane."[6] Newspapers reported otherwise: fifty thousand flu masks dispensed by the Red Cross, an acute nursing shortage, mansions converted into temporary hospitals.

Although the responsible microbe had not been identified, the New York City Health Department designed a control plan based on its experience with tuberculosis. This plan staggered business hours to diminish crowding on subways and elevated trains, suspended book circulation in public libraries, and encouraged theaters to sell only half their tickets, leaving a seat empty between patrons. An amendment to the Sanitary Code directed people to cover their mouths when coughing and noses when sneezing; spitting became a misdemeanor. Despite these measures, death notices filled the newspapers. Pictures of stalwart-looking young men in uniform and glowing young brides in wedding gowns added poignancy to the printed words. On October 12, in a defiant demonstration of patriotism, President Wilson and a crowd of twenty-five thousand paraded down New York's "Avenue of the Allies."[7] The next week, 2,100 New Yorkers succumbed to influenza.

Apprehension and grief pervaded the city. No one knew who harbored the influenza germ or who might fall ill; but everyone knew someone who had died. And there was no place to hide. Even if one had the means, leaving New York proved futile, since influenza was engulfing the country, terrorizing even the smallest towns. With no effective treatment, physicians felt helpless. This contagion was overwhelming the nursing force; many of the young and healthiest had already perished. If a visiting nurse was spotted on a street, a crowd surrounded her, begging for help. Desperate to ward off the illness, people wore camphor balls; others had their teeth extracted, believing they harbored the germs that caused influenza. Home remedies proliferated: red peppers, strychnine, whiskey, chloroform—all to no avail.

By the first week of November 1918, the death toll in New York reached 12,357.[8] The deluge of patients swamped the wards and hallways of every hospital. Covered in white except for their eyes and hands, nurses resembled angels, or ghosts, moving through a sea of the ill—groaning, writhing, struggling to breathe. Photographs from the time reveal makeshift infirmaries set up in armories, gymnasiums, and dancehalls, with hundreds of cots lined up, each occupied by a body—some alive, some still. Obituaries listed entire families dead. The air reeked of decaying flesh as days passed before a death cart collected the deceased. Undertakers ran out of coffins; packed morgues closed their doors. Two thousand corpses lay unburied in Queens until sanitary workers came to assist the gravediggers.

In desperation, some families buried their own. In a matter of months, an estimated twenty-one thousand New York children became orphans.[9]

Influenza traveled around the world with ferocity. Daily, the number of dead from the contagion almost equaled the tally of war casualties. The November 11, 1918, celebration over Germany's surrender was tempered by the scourge, which continued to stalk young adults worldwide. By the spring of 1919, the disease had run its course, killing more than thirty-three thousand in New York, 850,000 in the United States, twenty million worldwide. And still no one knew what microbe had massacred a generation or how to prevent its horrifying return.

※

BORN ON OCTOBER 28, 1914, in East Harlem, Jonas Salk was just a child when these two plagues preyed upon New York. Spared, he would one day play a major role in the prevention of both. Salk's work on the influenza vaccine would go largely unrecognized. His polio vaccine, however, would catapult him into a world of celebrity from which he could never extricate himself. When a waiting world learned on April 12, 1955, that his vaccine could prevent poliomyelitis, Salk, just forty years old, became a hero overnight. Born in a New York tenement and humble in manner, he had all the makings of a twentieth-century icon—a knight in a white coat. He had not anticipated the backlash from the scientific community, the one group whose adulation he craved. With the public awaiting his next medical triumph and his laurels tarnished by a cadre of academic naysayers, Jonas Salk had half a lifetime to prove himself.

Born to Serve

JONAS SALK'S MOTHER told him he had been born with a caul.[1] She said it meant he had special powers, that he was destined for greatness. And he believed her. "As I look back on my beginnings," Salk said when interviewed in his later years, "I'm aware of the influence my family had on me, my parents especially, and the circumstances that existed in the world at that time."[2] He revered his ancestors. None had leapt to fame; none had a brilliance that shone above others. Ordinary men and women, they worked hard, raised large families, and kept the faith. They were Russian Jews.[3] As their story unfolded, it sounded like a tale of persecution. To Salk, theirs was a story of perseverance.

◈

SALK'S MOTHER, DORA PRESS, came from Minsk.[4] Her grandparents, Elchana and Nachama Epstein, had raised their three daughters under the shadow of Tsar Nicholas I, a rigid, small-minded military man who loathed ethnic diversity. Most Jews lived in shtetls, or small towns, several families squeezed into one wooden shack. They heard themselves called *zhid*, a derogatory term for a Jew, connoting an enemy of Christ. Nicholas I forbade use of Yiddish in public documents and censored or destroyed Jewish books. Elchana owned a tavern where his two younger daughters met their husbands, soldiers in the Russian army, likely conscripted to meet the Jewish quota. His eldest daughter, Leah, born in 1849, married Hyman Moses Press, a dairy salesman also from Minsk. None of the family remembers how many children they had, only that eight survived. Dora, born in 1890, was their sixth.

The Presses raised their children during the reign of Alexander II, who tolerated the Jews and improved their status. A photograph from the late 1800s depicts the Presses as thriving, the six daughters in well-fitted dresses with puffed sleeves and cross-stitching, the two sons in frilly shirts and cutaway coats with watch bobs. Although the Press family fared better than most, life in Minsk was harsh, especially after a bomb killed Alexander II and his son took the throne.

Tsar Alexander III abhorred the Jews and renounced his father's reforms. One month into his reign, Russian youths looted the town of Elisavetgrad, destroying most of the businesses and homes of its fifteen thousand Jews. Streets were littered with smashed furniture and the bodies of children, men, and women, many of whom had been raped. A new vehicle for annihilation of the Jews had emerged: the pogrom, an organized massacre perpetrated by a mob of civilians. Over the next eight months, 160 villages and cities heard the dreaded cry—"death to the Jews."[5] The Jewish community hoped for relief in 1894 when Alexander III died from kidney failure. But his son and successor, Nicholas II, was weak and wavering. During his reign, atrocities intensified.

At the beginning of the twentieth century, weary from burying their slaughtered neighbors, one of every seven Russian Jews emigrated. And there was one place most wanted to go. "America was in everybody's mouth," a young Jewish woman wrote. "Businessmen talked of it over their accounts; the market women made up their quarrels that they might discuss it from stall to stall; people who had relatives in the famous land went around reading letters for the enlightenment of less fortunate folks [and] children played at emigrating....All talked of it, but scarcely anybody knew one true fact about this magic land."[6] Dora's older sister, Jennie, was the first in the Press family to emigrate. She and her husband left Russia in the mid-1890s. Her brothers, Joseph and Harry, followed. Joseph set up a dairy in Harlem and wrote his father suggesting he join him. Hyman Press immigrated to the United States in 1898 through Montreal and, as soon as he saved enough money, sent for Leah and his five other daughters. At age thirteen, Dora Press came to America.

The family settled on the Lower East Side among thousands of Jewish immigrants—the American version of shtetl living.[7] Tenement buildings filled every block, making it the most densely populated area in New York. Six or seven floors high, each tenement housed three hundred or more. Up rickety stairs, down a narrow dark hallway, a typical flat featured a parlor, living room, and one or two bedrooms in a line with all the light and air coming from the only room that had windows. Renters shared one water closet on each floor and privies behind the building. With the babble from shoppers, haggling in Yiddish and broken English; hungry babies crying; drays rumbling through the crowded streets, a moment of quiet was as rare as a breath of fresh air. Smells from communal sweat, overflowing privies, and rotting garbage were stifling. Although upper-floor apartments provided relief from the stench, climbing six flights of stairs challenged even the healthiest. The immigrants of the Lower East Side may have lived in appalling conditions, yet they slept without the fear of being rousted out of their beds and butchered.

The Press family persevered. Dora received no formal education, and although she learned to speak English and sign her name, she could read only Yiddish. To help support the family she worked in the garment industry, as did many female Jewish immigrants. Packed into overcrowded, poorly lit, unventilated rooms, these girls and women spent twelve hours a day bent over foot-powered sewing machines. They considered themselves fortunate to bring home four to seven dollars a week. But Dora didn't remain a sweatshop underling for long. Sharp-witted and with innate managerial skills, she became a foreman at age sixteen. Her father's naturalization card listed her as a "draper."

By 1910, the family earned enough to relocate to Harlem, known as "the aristocratic Jewish neighborhood of New York" because of its private homes.[8] Where the Presses lived, however, on East 110th Street between Central Park and the East River, tenements were springing up as tens of thousands migrated from the Lower East Side. Dora, her parents, and four other family members shared a small apartment. Although they lived in close quarters, they were moving up. Hyman Press achieved US citizenship that year, and the family never looked back. They considered America their home. A photograph from around 1913, taken at Leah and Hyman's anniversary party in a New York hotel, portrays a prosperous family of twenty-six. The men wear tuxedos, the women gowns covered with lace; none look underfed. A tall, good-looking man with thick, dark hair and a beautiful curve to his nose stands in the back row next to Dora. His smile sets him apart from the others. This is Daniel Salk, Dora's husband. They had married on December 21, 1912, both twenty-three at the time.

The Salk family had come from Lithuania, where they, too, suffered under the rule of the Russian tsars. In the late 1800s, Harris and Sophie Salk immigrated to New York, where they raised seven children. Daniel, born in 1890, was the oldest. An accomplished seamstress, Sophie passed on her talent to her children. Her daughter Murial sewed fine clothes for some of New York's wealthiest families, and Daniel, with only an elementary school education, became a superb lace maker and designer of women's neckwear.

Years later, family members puzzled over the attraction between Daniel and Dora. He was a natural-born American; she was an immigrant. He wasn't particularly bright, whereas she was smart and far from demure. Standing over six feet, Daniel looked dapper in his well-cut suit and fedora, a striking figure. Dora barely reached his shoulders. As a young woman, she appeared trim and stylish, but that didn't last. "Dora had the Press somatotype," her grandniece Harriet Press Brown said, "heavy-set, squat women, all five-feeters."[9] The two differed in temperament, as well. A gentle, placid man, Daniel stopped to talk with people on the street. Dora had no time for pleasantries.

Initially the newlyweds lived on the Lower East Side. When Dora became pregnant, she insisted they move to East Harlem to be near her family. The Presses had an incredible drive to become middle class. Although they came to America with nothing, they all acquired trades. And they appreciated the value of an education. Harriet Press Brown remembered her mother pointing out an inscription on Julia Richman High School on East 67th Street: "Knowledge Will Set You Free." "This was the theme in my family," Harriet said.[10] Eventually the Presses counted a large number of physicians, professors, and social workers among their descendants.

The siblings' lives centered on family—Shabbat dinners, bar mitzvahs, marriages, and funerals. Of Dora's five sisters, Fannie married well and was generous with relatives; her only child died at age thirteen. Rachel married her cousin, against her parents' wishes, and moved to Connecticut, the only sibling to leave the family circle. In her twenties, Rose died, leaving a one-year-old son. Dora's father succumbed to tuberculosis five years after he obtained US citizenship. Her mother lived with her and Daniel until she died from complications of diabetes seven years later. As the Press siblings had their own children, the get-togethers got larger. Yet it was always the Presses; Dora and Daniel seldom spent time with the Salk family.

※

THE FOURTEENTH YEAR of the twentieth century was a momentous one: The assassination of Austria's Archduke Ferdinand and his wife touched off a world war; the first passenger ship crossed the Panama Canal; a Belgian surgeon gave the first successful blood transfusion. That same year, the air conditioner was patented; Babe Ruth pitched his first professional game; and Paramount Pictures was formed. New literary works included Carl Sandburg's "Chicago" and James Joyce's *Dubliners*. And on October 28, 1914, Dora and Daniel Salk had their first child. They named him Jonas.

Dora persuaded Daniel to move from East Harlem to the Bronx. Their ground-floor apartment on Elsmere Place was four blocks from Crotona Park with its grassy knolls and native hickory, tulip, and sweet gum trees. A three-acre natural lake provided refuge for ducks and turtles. Seven blocks away was Bronx Park with its botanical gardens and zoo. Traveling libraries made books readily available. Dora had chosen an idyllic place to raise her son.

Jonas was a gentle child, docile like his father.[11] But it was his mother who molded him from the start. He described his early years as "the life of an only child, having full attention of a doting, controlling mother who wanted to be sure that her child is protected and will grow up to be a worthwhile person."[12] Stressing his education, Dora made certain her son learned to read early on. "Jonas was always in a book," recalled a relative.[13] When his cousin Helen coaxed him out to play tag or hide-and-seek, she occasionally extracted a laugh from Jonas. Although Salk's early childhood could have been tainted by the events surrounding it—a world war, a major outbreak of poliomyelitis, and the Great Influenza epidemic—all before he turned five, Jonas grew up unscathed, largely due to the efforts of his mother.

Thin, with a mop of curly hair and glasses, Jonas was among the smallest in his class at Public School no. 44, located on Prospect Avenue in the Bronx.[14] He pleased his teachers with his eagerness to learn and skipped several grades. Relatives likewise regarded him as highly intelligent. "Even as a kid," one noted, "when Jonas said something, you could put it in the bank."[15] He didn't talk much, however, and when he did, he spoke quietly, carefully selecting every word. "I tended to observe and reflect and wonder," he later said, although he didn't reveal his deliberations to others. "I kept pretty much to myself."[16] While neighborhood boys played stickball and marbles, Jonas read. Dora encouraged his intellectual growth over his physical or social development.

Before long, his quiet, orderly life was disrupted by the births of his brothers. Herman was born when Jonas was five. Talkative and gregarious, he pestered Jonas to play. His sense of humor and love of practical jokes seemed out of place in the Salk household. Lee was born seven years later. Socially adept, as he grew up he attracted a large number of friends, and he was the only person who could manipulate Dora with his charm. Jonas considered his brothers intrusions.

Dora ran her home like the foreman she had been in the garment industry. She cleaned the apartment, cooked and washed without the aid of modern appliances, and mended the boys' clothes so that they looked new. She nursed her sons through measles and mumps and guarded them against influenza and polio. She worked late into the evening finishing her housework and cooking for the next day so she could take her sons to the library or park. When other mothers complained they needed to go home and make dinner, she would announce, "I've already done mine."[17] Living in a community in which a woman's worth was measured by the cleanliness and orderliness of her home, the quantity and quality of the food she prepared, the clothes her children wore, and their scholastic achievements, Dora had no time for leisure. She soon looked older than her husband.

Dora was a tough taskmaster. Every night the dinner table resembled a battleground. She insisted the boys clean their plates, and when they finished, she piled on more. Herman defied his mother; Jonas, on the other hand, never rebelled openly. He tucked food in his cheeks, slipped away from the table, and spit it out. When it came to the boys' schoolwork, Dora expected perfect grades. That was easy for Jonas, who loved learning; Herman had difficulty reading and nearly failed. He was later thought to have dyslexia, though this was not understood at the time. His teachers attributed his poor performance to laziness. As a result, he and his mother regularly locked horns.

Daniel lacked his wife's tenacity. Although a talented lace maker and designer, he was a bit of a dreamer, in and out of work. Lee later likened his father to Willy Loman in *Death of a Salesman*, "beaten down in business but still believing that success would soon be his."[18] Worried about whether Daniel would make enough to cover the rent and food, Dora insisted he hand over his paychecks so that she could manage their finances. She squirreled away substantial amounts to cover those times when she could not count on her husband. Daniel was an affable man, content to sit in Central Park, chatting with strangers and feeding the squirrels and pigeons. "I think back on his innocent delight," Lee wrote, "as the pigeons would light and eat from his hand. I can vividly recall the feel of his whiskers and the smell when he would hug me or when he would pick me up and then lift me high into the air....And how I loved walking with him, holding onto his index finger...and how much he wanted to make me happy, even though he could scarcely afford even the simplest pleasures."[19]

Relatives don't remember Dora and Daniel fighting, nor do they recall much affection. If angry, Dora tightened her lips, and Daniel left. He could not bear quarrelling; besides, she always prevailed. When Jonas wanted to play an instrument, his father bought him a violin. Dora said they were not rich enough for violin lessons and made Daniel return it. When Dora decided Jonas needed a desk, he told his father he dreamed of one with a fold-down top, shelves on which he could arrange his books, and cubbyholes in which he could organize his papers. Daniel brought home a secretary, but Dora said it was too expensive and made him exchange it for a simple student's desk.[20]

Though not devout, the Salks were observant. In the Jewish tradition, a prayer is said at a child's birth, expressing the hope that his life will include Torah (symbolizing learning), *huppah* (the wedding canopy, representing commitment to family), and *ma'asim tovim* (meaning good deeds). In preparing for his bar mitzvah, a boy learns about the three types of *ma'asim tovim*—*tzedakah* (giving money to the poor), *gemilut hassadim* (acts of loving kindness), and *tikkun olam* (repairing the world). For Jews, acts of goodness define a person. For Jonas, *ma'asim tovim* was not an option; it was an obligation.

A number of childhood memories made lifelong impressions on Salk. As an adult, he remembered watching a parade in New York on Armistice Day in 1918.[21] Although only four at the time, he was struck by the soldiers missing an arm or leg. That same year, when influenza almost decimated New York, he recalled standing on the sidewalk watching horse-drawn wagons filled with coffins pass by. In the schoolyard, he saw children wearing leg braces. Those early childhood images of amputees, crippled children, and coffins—images that evoked fear and loathing in others—settled in Salk's soul. "I became aware of a desire to do something in life that would help relieve some of the suffering," he later said.[22] Inspired by reading about Moses and Lincoln, young Jonas set out to fulfill his duty of *tikkun olam*. Every day he prayed he would do something good for mankind. His brothers called him "Little Jesus."[23]

During Jonas's later childhood, Daniel spent less time at home. Dora didn't seem to care. She expended her energy on her sons, especially Jonas. They spent hours at the kitchen table talking about the daily news, the family budget, and his future. As the first child, he bore the burden of her expectations. She set the bar high, and once Jonas cleared it, she raised it higher. "With Dora," her grandson Jonathan said, "you weren't allowed to be yourself. You had to be what she wanted you to be."[24] Jonas complied with her wishes and performed his duties well, if joylessly. He never crossed her, as his brothers did: "I tended to be yielding and more obedient than rebellious."[25] Like his father, Jonas found confrontation disquieting. Instead of slipping away, he learned how to maneuver around his mother, a skill that would help him later in his career.

Jonas had few fond memories of childhood. He longed for privacy, but his mother hovered; her rules suffocated him. Living in cramped quarters, forbidden to go out alone, Jonas had nowhere to escape, even to reflect. "Someday I shall grow up and do something in my own way," he recalled thinking, "without anyone telling me how."[26] By the time Jonas entered high school, he was driven and focused. "He was basically born an adult," his son Peter said. "He didn't have the freedom to be a child in the constellation of his family."[27]

In many regards, Salk's early life typified that of New York Jewish immigrant society. Dora retained the power in the family, as did most housewives of the time. "She often used this power with legendary self-lessness," one historian wrote of the archetypal Jewish mother. Yet it could transform her into the "brassy-voiced, smothering, and shrewish mama upon whom generations of unsettled sons would blame everything from intellectual sterility to sexual incompetence."[28] Jonas blamed none of his shortcomings on his mother. She may have been controlling, to the point of being tyrannical, but he loved her. He inherited her work ethic, which would serve him well, and he mastered the art of hiding his true feelings behind an agreeable, subdued persona. Dora planned for her sons to succeed in school, go to university, and enter a profession such as medicine or law. Like many Jewish mothers, she looked to her sons to fulfill her aspirations for a better life. "She wanted her children to have more than she had," Jonas explained. "She lived her life through her children."[29]

What distinguished Jonas Salk from the thousands of others born into New York Jewish immigrant society was that many found their parents' expectations to be a burden; he considered them a kind of beacon. Jonas believed that one day he would perform some noble service to humanity. Yet it seemed improbable that this first-generation Jewish boy—small for his age, bright but not brilliant, physically inept, reserved in speech and manner, and comfortable with solitude—could fight for justice, help repair the world. He was no fearless explorer, no golden-tongued orator, no inspirational leader, no swashbuckling hero. "I knew I was competent," Salk told a journalist years later. "I had proved it by achieving that which I was supposed to achieve, time and again. The remainder of childhood was for me a period of patient waiting," waiting for the time he could perform his good deeds, his *ma'asim tovim*.[30] Haunted by the images of caskets and crutches, inspired by Moses and Lincoln, committed to *tikkun olam*—repairing the world—and imbued with the perseverance of his ancestors, he would. Jonas Salk trusted in his destiny. After all, he was born with a caul.

Finding His Place

TWELVE-YEAR-OLD Jonas enrolled at Townsend Harris Hall, an all-boys college preparatory high school located on the campus of the City College of New York.[1] Perched on Saint Nicholas Heights, overlooking Harlem, its main quadrangle was surrounded by four majestic neo-Gothic buildings with vaulted roofs, buttresses, and spires. Across the street, Shepard Hall, the campus centerpiece, resembled a medieval cathedral. In 1847, Townsend Harris, a leading New York merchant and president of the Board of Education, had persuaded the state legislature to establish City College, which worthy students could attend at no charge, giving sons of immigrants their only chance for a college education. Hundreds vied for admission to its affiliated high school, the positions filled mostly by boys from working-class Jewish families, with a few Italians and Irish intermingled.

At Townsend Harris, Jonas found himself among classmates just as smart and even smarter than him. Students voted the *New Yorker* their favorite magazine, Aristophanes' *Lysistrata* their favorite play; they published a school newspaper in Latin.[2] Although they had competed for admission to Townsend Harris, taking a difficult entrance examination, once admitted they found the mantra to be individual growth—surpassing oneself, not others. The school could boast of many lawyers, writers, and civic leaders among its graduates. College faculty taught several courses at Townsend Harris, ranking it with Stuyvesant and Brooklyn Technical, both of which spawned future scientists, engineers, and mathematicians. A magnet school for the humanities, Townsend Harris had only one token science course—physics. Conversant with the great books, students remained unschooled in chemistry or biology. That suited Jonas. "I was not interested in science," he recollected. "I was merely interested in things human."[3]

Classmates described Jonas as modest and affable. He didn't stand out like his friend Harold Goldstein, a champion debater, voted "most conscientious," or his best friend, Murray Nathan, the student body president, voted "most popular."[4] He wasn't outspoken like war resister Ralph DiGia, and he couldn't write as well as James Wechsler, who later became editor of the *New York Post*. Academically he was just one of many excellent students. "There were several others I'd call geniuses," Nathan said, "but not Jonas."[5] Although not strikingly handsome like classmates Charles Schlang and Nathaniel Fensterstock, Jonas was nice-looking with almond-shaped eyes, thick, curly hair, and a slender build. What did stand out was his attire. "He was impeccably dressed," recalled Herbert Fabricant, "while the rest of us looked like ruffians."[6] His mother made sure of that.

Although Jonas dutifully mastered Latin and French, he relished his literature classes. The lessons he learned about individualism from Emerson, Thoreau, and Lincoln remained lodestars throughout his life: "Nothing is at last sacred but the integrity of your own mind," he read in Emerson's "Self-Reliance."[7] He came across a similar theme in one of Lincoln's addresses. "I desire so to conduct the affairs of this administration," Lincoln had said in 1864, "that if in the end, when I come to lay down the reins of power, I have lost every other friend on earth, I shall at least have one friend left, and that friend shall be down inside of me."[8] Francis Bacon's metaphysical writings would resurface years later when Salk took up the philosophical banner of metabiology.

Townsend Harris encouraged leadership and a sense of community through its clubs. In the late 1920s, Tammany Hall still controlled New York under Mayor Jimmy Walker. The stock market crashed the day after Jonas's fifteenth birthday. Picketing, breadlines, bankruptcies, and suicides clarified his sense of destiny: he planned to become a lawyer and fight injustice, or perhaps a congressman, so that he would gain the power to effect change. He never voiced his aspirations to Harold Goldstein on their streetcar ride home each day, or to his friend Murray Nathan. Yet his choice of clubs reflected his ambition: as vice president of the Current History Society, he arranged talks by local officials and visits to city courts; a member of the Law and Debate Society, he won first prize in a current events contest.

Encouraging leadership and a sense of community at Townsend Harris did not include athletics. Jonas dabbled in boxing but mainly limited his athletic endeavors to the required two hours of weekly calisthenics. Intellectually precocious, socially inept: that defined most Townsend Harris youths. Leisure time was taken up with "work, work, work," Stanley Gitenstein recounted.[9] Not that they weren't interested in girls. "There were no girls in sight," Murray Nathan bemoaned.[10] "The presence of a girl mutes his mighty debating tongue with fear and raises up a scarlet tinge behind a trembling ear," the yearbook teased elocutionary champion Harold Goldstein.[11] Jonas enjoyed dancing, but the school held no co-ed parties. He didn't even meet girls working summers in the Catskills; he was a counselor at an all-boys camp.

One of sixty-four seniors, Jonas served as class secretary, advertising manager for the yearbook—*Crimson and Gold*—and assistant business manager of *Stadium*, the student newspaper. He worked hard to overcome his inherent shyness and got his first taste of popularity when a cartoon in the yearbook depicted him with a bowler hat perched jauntily on his head, dubbing him one of nine "Big Shots."[12] And among pictures of five studious "Seniors at Work" was one of Jonas in a three-piece suit, feet propped up on an executive desk, thumbs in his vest pockets, smiling broadly at the camera, looking like a successful lawyer or future congressman.[13] His friends assumed he would be elected to Arista, the elite organization of students notable for their "conscientious endeavor to attain the best results, not only from scholarship, but in growth of character as evidenced by sincerity, fidelity…and service."[14] But he wasn't. Murray Nathan thought his exclusion a glaring omission, as did one of the editors of *Crimson and Gold*, who wrote, "In the society of the chosen few, Jonas should have been chosen, too."[15] As he would throughout life, he bore his disappointment in silence.

Townsend Harris may not have launched Salk's career in science, but it did foster his dreams of performing service to humanity. All Townsend Harris students recited the Ephebic Oath, taken by boys in ancient Athens when they reached manhood, vowing to be good citizens and leave their city better than they found it. Jonas's favorite teacher, Robert Chastney, wrote to the graduating class: "Yours is the task to reflect credit upon yourselves and thereby upon your institution by devoting your lives to high ideals and to the best service of your fellow man."[16] That is just what Jonas Salk set out to do.

Before his sixteenth birthday, Jonas began his collegiate studies at City College along with three-quarters of his classmates. The first in his family to attend college, he didn't even contemplate other choices. City College prided itself in being the first free public institution of higher education in America.[17] Jonas only had to pay for books and streetcar fare. Top students from Townsend Harris, Brooklyn Technical, Stuyvesant, and the new Bronx Science competed for positions there. "We knew it as gospel truth," a graduate wrote, "that this plain College was for each of us a passport to a higher and ennobled life."[18] With a student population comprising at least 80 percent Jews, City College gained a reputation as "the haven of Jewish minds."[19]

The administration recognized that to gain acceptance into professions populated by Harvard and Yale graduates, these rough-hewn young men needed to be smoothed and polished. Once a week the entire freshman class assembled in the Great Hall, its high curved ceiling and stately columns creating an aura of nobility and civility, where they heard lectures on art and music. They sang traditional European university songs, such as "Gaudeamus Igitur" (Let us rejoice). "They were trying to instill some culture into these unwashed, immigrant children," Goldstein said.[20] Sometimes, however, efforts to transform them into proper gentlemen seemed hopeless. Goldstein recalled a lecture on Greek art during which every slide displaying a statue of a bare-breasted woman evoked a round of catcalls.

The high percentage of prelaw and premedical students pushed the academic competition to a level Jonas had not experienced at Townsend

Harris. A D in French; Cs in Chemistry, Math, and English; Bs in History and Social Studies—his first semester grades hardly predicted a distinguished career. Determined to succeed, Jonas persevered and subsequently achieved a string of As, except in those courses requiring natural ability, such as Music, Public Speaking, and Hygiene (physical education).[21] The caption under Jonas's picture in *Microcosm*, the yearbook, was strikingly blank—no clubs, no leadership positions, no honors, no witty entry to indicate any engagement beyond his studies.[22] And he developed few close relationships. "He was awfully difficult to know well," a classmate said. "Not that he wasn't agreeable and companionable, but he hoarded his being more than most people do, as if he had walled it up for safekeeping in a sanctuary surrounded by a labyrinth and moats.... You somehow got the sense that perhaps he was holding back...because he was preoccupied with something."[23]

That "something" was his future. When Jonas disclosed his intent to study law to his mother, she objected. "My mother didn't think I would make a very good lawyer," Salk said. "I really couldn't win an argument with her."[24] Doubtless she was right; Jonas avoided altercations. So he switched to premedical studies, although he had taken only one science course in high school and was now competing with Bronx Science and Stuyvesant students who had grown up on science. Surprisingly, he liked these courses, especially chemistry, despite having gotten a grade of C in Chemistry I. The orderliness appealed to him, and the subject matter fascinated him. His mother once again objected to his choice, believing him to be too weak physically to be a doctor. She pronounced teaching a more suitable career for someone of his intellect and stamina. For the first time, he defied his mother and applied to medical school.

As Jonas approached the end of his senior year with no letter of acceptance, his mediocre grades—an overall B- average—along with the tacit Jewish quotas were barring his admission to medical school. One item on his application, however, differentiated him from thousands of others. "I didn't see myself practicing medicine," he said, as was the usual career for most medical school graduates. "I saw myself trying to bring science into medicine."[25] Why Salk chose a different path is unclear. He later recollected how inspiring he had found Louis Pasteur's biography.[26] And at Townsend Harris, his physics professor had challenged students to conduct independent research in their chosen field. What was clear, though, was his passion and resolve. In his medical school interviews, Salk remembered some doubt about the veracity of his avowed intent. When a professor at New York University's medical school warned him he'd never get rich doing research, Jonas had replied, "There is more in life than money."[27] Before long, he received his first and only letter of acceptance.

⑂

IN 1934, SALK matriculated at University and Bellevue Hospital Medical College, soon to be renamed the New York University College of Medicine. Nearing its centennial year, the school took pride in its alumni: Walter Reed had discovered the transmission of yellow fever by mosquitoes; William Gorgas had destroyed mosquito breeding grounds in the Panama Canal Zone, enabling construction of the canal; Hermann Biggs had established the New York Board of Health Laboratory to control tuberculosis, diphtheria, and venereal disease.[28] Although the school's facilities—three unremarkable buildings along First Avenue—were unimpressive, its association with the venerable Bellevue Hospital, the country's oldest public hospital, boosted the school's reputation.

The traditional four-year curriculum consisted of two years devoted to the basic medical sciences, the other two to clinical rotations. Salk's class numbered 124 men, most of whom had graduated from City College or New York University, and thirteen women, most from prominent women's colleges such as Smith and Vassar.[29] First-year students spent forty hours a week in the lecture hall or laboratory, learning anatomy, biochemistry, and physiology, then studied late into the night. Within the year, the relentless pace and enormous workload eliminated a number of them.

Few students remembered Jonas. John Stetler, whose name followed Salk's alphabetically, sat next to him in every class, yet they rarely spoke.[30] When called upon, Jonas did not distinguish himself, unlike Sol Sherry, who many classmates predicted would become a department of medicine chairman or dean someday. "Jonas was not very verbose," said Walter Kees, "not a social man."[31] He rarely attended a class dinner or joined his fellow students in the standing game of hearts. "He was already engaged in the academic and scientific," Isidor Bernstein recalled.[32] That wasn't the only reason. Jonas had taken a part-time job to help pay for tuition, books, a microscope, and medical instruments, and he still lived at home.

Jonas did enjoy spending time with Karl Paley, the son of Russian Jewish immigrants.[33] Assigned to the same class section, they shared laboratory experiments and a reverence for research. Jonas regularly joined Karl for lunch along with his anatomy dissection partners, Olga Frankel and Frances Bailen. His manners and modesty impressed Bailen. She knew he must be smart, since he was exempted from many of his final exams. Over lunch the four conferred about their cadavers and complained about the cafeteria food. If one of the girls had attended an art show or concert, the others enjoyed it vicariously.

Most of Jonas's classmates planned to practice medicine and would go on to do so. Isidor Bernstein became a psychiatrist, Herman Zuckerman a radiologist, Rudy Drosd a general surgeon. Walter Kees practiced family medicine in rural Pennsylvania for fifty years; Frances Bailen-Rose practiced cardiology until age eighty-seven.[34] Jonas charted a different course, beginning in his first-year biochemistry class when his professor, R. Keith Cannan, tapped him on the shoulder and asked to see him in his office. Jonas worried that he had failed the recent exam. To his surprise, Cannan complimented him on his analysis of a test question that had no correct answer. He offered Jonas a year's fellowship to conduct research in his lab and teach biochemistry. Although this meant taking a leave from his medical studies, Jonas would receive a stipend to help finance his medical education. "After much agony [about] leaving my class," he said, "I decided that I would do so....I was going to be different from others. I just had to accept that."[35]

Jonas's first project involved extracting albumin from hen eggs and heating it until it solidified.[36] His task was to determine whether the observed physical change was accompanied by a specific chemical change—an attempt to decipher the process called denaturation. Even though his research was not directly applicable to disease, Jonas considered that year a turning point. Surrounded by beakers, pipettes, and Bunsen burners, he resolved to make scientific investigation his life's work.

His second project did have clinical relevance. Cannan asked him to inoculate rabbits with streptococcus, the bacteria responsible for scarlet fever, and then to test the antibody response. The study required large quantities of bacteria, which had to be separated from the culture broth in which they were grown. This laborious process entailed rotating the broth at high speed in a centrifuge and removing the layer of bacteria that collected at the bottom. Before long, Jonas sought a faster method to perform this tedious task. He postulated that if he chilled the culture broth to the freezing point, the bacteria would concentrate into a mass which could be more easily extracted. Using the same technique his mother used to make ice cream, Jonas put a can of culture broth inside a larger container and packed it with ice, adding calcium phosphate to depress the freezing point. At first, nothing happened. He then added a small amount of alcohol, hoping to enhance the process. To his delight, the bacteria clumped instantaneously.

When he tried to demonstrate this phenomenon to Cannan, however, it didn't work. Instead of abandoning his idea, Jonas meticulously repeated each step and found that the aggregation of bacteria had not been induced by freezing or adding alcohol. A small amount of calcium phosphate had leaked into the culture media, forming a precipitate. Bacteria had adsorbed to the precipitate and dropped to the bottom of the container. Siphoning off the clear liquid, he could easily recover the bacteria. "It worked at will," he later recalled.[37] Remarkable for its simplicity, his discovery allowed scientists to separate bacteria from twenty liters of culture broth in less time than that required for three liters using the standard method. Just twenty-two, Salk saw his first paper published in the *Proceedings of the Society of Experimental and Biological Medicine*.[38]

Impressed with the ingenuity of this blooming scientist, Cannan suggested Jonas obtain a PhD instead of an MD. He declined. He perceived how easily one could become absorbed in some chemical puzzle and lose sight of the human element. And that is what drove him. He did accept Dean Currier McEwen's invitation to attend the weekly faculty research symposium. The dean noticed that this young man, already sophisticated in the basic sciences yet earnest and humble, came not to fraternize with him, as did other students, but to learn how scientists think.[39]

In the fall of 1936, Jonas returned to his medical studies, spending thirty hours a week in the lecture hall learning pathology, bacteriology, immunology, and pharmacology. Instead of practicing the customary rote memorization, he mulled over the material, digesting it. Through such critical thinking, he became intrigued by a seeming paradox. In one lecture he was told that it was possible to immunize against tetanus and diphtheria using the toxins produced by these microbes once they were rendered harmless by chemicals. In the next, he was told that immunization against viral diseases required actual infection with live virus; vaccines made from killed viruses wouldn't work. Salk thought those two statements couldn't both be true.[40] When his professor couldn't explain the discrepancy to his satisfaction, he determined to explore the contradiction.

During the last year of medical school, Jonas got his chance. New York University had recently recruited as chairman of the Department of Bacteriology Thomas Francis, Jr., who had gained renown for discovering a new type of influenza virus. When Jonas first sought his mentorship, Francis found him "a well-groomed, dark-haired youngster with time to spare."[41] But as Jonas talked about his work with Cannan, Francis realized he wasn't a student who just wanted to dabble in the lab for a few months. "There was something appealing," Francis recalled, "about the pleasantly energetic way in which he kept impressing you with his desire to do research."[42] Not just any research; Jonas wanted to test the hypothesis that one could kill a virus, destroying its infectivity, while retaining its ability to stimulate antibody production. At that time, the three available antiviral vaccines—smallpox, rabies, and yellow fever—relied on live, weakened virus, in keeping with the prevailing belief that only by inducing a mild infection could one prevent a deadly one.

Francis put his young mentee to work vaccinating mice with killed influenza virus. To begin, Jonas removed the lungs from mice infected with influenza, extracted the virus, and rushed the specimens forty-two blocks to the Rockefeller Institute, where a collaborating scientist inactivated the virus with ultraviolet light. He then carried the dead virus back to Francis's laboratory, injected it into mice, and measured antibodies against influenza.[43] By the time he left Francis's lab, Jonas knew there was no paradox—a killed virus could impart immunity.

Jonas was far from just a "lab rat." He excelled at the bedside as well. Showing the stamina his mother thought lacking, he completed clinical rotations in medicine, pediatrics, surgery, and obstetrics with such proficiency he was elected to the elite honor society, Alpha Omega Alpha, the medical equivalent of Phi Beta Kappa. The caption under his 1939 graduation photograph in the student yearbook noted that he seemed to have conducted research in every laboratory on First Avenue. "[He] can probably call more faculty members by their first name than anyone else in school," it read. The prediction: "At present rate, will be professor of medicine in about 2 years."[44]

On June 8, Jonas Salk received his MD degree. The next day he got married.

A Wedding and a War

WHEN JONAS SALK first spotted Donna Lindsay on the beach in Woods Hole, Massachusetts, he saw much to attract him. As he got to know her, he discovered much more. And he resolved to marry her.

The summer before he graduated from medical school, Jonas was working in Woods Hole at the Marine Biological Laboratory. An international center for research in biology and ecology, it served as a breeding ground for young scientists. Donna was vacationing in the area with her family. Jonas thought Donna was stunning. Five feet ten, she stood an inch taller than him, with full red lips, fashionably arched eyebrows, deep-set eyes, and thick, wavy hair in the sleek, upswept style of the thirties. Her halter top accentuated her broad shoulders, and her tennis skirt revealed shapely legs.[1] Inquiring about her, Jonas found out she came from an affluent New York family, had graduated from Smith College, and was studying for a Master's degree at the New York College of Social Work. Jonas was smitten; Donna wasn't. "He seemed a little boyish," she admitted, but she agreed to a date.[2]

Jonas had never met a woman like Donna—versed in the arts, fluent in French and German, conversant with current events, her observations peppered with a sharp wit. Whether playing the piano or swimming in the ocean, she did everything well, with seeming ease yet with no conceit. "Donna outshined Jonas in so many ways," a relative said, "but she never made anything of it."[3] And she was a good listener. When Jonas was speaking, she focused on him, never fidgeted. "Elegant in repose" is how her niece described her.[4]

Although she rarely talked about herself, Jonas learned more about Donna with time.[5] She was born in White Plains, New York, on February 3, 1917, to Elmer and Florence Lindsay. Her grandfather had emigrated from Hungary and upon reaching the New World changed his name from Schoenfeld to Lindsay, shedding outward signs of his Jewish heritage in an attempt to assimilate. Her father, Elmer Lindsay, became a successful Manhattan dentist whose clients included movie star Tyrone Powers, the Phillip Morris midget bellhop, and dance-instruction maestro Arthur Murray. A debonair man, Lindsay sported a stylish cane, monocle, and top hat. His grandson Jonathan described him as "a bit of a dandy" who fancied himself part of high society.[6] His wife, Florence, patient and caring, provided a good balance.

Donna and her younger sister, Margot, grew up in an artistically vibrant family. Elmer was a concert baritone, and Florence, a talented pianist, accompanied him as he practiced his arias. Florence's sister, Rose Franken, was an internationally known novelist and playwright, considered one of the most influential Jewish women writers in the early twentieth century. Her Broadway play *Claudia* ran for 722 performances before she sold the rights to Hollywood, resulting in two hit movies. She counted Lillian Hellman, William Faulkner, and F. Scott Fitzgerald among her acquaintances.

The Lindsays lived in an upscale Manhattan apartment, and the girls attended private schools. Donna studied psychology at Smith, her outstanding performance recognized by a summa cum laude degree and election to Phi Beta Kappa. Celebration of her success, however, was overshadowed by her mother's death from metastatic colon cancer.

Jonas made up his mind to marry this beautiful, cultured, and talented woman whose family enjoyed wealth and social position. Although those attributes may have attracted him to Donna, what bound him was her heart. An avid humanitarian, she cared deeply about others. And she made Jonas feel good about himself. Donna was not swept away by Jonas.

He wasn't strikingly handsome, although she liked his graceful hands. "He was a good dancer," she recalled, "an amusing and exciting conversationalist, and as different from the stereotype of the one-track scientist as anyone could possibly be."[7] As they talked, she learned that Jonas shared her zeal for social justice. While at Smith, Donna had supported several left-wing causes. "My mother was an activist," her son Darrell explained. "Part of it was based on her passion for the underdog, and part, I suspect, was a rebellion against the life of privilege she had led."[8] Jonas still lived at home, dominated by his mother, oblivious to the latest Broadway shows or gallery openings, barely able to afford dinner at the local deli. Yet like her, he wanted to make a difference. And when he spoke about his desire to better the world, she couldn't help find him endearing.

Woods Hole provided the perfect backdrop for a summer romance. An old New England seaport, the village lay a ferry ride away from Nantucket. A hike along Church Street took Donna and Jonas to Nobska Lighthouse with its breathtaking views of Vineyard Sound, Martha's Vineyard in the distance. Ambling along the waterfront, they reached Spohr Gardens and the peaceful Quissett Harbor. And climbing the path to the Knob rewarded them with a romantic sunset over Buzzards Bay. Jonas was in love. He called classmate Frances Bailen and asked her to take the train to Woods Hole. "I've met the girl I'm going to marry," he announced, "and I'd like you to meet her."[9] Their courtship was brief. No one recalled Donna swooning over Jonas or blushing in his presence. She was a practical woman. Already in her mid-twenties, Donna had passed the time when most women wed; her younger sister, Margot, would soon marry and move to Missouri. Donna respected Jonas's ambitions and admired his intellect. So when he proposed, she accepted.

The reaction from their families was tepid. Although her son was marrying into an upper-middle-class Jewish family, Dora Salk did not seem pleased. Donna didn't fit the picture of a good Jewish wife: she didn't keep kosher; she didn't celebrate the Jewish holidays; and her family put up a Christmas tree. "When he married my mother," their son Jonathan said, "it was the closest he could get to marrying a gentile without marrying a gentile."[10] Donna's father wasn't happy with the match either; he treated Jonas like an outsider. He never expected his daughter to marry a struggling student from the Bronx, slipping back into the Jewish immigrant social stratum above which he and his father had risen. He agreed to the marriage on two conditions: First, Donna's fiancé had to take a middle name. Jonas Salk sounded a bit pedestrian; "Edward" would lend some dignity. Second, the marriage had to take place after Jonas graduated so the wedding announcement would read "Jonas Edward Salk, M.D."[11] To Jonas, those seemed small concessions.

Elmer Lindsay may have anticipated a lavish social event with champagne flowing, his daughter in a chic white gown. Donna, however, shied away from the spotlight and railed against anything that displayed her family's wealth. Dora may have expected her son to be married under a huppah, surrounded by the Press clan, but Donna planned a simple wedding in her father's apartment, keeping the guest list small.[12] On June 9, 1939, Donna Lindsay married Dr. Jonas Edward Salk.

THE NEWLYWEDS MOVED into an apartment at 308 East 79th Street. Donna went to work at the Jewish Child Care Association, and Jonas prepared to begin his two-year internship. He felt fortunate to be one of twelve selected for the 1939–40 class at Mount Sinai Hospital, which to this day remains among New York's most esteemed teaching hospitals.[13] "To be an intern at Mt. Sinai," one physician said, "was like playing ball for the New York Yankees."[14] In order to intermix experienced and unseasoned interns, the hospital staggered the start date. Assigned the third rotation, Jonas had nine months to get acquainted with his new wife and finish his research with Thomas Francis.

On March 1, 1940, Salk began his internship. The 850-bed Mount Sinai Hospital, located on 98th Street and Madison Avenue, served Harlem and the Upper East Side. Patients were housed on large open wards where curtains provided the only privacy. "The old building hadn't been touched by modernization," a former intern said, "except for a lot of new signs."[15] Over the next two years, Jonas rotated through the medicine, pediatrics, neurology, and surgery services, working his way up from wardsman to junior to senior to house physician. He started on the medicine service under house physician Arthur Seligmann, who, having heard Jonas planned a laboratory career, expected a detached academician. Instead, Seligmann found Jonas to be tender with patients, courteous to nursing staff, willing to help other interns, and uncomplaining about the chronic sleep deprivation from being on duty thirty-six hours straight. At midnight meals, Jonas became acquainted with the other interns. Their spouses joined them for Sunday lunches. "At first, the entire conversation would be about medicine," Seligmann recalled, "but then the wives joined in, and we started talking about the diaper service."[16] Attempting to be part of her husband's world, Donna often ate dinner with him in the hospital cafeteria and read cases published in the *New England Journal of Medicine*.

On the medical wards, Jonas treated patients with diabetes, pneumonia, and heart failure. Polio patients were admitted to a convalescent hospital; cancer patients were shipped to a Long Island facility. As the wardsman on his service, he performed most of the procedures—drawing blood, staining sputum for tuberculosis, examining stool for parasites, performing lumbar punctures. On the surgical service, he arrived before dawn to ready patients for their operations. Later he sewed up lacerations and performed circumcisions and appendectomies. He displayed such impressive surgical skills that one of the staff surgeons asked him to join his practice.[17] The most relaxed rotation was the dermatology service; most intimidating was the emergency room. "Saturday nights in the South Bronx could be wild," Seligmann recalled.[18]

As compensation, interns received six uniforms, room and board, and twenty-five dollars at the completion of training. Some interns agitated for a monthly paycheck; others complained about the hours. Not Jonas. He seemed to personify equanimity, leading to his election as president of the intern group. Several recalled the time he stood up to the hospital administrator who had banned interns from wearing "Bundles for Britain" buttons in support of the New York organization that sent knitted goods to Great Britain. When the administrator threatened to deny Jonas a future staff position at Mount Sinai, he respectfully and repeatedly cited his constitutional rights. Exasperated, the administrator eventually backed down, and Jonas became a demi-hero among the interns.[19] At their end-of-the-year party, the nurses voted Jonas and John Dehoff "most popular interns."[20] Staff physicians, fellow interns, and nurses all considered Jonas an outstanding clinician, a leader, and a gentleman—a guaranteed success in practice. But he had other plans.

During the second year of his internship, Jonas received notification that the work he had done in medical school on the calcium phosphate adsorption technique had been selected for presentation at a meeting of the Society for Experimental Biology and Medicine. Initially he had conceived of the procedure to facilitate collection of bacteria from culture broth. In Francis's lab, he had used the technique to purify influenza virus, and he believed calcium phosphate might increase the immunizing effect of the virus. He planned to introduce this possibility in his ten-minute presentation, although he had no data to back up his conjecture.

In the audience sat Francis and Joseph Smadel, a microbiologist whose research had led to the cure for typhoid fever and typhus. An impatient man whose formal portrait showed a knitted brow and pressed lips, Smadel had a reputation as a crusader against shallow thinking.[21] When Jonas finished his presentation, Smadel disparaged his work, and Francis didn't come to his rescue. "I don't remember what he said, it shocked and upset me so much," Salk later recounted. "I was only an intern with a lot of ambition, and here this guy gets as nasty as if I had committed a crime against science. I was crushed."[22] He planned to be a virologist, and a giant in the field had just filleted him in public, giving him his first inkling of how unwelcoming the elite clique of academic virologists could be to those attempting to join their ranks. Other aspiring scientists might have packed up their lab coats and taken positions in private practice. Jonas wrote to Smadel, repeating his key points with deference, giving further explanation in case he had not been clear. Smadel never replied.

Toward the end of internship, Jonas began applying for research positions, detailing his plans to investigate immunization against viral diseases. His impressive curriculum vitae—a research fellowship at NYU, election to AOA, internship at Mount Sinai, a presentation to the Society for Experimental Biology and Medicine, two publications and another in preparation—practically guaranteed acceptance to his first choice, the Rockefeller Institute. Research fellows from the Rockefeller went on to fill almost half of the major academic positions in internal medicine. Salk, however, faced two obstacles: He didn't have an Ivy League pedigree, and he was Jewish. Thomas Rivers, chief of the Rockefeller Institute's hospital, who referred to Jonas as "a young Jew," replied that all of their positions were filled.[23] Several other institutions, including Columbia University, turned him down as well. Undeterred, Jonas looked to Thomas Francis, Jr., who had just accepted the chairmanship of the Department of Epidemiology at the University of Michigan's new School of Public Health.

He first inquired about a position with Francis in March of 1941. Six months passed before Francis responded. "If you would like to come to Ann Arbor," he wrote, "I should be glad to see you, but I would not urge you to come if the matter of expense is important."[24] Sensing from Jonas's reply that he had hurt his feelings, Francis later wrote: "I did not want you to interpret my comments as indicating lukewarmness on my part."[25] Jonas construed that to be a tacit acceptance. When Francis suggested he apply for a fellowship from the National Foundation for Infantile Paralysis (NFIP), which was funding immunology research, Jonas replied, "It is hard to express sufficient appreciation for the help you are extending in my behalf toward the realization of this plan which is now emerged as the clear expression of hitherto undefined hopes."[26] Though he had no guaranteed salary, Salk prepared to move to Ann Arbor after completion of his internship.

Then, on December 7, the Japanese attacked Pearl Harbor. Four days after the United States declared war, Salk wrote Francis: "At the very moment I heard the news, my first reaction was to write to you....I feel that my greatest contribution now is on utilizing the training I had with you, since it is in a field that has such special implications and significance in war time."[27] During World War I, almost as many US servicemen died from influenza or associated pneumonia as were killed in battle. Concerned about the repetition of such a military disaster, the secretary of war formed the Commission on Influenza with Francis as director. Salk told Francis he was prepared to resign his internship and assist him: "I am at your disposal."[28] A week later he received Francis's reply: "I have delayed in answering your letter simply because you needed a cooling-off."[29] He urged Jonas not to interrupt his internship; he would always regret it. A month later, Jonas wrote that he had requested a draft deferment and was moving to Ann Arbor as soon as his internship ended. Francis was taken aback. Jonas would soon be at his doorstep without a source of salary or a deferment.

Shortly thereafter Colonel Kopetzky from Selective Service Headquarters informed Salk they were denying his request to work with Francis. They could consider the "luxury of research," he wrote, only if they won the war, and if they didn't, "neither you nor anybody else within his lifetime will do any research."[30] He ordered Salk to report for a physical. Jonas pleaded with Francis to intervene, and Francis appealed to the Selective Service Local Board no. 45 in New York, calling his influenza studies critical for national defense and Salk's assistance indispensable.[31]

On March 5, 1942, a notice arrived from the University of Michigan, informing Salk of his appointment as a research fellow in the Department of Epidemiology effective April 1 without salary.[32] The same day, the NFIP awarded him a $2,100 fellowship.[33] Two weeks later, Local Board no. 45 classified him IIA, meaning his draft was deferred in support of national health.[34] Jonas and Donna left for Ann Arbor.

Joining the Fight Against Influenza

Of the 1918 influenza epidemic, Jonas Salk had just a vague memory of horse-drawn wagons filled with coffins. If he or any of his immediate family were stricken, as five thousand were every day in New York, none had died. His mother understood the threat. She could see quarantine signs in the neighbors' windows, followed a few days later by a death cart; she could smell the uncollected garbage mixed with the stench of decaying flesh; she could read about the disturbing number of orphans, or worse yet, of entire families gone. She successfully shielded Jonas not only from the contagion but also from the terror pervading the Bronx.

Only later, in medical school, did Salk learn about the disease, its name derived from the Italian word *influenza*, as early astrologers blamed epidemics on the influence of heavenly bodies.[1] Every few years, influenza spread throughout entire communities, but physicians considered it a temporary nuisance, not in the same league as smallpox or typhoid fever. So the initial US cases reported in the spring of 1918 didn't alarm public health officials. What later became known as the first wave spread across the world in five months. It acquired the name "Spanish influenza," as Spain was the first country to report a high number of victims, including King Alfonso XIII who, though gravely ill, survived. Most infections were mild, and by summer, the contagion seemed to have vanished. When it resurfaced in late August, it had changed its character and become vicious.

Johns Hopkins pathologist William Henry Welch and Rockefeller Institute microbiologist Rufus Cole had been sent by the surgeon general to investigate an outbreak at Camp Devens outside Boston.[2] On September 7, 1918, a soldier had come to the infirmary complaining of headache and fever. He died so quickly medics diagnosed meningitis. The next day, a dozen recruits came in with the same symptoms, and before long medical officers suspected they were dealing with a highly virulent contagion. By the time Welch and Cole reached Camp Devens on September 23, more than twelve thousand recruits and officers had become ill. What they saw horrified them.

"It was cold and drizzling rain," Cole recalled, "and there was a continuous line of men coming in from the various barracks [to the hospital], carrying their blankets, many of the men looking extremely ill, most of them cyanosed [blue] and coughing."[3] The course of the disease astonished them. Although it had all of the usual characteristics of influenza—rapid onset, headache, fever, muscle aches—it differed in two major respects. First, this influenza caused an inordinate number of pneumonias. Men were coughing up blood, drowning in their own secretions; a bluish-purple discoloration of the lips and face forecast imminent death. Second, it had a preference for young, healthy adults. Sixty-three died the day Welch and Cole arrived. "Owing to the rush and the great numbers of bodies coming into the morgue," Cole reported, "they were placed on the floor without any order or system, and we had to step amongst them to get into the room where an autopsy was going on."[4] When the prosector opened the chest, they saw "blue, swollen lungs" with "wet, foamy surfaces"—quite different from bacterial pneumonia, which involved one or two lobes of the lung. This organism could destroy both lungs in a matter of hours. They had never seen anything like it. "This must be some new kind of infection or plague," Welch told the team.[5] Looking at the lung tissue under the microscope, however, they detected no microbe. Some elusive agent killed almost eight hundred at Camp Devens.

Barracks and troopships with their crowded quarters facilitated rapid dissemination of the disease within the armed forces. One sneeze could infect an entire platoon. Influenza soon spread to civilians. At San Francisco's city hospital, three-quarters of the nurses fell ill; dental students served as doctors. In Providence, Rhode Island, as evangelist Billy Sunday exhorted a crowded assembly to "pray down the epidemic," congregants collapsed around him.[6] Steam shovels were used to dig mass graves in Philadelphia's potter's field. When a quarter of the citizens of Brockton, Massachusetts, lay ill, the local health commissioner said he felt like he was "fighting a ghost."[7] Transport of troops overseas hastened its dissemination. From Africa to Canada, no town seemed immune, no person safe. Influenza traversed the world with fury, killing 25 percent of the Samoan population, obliterating entire Eskimo villages, leaving streets throughout the Punjab Province littered with bodies. In six weeks' time, the scourge devastated a city and moved on. President Wilson, one of the last afflicted, almost died. By the spring of 1919, it had dissipated, leaving twenty million dead. Between influenza and the war, a generation of young adults had been annihilated. And still no one had found the responsible microbe.

It wasn't until 1931 that Richard Shope of the Rockefeller Institute provided the first evidence that a virus caused influenza, at least in animals, when he transmitted the disease from one pig to another.[8] Two years later, during a London epidemic, three British researchers set out to prove a virus underlay the human disease. When one of them contracted influenza, they swabbed a filtrate from his throat washings into the noses of ferrets. The animals developed all the signs of influenza and made anti-influenza antibodies, protecting them against a second infection. Although it would be almost a decade until the invention of the electron microscope allowed scientists to actually see the viral structure, its identification as the responsible organism meant scientists could attempt to make a protective vaccine. Among the first to try was Thomas Francis, Jr.[9]

⚜

FRANCIS WAS EIGHTEEN at the time of the 1918 pandemic, working at an Army Training Corps infirmary. If he didn't see enough influenza there, he likely later heard Cole's harrowing stories while at the Rockefeller Institute. Francis was born in 1900 in Gas City, Indiana, to Welsh immigrants.

Shortly thereafter, the family moved to New Castle, Pennsylvania, where his father sought a better living working in the steel mills. There young Tommy enjoyed riding with the family doctor in his buggy to make house calls and looking at samples of blood and urine under the microscope. After graduating from Allegheny College in 1921, prompted by his surgeon brother-in-law, he studied medicine at Yale University. The chief of medicine recognized Francis's potential and recommended he pursue research training at the hospital of the Rockefeller Institute. When Francis arrived on a Sunday in 1928, he found the gates locked. Undeterred, he threw his bag over the fence and scaled it.

Initially Francis conducted studies on pneumococci, bacteria that commonly cause pneumonia. But a chance occurrence shifted his attention to a different microorganism. On a train ride from New York to Princeton, New Jersey, he happened to sit with two leading scientists and listened to them talk about the new field of virology. By the time Francis reached Princeton, he had become intrigued by these smallest of microbes.

After ten years at Rockefeller, Francis became the chairman of the Department of Microbiology at New York University, where Salk, a medical student at the time, sought his mentorship. Not content with lab work alone, Francis delved into the new field of epidemiology, the study of disease transmission within populations. The breadth of it appealed to him, and, when offered the chairmanship of the University of Michigan's new School of Public Health, he accepted. In Ann Arbor, Francis and his wife, Dorothy, frequently entertained scientists, who were impressed by their colleague's knowledge of art, music, theater, and Michigan's athletic teams. His refined speech, brush mustache, and tailored dress belied his origin. A short, somewhat pudgy, proper man, Francis had many devoted trainees. Although nurturing, he was tough—"fussy,"[10] one junior colleague called him; "pitilessly critical," another said.[11] The dean of the School of Public Health described him as "a combination of articulateness, humor, wisdom, and sound criticism—yoked to friendliness."[12] What attracted Salk was the boldness and determination with which Francis attacked disease.[13]

Francis was the first American to isolate a human influenza virus. While at the Rockefeller Institute, he was investigating a Puerto Rican epidemic when he found the infecting agent to be a variant of the British strain. He called it PR8.[14] Soon thereafter, he and his colleague Thomas

Magill found another strain in a Philadelphia outbreak. So closely related were the viruses that animals infected with either of them produced antibodies that conferred immunity against infection with the other. Francis and Magill categorized them as Type A influenza viruses.[15]

Then in 1940, Francis made a startling and disquieting observation. At a convalescent home in Irvington, New York, children recovering from rheumatic fever fell ill with an infection resembling influenza. The antibodies in their blood, however, did not react with any of the Type A influenza strains. By infecting ferrets with throat washings from the children, Francis isolated an entirely new type of influenza virus, which he called Type B.[16] Other virologists were incredulous; this finding meant that, unlike rabies or smallpox, not all influenza infections were caused by one virus. That explained why one episode of influenza did not confer lifetime immunity, as did a case of measles or mumps. Prevention through vaccination would be a more complex undertaking than they had thought.

When the United States entered the war in December 1941, military leaders feared another pandemic would wipe out their troops. As the director of the Commission on Influenza, Francis was charged with investigating suspected cases, providing assistance in the event of an outbreak, and developing an influenza vaccine—a formidable task. He needed to anticipate which viral strain would emerge in any given year, make a vaccine against that particular strain, substantiate its safety, prove it prevented influenza, oversee the manufacture of large quantities of vaccine, and decide when and how to inoculate the troops.

At that time, only three vaccines had been constituted against viral diseases.[17] Smallpox had plagued the world until 1796, when English physician Edward Jenner performed a daring experiment. For years he had heard that milkmaids infected with cowpox—akin to but far less virulent than smallpox—seemed immune. When dairymaid Sarah Nelms developed fresh cowpox on her hands and arms, Jenner inoculated eight-year-old James Phipps, his gardener's son, with pus from her lesions. The boy developed fever and a pustule at the inoculation site. Then six weeks later, Jenner did the unthinkable—he injected the boy with pus from a smallpox lesion. The boy remained well, resistant to infection with the deadly microbe. Jenner called this substance a "vaccine" after the Latin word for cowpox—*vaccinia*.

In the late 1800s, Louis Pasteur concocted a rabies vaccine from the saliva of a rabid dog. He knew that following a bite the rabies virus spread from the wound along nerves to the brain, taking several weeks to reach its target. At that point, the victim developed severe pain, violent jerking movements, high fever, and impaired swallowing, causing hydrophobia (fear of drinking) and foaming at the mouth. Coma followed, then death. Pasteur had been cultivating the virus in rabbit spinal cord when nine-year-old Joseph Meister, mauled by a rabid dog, was brought to his laboratory. Pasteur inoculated the boy with a small amount of the live, weakened rabies virus daily for two weeks. Instead of dying in agony, Meister survived.

Unlike bacteria, which could be cultivated in what is known as broth, media that contained essential nutrients, virus could only be grown in living cells, requiring large numbers of laboratory animals in a cumbersome, prolonged undertaking. Finally, in 1931, when pathologist Ernest Goodpasture developed a technique for growing viruses in chick embryos, he provided a major tool for viral vaccine preparation. Six years later, South African microbiologist Max Theiler announced a successful vaccine against the yellow fever virus.

Francis had already made some headway on an influenza vaccine when the war broke out. In 1935, he and Magill had made a crude vaccine and began testing human volunteers for antibody response following inoculation. The method was tedious, as they had to measure how well serum from the subject's blood protected mice from infection after exposure to influenza. Then in 1941, Rockefeller virologist George Hirst made an observation that revolutionized the field.[18] While he was harvesting some influenza-infected chicken embryos, he accidentally spilled a drop of blood on one, and the red blood cells clumped, a process known as hemagglutination. It appeared the virus had caused red blood cells to stick together. Hirst found that if he added serum from immunized mice, their antibodies blocked the clumping. By measuring the amount of clumping, he could determine antibody levels rapidly and accurately.

Now Francis could proceed at a faster pace.[19] Although he had demonstrated the presence of influenza antibodies in volunteers, that didn't prove they had protection against the disease. This required a field trial—vaccinating a large number of individuals and comparing their rate of infection to that of a control group who did not get the vaccine. A proper field trial required a stable population of subjects, a team of experienced personnel, and a pharmaceutical company capable of manufacturing large quantities of vaccine. The task seemed almost insurmountable, especially since Francis was busy traveling to suspected sites of outbreaks around the world. In addition to that, he faced the constant pressure of time: the 1918 pandemic had erupted shortly after the troops had been mobilized. His University of Michigan team included just a couple of laboratory investigators, by no means enough manpower to complete the monumental undertaking. Then, in April of 1942, Jonas Salk arrived.

Salk made a wise choice in attaching himself to this highly respected physician-scientist. Francis would provide him with many of the elements necessary for success—laboratory space, an opportunity to participate in the country's largest vaccine trials, credibility in the cliquish field of virology, a steadying hand for his overeagerness, wisdom for his naiveté, and a stepping stone for his academic career. Salk didn't consider these when he moved to Ann Arbor shortly after the United States entered the war. He joined Francis to help prevent a disease that could decimate their troops and change the course of history.

Vaccine Neophyte

THE SALKS FOUND Ann Arbor, Michigan, quite a change from Manhattan's Upper East Side. In this peaceful college town, with its population of thirty thousand, the June Flower Show was considered a major annual event; *Yankee Doodle Dandy* and *Bambi* played at the local movie house; parking meters were nowhere to be found; children swung on tires over the Huron River.[1] When America went to war, everyone pitched in. No one complained about the Ration Guides or waiting in line at Cunningham Drugs for an hour to buy a pack of cigarettes. The Boy Scouts ran a paper collection drive; residents converted their backyards into victory gardens.

Donna and Jonas rented an old farmhouse on the edge of town. It was heated by a cast-iron stove. Chopping wood, at first novel, proved burdensome as winter dragged on. "The last human being I expected to see using a wood burning stove was Donna Salk," a friend remarked.[2] With a lawn to mow and a sizeable garden to maintain, the couple made their first visit to a nursery. Jonas learned to till the soil, Donna to can vegetables. They took long walks in the countryside and bought their first car, a used Pontiac with a hand crank to start the motor.[3] Donna worked at Family and Children's Service, supplementing Jonas's $120 monthly paycheck.[4]

Among their Ann Arbor friends were June and Walter Mack. During the summer, the two couples enjoyed Sunday picnics on the Huron River; in the evenings, they often met for ice cream. Mack also worked in Francis's lab, and he and Salk always seemed to be discussing science. His research on polio fascinated Salk, and before long Donna and June were going to the movie house together while their husbands returned to the laboratory. Mack taught Salk how to examine infected monkeys for signs of paralysis, how to dissect the brain and spinal cord to recover poliovirus. Sometimes they didn't return home until two in the morning.[5]

Ann Arbor friends described Salk as "mild-mannered,"[6] a "jaunty fellow."[7] It was Donna who impressed them. The first time scientist Paul Stumpf joined the Salks for dinner, he thought Donna was striking— taller and more sophisticated than Jonas and more perceptive about society's problems and their possible solutions. "I've heard people say she was the brains of the outfit," June Mack said.[8] Yet Donna seemed content with a supporting role, second to her husband's career. "Jonas is going to be a big guy someday," she told June.[9]

When Salk joined the Francis laboratory, it included just three other people—surprisingly small given its responsibilities. From the start, Salk bonded with Francis's secretary, Stella Barlow. Her organization and sense of humor helped steady Francis, who was directing Michigan's new epidemiology department while serving as watchdog for influenza outbreaks worldwide. Now Secretary of War Henry Stimson had charged him with developing an influenza vaccine expeditiously. "Jonas was a blessing in those days," Francis admitted.[10] The neophyte whom he had initially discouraged brought to his lab unflagging energy and a determination that exceeded his experience.

Having been away from the lab for two years, Salk needed to master the latest technique for growing influenza virus. Starting with eleven-day-old fertilized eggs, he sprayed the shell with germicide, punctured the top with a hypodermic needle, located the small membranous sac surrounding the embryo, and introduced a drop of viral suspension. After two days of incubation, he burned the top of the shell with an acetylene torch and gently lifted it off. Using sterile instruments, he pushed aside the embryo and drew fluid from the membranous sac, now teeming with virus. To obtain a pure specimen, he had to separate the virus from the embryonic fluid in which it had grown—a tricky and time-consuming process. But Salk had a talent for recognizing how another scientist's discovery could be applied to a task in order to perform it more efficiently. In this case, he devised a simpler technique for extracting the virus based on Hirst's observation that influenza virus caused red blood cells to clump. Salk disrupted some of the embryonic blood vessels with a needle just prior to removing the suspension. Virus stuck to the red blood cells, and when he put the suspension in a flask, the blood and virus formed an aggregate which settled on the bottom. He removed this pellet and washed off the blood cells. A pure solution of live virus remained, which he inactivated with a chemical and stored in a sterile vial. This was the influenza vaccine.[11]

The procedure took months to perfect, requiring considerable patience. Salk faced numerous pitfalls: scores of eggs broken, a pellet that disintegrated upon removal, a vaccine that still contained live virus. It was hazardous working with a microbe known to be highly infectious and potentially deadly. Gloves and masks provided his only safeguard.

By the 1940s, it was well-established that in response to vaccination, the human body produced antibodies against microbes. The ultimate proof of a vaccine's merit, however, was prevention of human infection. That required a field trial, one in which half the subjects received vaccine and half received saline as a placebo, after which the incidence of influenza in the two groups was compared. For such a trial, Salk and Francis needed a readily available group of human subjects. Eloise Hospital for the Insane, located outside Detroit, housed thousands of patients. Beyond an iron fence stood a vast compound the public considered the place of last resort for the mentally ill.[12] Seven thousand unnamed residents were buried in the Eloise Cemetery. Ypsilanti State Hospital, a three-story brick building with gracious white columns and barred windows, held up to 4,000 of Michigan's most severe psychiatric cases at any one time. It was one of the first institutions where surgeons performed lobotomies on combative patients who did not respond to psychotherapy. The asylum was described as a human warehouse "designed for custodial care of the insane."[13] It was at these two state institutions that Francis and Salk planned to conduct their studies.

In the fall of 1942, with Salk taking the lead, the first influenza vaccine trial commenced. In one week's time, he and two other physicians inoculated eight thousand psychiatric patients at the two hospitals. They collected blood samples before and after immunization. Salk found a rise in antibody level in 85 percent. The trial was inconclusive however; no influenza outbreak occurred that winter. They would have to simulate one. Salk returned to Ypsilanti State Hospital, where he inoculated two hundred male residents—half with vaccine, half with saline. In May of 1943, two weeks after the last inoculation, they exposed inmates to influenza, spraying mist made from dried, infected mouse lung tissue into their nostrils. Deliberately infecting institutionalized patients was accepted practice at the time. It wasn't until 1947, following the Nuremberg Trials, that human subjects were protected by a set of ethical principles. One only can guess that Salk felt the prospect of fifty thousand or more young soldiers dying from influenza justified their actions.

The staff at Ypsilanti examined the patients twice daily for signs of influenza. To prevent bias, Salk and Francis blinded the trial; no one knew who had received vaccine and who the placebo. When they broke the code, they found that just 16 percent of those inoculated with vaccine became ill, whereas almost half of the control subjects who had received placebo contracted the flu. They concluded that their vaccine had protected against experimental infection with influenza virus.[14] The question remained whether it would be potent enough in a true epidemic.

That summer, Salk was dispatched to investigate a probable outbreak of influenza at Fort Custer in Augusta, Michigan, where thousands of troops were preparing for combat.[15] Three hundred soldiers had just been hospitalized. He discovered the cause to be a strain of Type A (Weiss) never before associated with an epidemic and thus not included in the vaccine they were preparing for widespread use. Although a Type A strain, the Weiss virus was not related closely enough to the other Type A strains for them to confer immunity. The episode served as a warning: an influenza viral strain could change its stripes, making the prospects for a single vaccine remote.

Salk was rushing between Ypsilanti, Eloise, and Fort Custer, identifying the viral strain from hundreds of throat washings, testing antibody levels in blood samples, and gearing up for a trial to be conducted by the

Commission on Influenza during the coming flu season. At the same time, he was working to improve the vaccine's efficacy in the laboratory and trying to publish their results so that he could begin gaining academic credibility. He started spending evenings and weekends in the lab. Gone were the country walks and weekend picnics. Even his hard-working colleague Walter Mack thought Salk left Donna alone too much. Yet she never complained. It was wartime, and at least her husband was fighting on the home front.

If he appeared "mild-mannered" and "jaunty," Salk concealed his feelings well. His sleep interrupted by his overactive mind, he kept at his bedside a notebook in which he jotted his thoughts and concerns which he would later refer to as his "night notes." He began having chest pains, which he told his physician came on with "emotional upsets and periods of frustration" as a result of having too many things to do and not enough time in which to do them. She found no evident heart disease and suggested psychoanalysis. "I've toyed with the idea of an analysis for some time," he wrote to a Detroit psychiatrist. "I think it would be foolish to put the question off any longer."[16] Responsibility for the health of the military hung over him.

Although no influenza outbreak had materialized in 1942, the Commission expected one in the winter of 1943 and initiated its first major prevention trial under Francis's direction.[17] This would be the largest to date: 12,500 men from the Army Specialized Training Program at eight universities and five medical colleges. Subjects, housed in large dormitories, would receive either vaccine or placebo. Three pharmaceutical firms assumed responsibility for preparation of the vaccine, which consisted of two strains of Type A virus and one of Type B. Fifteen investigators from across the country participated in the trial. The inoculations completed, they waited for signs of an outbreak.

On November 17, several University of Michigan students showed up for sick call. Throat washings identified a Type A influenza virus. Five days later, Francis received a wire from Saint Louis University reporting a hundred new cases. Within six weeks, an epidemic spread across the United States, infecting more civilians than in any other outbreak since the 1918 pandemic. Fortunately, this virus did not attack the lungs, and the death rate remained relatively low. When the commission analyzed their data, they found that only 2 percent of the vaccinated group had contracted influenza. "SOLDIERS WILL BE VACCINATED IF INFLUENZA THREATENS, ARMY ANNOUNCES. TRIALS SHOW 75% REDUCTION IN CASES AMONG VACCINATED," Science Service reported to newspapers nation-wide.[18] Francis and Salk had made a vaccine that could prevent influenza. This was an impressive accomplishment for the twenty-nine-year-old. And they had averted an infection with a killed-virus vaccine.

Salk had set out to disprove the prevailing scientific dogma—that only a live-virus vaccine could provoke lifelong immunity by simulating a natural infection. Such had been the case with smallpox, yellow fever, and rabies. Most microbiologists believed that protection following inocula-tion with a killed virus would be fleeting, lasting weeks to months at most. So Salk pushed the point further. He showed that antibody levels in University of Michigan students who had received killed-virus vaccine were as high as those who contracted influenza.[19] Next he went back to the Ypsilanti and Eloise hospitals, where outbreaks of influenza were raging. He reported no cases of infection among those inmates vaccinated back in 1942. They still had elevated anti-influenza antibody levels more than a year after immunization. Salk and Francis noted something else in their field trial, which had major implications for future widespread im-munization: The incidence of influenza among other students on campus was lower than that in the general population. Since fewer students had gotten the flu as a result of vaccination, there were fewer infected students to spread it to others, a consequence they called the "herd effect."[20]

On April 4, 1944, the surgeon general ordered Salk to report to Washington, DC. Based on the commission's findings, he had decided to vaccinate the entire army in the fall of 1945. Salk volunteered to consult with seven manufacturers on procedures and production.[21] Within a month, he reported back the number of doses prepared daily by each, comparison of potency among strains prepared by different firms, and some sterility issues. These interactions introduced Salk to a new world, that of the large pharmaceutical companies. His respect for their work and willingness to collaborate seemed refreshing compared with the attitude of most aca-demic scientists, who considered pharmaceutical researchers second-class.

Salk soon appreciated the mutual advantages. His monthly salary of $300 barely covered food and rent.[22] Donna, now pregnant, planned to quit her job once their child was born. Without consulting Francis, Salk signed an agreement with Parke, Davis and Company by which he would give them access to any new process he devised for producing vaccine, including "full information concerning the product, all laboratory data and formulae, [and] copies of all letters and patents."[23] The company would have the exclusive right to manufacture and sell the product. In return, they would pay Salk royalties based upon sales. A year later, he agreed to serve as a consultant to the company, for which he received a stipend of $100 each month.[24] Salk could barely believe his good fortune. Francis could barely believe his presumptuousness. Salk had strayed off the straight and narrow path of academia, and it hadn't gone unnoticed.

In the fall of 1945, the army vaccinated eight million soldiers, shortly before an epidemic of influenza B spread across the United States. Immunization reduced the attack rate by 92 percent. "Incontrovertible evidence is now available," Salk and Francis concluded, "that the resistance of man to infection by the viruses of influenza A and B can be enhanced."[25] For his pioneering work, as well as his leadership of the Commission on Influenza, Francis was awarded the Medal of Freedom and elected to the National Academy of Sciences.

While Francis traveled around the world to advise on international infection control, Salk served as acting director of the Commission on Influenza. In this role, he assumed a myriad of new tasks, such as analyzing influenza cases at Lowry Air Force Base, identifying a new Type B strain at Fort Benjamin Harrison, examining German prisoners at Camp Atterbury, and investigating the death of a soldier at Buckley Field nine days after vaccination.[26] Each required a full report to the surgeon general; a letter of commendation usually followed. "The speed, skill, and accuracy with which you got at the nature of this outbreak," the surgeon general wrote on one occasion, "was a marvel to me and will always be an admirable example of the work of an expert who can handle not only technical details but also a large and complex situation."[27] At the same time, Salk oversaw the University of Michigan's virology laboratory and taught several epidemiology courses. When he got his 1945 appointment notice, although his salary had increased to $4,750, he remained in a staff position with no faculty appointment forthcoming.[28]

Nonetheless Salk was starting to make a name for himself, being elected to membership in several research societies and invited into

virology circles. Albert Sabin of the Rockefeller Institute sought his
advice on inactivating virus.[29] The chief of the Biologics Control Laboratory in Washington, DC, requested he critique a memorandum on
vaccine preparation.[30] He was asked to present a paper at the International Congress for Microbiology and to attend the National Research
Council's conference on vaccines.[31] A leading virologist requested that
he join a round-table discussion on influenza at the meeting of the
Society of American Bacteriologists.[32] The list of participants suggested he was gaining stature. "It was the dawn of his professional prom-
inence," Richard Carter, author of *Breakthrough: The Saga of Jonas Salk*,
later wrote.[33]

Meanwhile, in the laboratory, Salk was seeking ways to increase the
vaccine's strength by adding adjuvants, chemical agents to enhance vaccine effectiveness. Adjuvants would allow him to use a smaller dose of
virus in each vaccine. The approach worked in mice, and he proceeded to
vaccinate 369 prisoners committed to Ionia State Hospital, an asylum for
sexual psychopaths and convicts with homicidal tendencies.[34] Although
adjuvants failed to strengthen the vaccine in these subjects, he didn't give
up. The death of a three-year-old girl gave impetus to his work.[35]

A physician in Hempstead, New York, had vaccinated a family
against influenza. Four hours later, the youngest child complained of
stomach pains and began convulsing. Her temperature reached 109° F;
her lips turned blue, and she began bleeding from the mouth and vagina.
Within hours, she was dead. The chief medical examiner attributed her
death to an undetected egg allergy and called for allergy testing prior to
all inoculations. After reviewing the case, Salk concluded the child had
not suffered an allergic reaction; the high concentration of virus in the
vaccine had killed her.[36] Now more convinced of the need for adjuvants
with which he could reduce the viral content in vaccines, Salk intensified
his search for an effective agent, a line of research that would pit him
against some of the world's most powerful virologists.

As the 1946–47 flu season approached, the commission, on Francis
and Salk's advice, recommended the army vaccinate troops with the preparation used the prior year. The winter passed without incident until
April, when Salk was called to Chanute Field, Illinois, where more than 500
had been hospitalized for influenza. He found the vaccine had failed to

protect them because yet another new strain had arisen.[37] Discouraged, commission members wondered how they could ever keep up with the emerging variants of the influenza virus. Approaching the problem like an epidemiologist, Francis maintained that they could make a vaccine against any viral strain; they just needed to predict which strain would cause the next epidemic. Approaching the problem like an immunologist, Salk said that the 1947 epidemic underscored the importance of his adjuvant work. "To avoid the failures," he concluded, "you must cram your vaccine with every strain you can lay hands on."[38] There was a limit, however, to the amount of virus that could be included in each dose. He calculated that adjuvants could reduce the quantity of virus to one-hundredth of that required for the standard vaccine, yet he remained a lone advocate for this approach.

⁂

IN THE FOUR YEARS since Salk had joined Francis, they had made significant progress, considering the effort each field trial required. Thousands of subjects had to be inoculated and examined, blood samples and throat washings had to be collected and tested, data from tens of thousands of punch cards had to be analyzed. In large part, they had accomplished all this because Salk was able to enlist the help of army medical officers, physicians from prisons and mental institutions, wardens, hospital directors, nurses, and technicians. He created a sense of urgency; they were doing patriotic work. As well, he had developed close associations with research directors at Parke, Davis and Company and Sharp and Dohme, who provided vaccines at minimal charge.

Salk recognized individuals for their vital roles in the race to prevent another catastrophic epidemic and those who had been kind to him along the way. To the warden of the Michigan State Reformatory he wrote, "Without your generosity and the invaluable assistance given us by your nurses, we would not have been able to accomplish so large a task in so short a time."[39] His thank-you note to the wife of Ionia State Hospital's warden began, "You have spoiled me so that it will take a while for me not to expect fluffy pancakes, wild duck and cheesecake fit for the gods at every meal."[40] When he returned from Fort Custer, he wrote Lieutenant Colonel Slevin, "I want to express my sincere appreciation for the hospitality and courtesy shown me and for the cooperation of the personnel."[41] The next time he needed specimens or wanted to test a new vaccine, they readily obliged. And he didn't forget to thank the participants. He wrote an article for the Michigan Reformatory newspaper, notifying inmates about the study in which they had taken part, calling it an "aid in the conquest of this dreaded disease."[42] Sincere in expressing his gratitude, Salk was beginning to appreciate that his courtesy generated allegiance.

At the same time, Salk learned the power of the press. "VACCINATION AGAINST 'FLU ADVISED ON BASIS OF ARMY EXPERIENCE" read a news release summarizing Salk's presentation to the American College of Physicians.[43] When it made headlines across the country, Salk got his first taste of celebrity. But when he wrote an article on influenza immunization for *Parents Magazine*, some thought he had gone too far.[44] Salk believed experts had an obligation to educate the community. That article, however, spawned the belief among some scientists that Salk sought the public's attention.

It was true that Jonas Salk had great aspirations. "My striving was strong and unconcealed," he admitted years later.[45] He wanted to direct his own laboratory, but to do that he needed an academic appointment, and to obtain an academic appointment he needed to show independent thought. The first author listed on his early papers was Francis. Although he had designed many of the trials, Salk did most of the work. He wanted to be first author. "Everyone knows who you are," he told Francis. "It doesn't matter if your name is first or last."[46] Salk had been at the University of Michigan for four years before he received his first academic appointment in July of 1946 as assistant professor. He wanted to progress more rapidly than that. "You've got to admire ambition," Francis said, "especially when it's combined with the kind of ability this fellow had."[47]

With time, the relationship between the novice and mentor developed an edge. Salk did not always conform to the standard scientific way of thinking. Researchers in Francis's lab noted an overt tension between them. "Damn it all, Salk," Francis was heard to say, "why can't you do things the way everyone else does?"[48] Sometimes Salk's creativity paid off, such as when he devised a simplified procedure for recovering virus from chick embryos which proved quicker, less expensive, and more accurate. Sometimes it didn't. His insistence on trying to increase immune potency with adjuvants had not panned out. And then there was the issue of credit. Biochemist Paul Stumpf rarely saw Francis in the laboratory. He always seemed to be at a committee meeting or out of the country. "Jonas was doing all the work," Stumpf said, "and Tommy was getting all the fame, so that caused an obvious friction."[49] Increasingly Salk felt stymied by his boss. He had agreed to present a paper at the International Congress of Microbiology in Copenhagen, but Francis refused to cover his travel expenses. Salk wrote to the surgeon general's office, asking if he could board an army transport going to Europe: "I would be willing to work my way across or do anything necessary to justify transportation from this country across the Atlantic and back."[50] His request denied, Salk had to cancel his presentation.

The friction between Salk and Francis had a deeper source—their basic ideological differences. Francis approached disease as an epidemiologist, Salk as an immunologist. Francis was a traditional academician; Salk wasn't and never would be. His relationships with pharmaceutical companies and the press were unconventional for a scientist at that time and were thought unbecoming for a professor. Francis solved problems empirically; Salk let philosophical musings enter his deliberations. "I was not functioning in the expected way," he conceded years later. "I engaged in extrapolation because I had always felt that it was a legitimate means of provoking scientific thought and discussion. I engaged in prediction because I felt it was the essence of scientific thought."[51] As a result, his papers tended to be speculative, less data-based, rambling. "I view with some alarm," a friend teased, "the extent to which your prose has come to have a style of academic pontifications."[52] Whereas the report of the commission's pivotal vaccine trial involving fifteen investigators ran three pages, Salk's analysis of his site spread over thirty-seven. Top medical journals rejected several of his manuscripts because of length.

Salk became more difficult for Francis to rein in. Once, after reading a paper Salk had just written, Francis told him he didn't have enough data to substantiate his conclusions. "The inferences were warranted by reason," Salk replied, "if not by hard data."[53] When Francis frowned, Salk said others published without providing complete data. Francis told him that wasn't the kind of work expected out of his department. Salk said he thought he'd submit it for publication anyway. "I told him if he did," Francis recalled, "he had better go with it."[54]

Throughout 1947, Salk was investigating influenza outbreaks at army airfields across the country while continuing his work on vaccine dose and formulation at the Ionia State Hospital and Jackson State Prison, forty miles from Ann Arbor. Donna was pregnant with their second child. Their son Peter had been born in 1944, and in April of 1947, they had another boy, Darrell, making their financial situation even more precarious. Salk was getting restless. He began to seek an academic position elsewhere, even though Francis told him he was not ready to run his own laboratory. He inquired about open positions at Berkeley, UCLA, the University of Kansas, and Washington University in Saint Louis but received no offers. Then in May of 1947, virologist Max Lauffer at the University of Pittsburgh contacted Salk about a position as chief of their animal virology laboratory.[55]

None of Salk's colleagues could understand why he even looked at this undistinguished medical school with its aging faculty. "The school was seriously underfunded," a historian wrote, "its curriculum outmoded and its physical facilities crumbling and out of date."[56] A colleague warned him to be cautious; he had just heard that a promising researcher was leaving Pitt "presumably because he was totally unable to overcome the indifferences and lethargy which surrounded him on all sides."[57] Still Pittsburgh offered Salk a secretary, technician, laboratory, an associate professor title, and a salary of $7,500.[58] In addition, Dean William McEllroy, a gracious man with a laissez-faire leadership style, spent much of his time fundraising and gave faculty the freedom to make decisions. This had great appeal for Salk. "What's in Pittsburgh, for heaven's sake?" someone asked. "I guess I fell in love," he replied. "What I was in love with, of course," Salk added years later, "was the prospect of independence."[59]

By the time Salk left Ann Arbor in October of 1947, he and Francis had developed a vaccine that could prevent influenza. They had shown that a killed-virus vaccine could confer the same immunity as a natural infection and had described the herd effect. In addition, Salk had begun testing adjuvants as a means to enhance immunity. All this he had accomplished in just five years. "En route to this achievement," historian Richard Carter observed, "Salk acquired the administrative polish, the technical virtuosity and, above all, the philosophic grasp of viral disease that later enabled him to cope with polio."[60]

Pittsburgh's Virgin Territory

WHEN MAX LAUFFER showed Jonas Salk his new laboratory, he was shocked to see that it consisted of forty square feet in Municipal Hospital's basement, in what had previously been the morgue.[1] Salk had come to the University of Pittsburgh eager to move ahead with his influenza research, convinced he had a strategy to halt this protean disease. "The position at Pittsburgh suits my desires perfectly," he had written a friend, touting its "infinite potentialities."[2] No longer subject to Francis's control, he called Pitt's infectious disease program "virgin territory."[3] As he looked at his new lab, however, his exuberance faded.

❖

PITTSBURGH—THE "STEEL CITY"—one of the nation's greatest industrial centers, stands on a triangle of land where the Allegheny and Monongahela Rivers join to form the Ohio. For much of Pittsburgh's existence, warehouses, glass factories, and steel mills lined their banks. A city of contrasts, it boasted a symphony, ballet, art museum, zoo, several colleges and universities, yet had among the most dilapidated urban housing nationwide. While generating prosperity, manufacturers had created considerable pollution. "Pittsburgh was suffering from years of benign neglect," one historian wrote in the late 1940s. "Its buildings were decaying, slums blighted the historic Point District, and a thousand mill stacks and coal-burning furnaces, running full tilt during the wartime boom, smothered the city in a dense smog that turned day into night. Streetlights went on at noon, and buildings were blackened by the soot."[4]

When the Salks moved to Pittsburgh in the fall of 1947, the city had just launched a smoke-control program and an urban renewal project, cleaning the long-accumulated grime off buildings, clearing slums, widening streets, and starting to replace downtown warehouses with sleek skyscrapers. The New Deal's Public Works Administration had built the modern Municipal Hospital to house patients with contagious diseases. Donna and Jonas sought the same country living they had enjoyed in Ann Arbor and settled in the suburb of Wexford, surrounded by woods and fields, where Donna could garden and three-year-old Peter and infant Darrell could breathe clean air.[5] Salk had to remind himself of these benefits while he spent an hour and a half commuting each day. His brother Herman and sister-in-law Sylvia moved into a farmhouse three miles away with their two children. A veterinarian, Herman managed the two-hundred-acre Shalom Research Farm, which supplied animals for laboratory research.

In his new position as associate professor of bacteriology, Salk directed the Virus Research Laboratory, one of three that comprised the Virus Research Program under the direction of Max Lauffer. A plant virologist, Lauffer did not seem to understand the requirements for animal studies and clinical trials. In his rush to accept the offer, Salk had failed to stipulate specific arrangements. It was not until he arrived at Pitt that he realized Lauffer had assigned him a lab that was incommensurate with his position and inadequate for his work. In addition, the lab needed substantial renovation to be functional, requiring funds that Salk didn't have and Lauffer didn't offer. "You don't appreciate what you have until you don't have it," he bemoaned to Stella Barlow, Francis's secretary back in Ann Arbor.[6] Anxious to be independent, Salk now missed Francis. "It was good to talk to you on the phone," he wrote soon after moving. "I was really feeling quite homesick."[7]

His loneliness was mitigated somewhat when he hired his first secretary, Lorraine Friedman. In her twenties, Lorraine had no science background, had not worked at a university, and had never set foot in a laboratory. Perhaps the words in her *Pittsburgh Press* want ad—"willing to work long, hard hours"—caught Salk's attention.[8] Lorraine's Hungarian Jewish immigrant family had a strong work ethic. The first of them to attend college, she had enlisted in the navy when the war broke out. Once back in Pittsburgh, she took a job in a home-improvement firm, but she was seeking something more interesting than furnaces and water heaters when she put her ad in the paper. Lorraine liked Dr. Salk immediately. Resolute yet friendly, he spoke passionately about his work. For his part, Salk saw a presentable young woman wearing a straight skirt, sweater, and pearls. Big-boned with short, curly brown hair, which did nothing to soften her prominent facial features, she stood almost a head taller than him. Lorraine might not have known the difference between a beaker and a graduated cylinder, but she was a self-possessed, personable young woman with a whimsical sense of humor who didn't appear to be biding her time until she found a husband. Friedman stayed with Salk the rest of her career.

Before long, Salk began to chafe under university restraints. Although he no longer had to answer to Francis, now he had to seek permission from Lauffer for everything from grant proposals to buying a bookcase, and he had to account for and justify each dollar he spent. Lauffer required a formal letter of request to hire new employees, and he set their salaries. The original attractiveness of the University of Pittsburgh had been its openness, but that openness was proving to be illusory. Salk had come there seeking autonomy; instead, he said he felt "bound and gagged."[9] Although Pitt wasn't any more restrictive than most universities, Salk considered its rules and regulations "administrative bondage."[10] At one point he asked the university bursar, "Can we not consider forgetting the customary routine and the rules...[and] modify what seems to be a rigid university policy?"[11]

Rules and regulations may have exasperated him, but Salk never faltered. He had a mission to accomplish, so he began to maneuver around the blockades. He started at the top with Dean William McEllroy. His modus operandi—flattery and persistence—had proved successful in his influenza fieldwork. Writing to McEllroy, he commended the dean on a recent address, mentioning his "courage of action,"[12] and sent an outline of his research agenda, excitement emanating from every page.[13] This

resonated with McEllroy, who aspired to build a research-oriented medical school. Having laid the groundwork, Salk told the dean that a
shortage of space impeded his efforts. He had been wandering around
Municipal Hospital and thought the conference room could be converted into a lab with minimal effort; a second-floor storeroom could
house his research animals. He sent his own drawings of the renovated
space for the dean's consideration.[14] When McEllroy told Salk he didn't
have authority over Municipal Hospital space, Salk started courting the
director of the Public Health Department, I. Hope Alexander, who did.

Salk invited Alexander to visit, showed him his current space, and laid
out his plans for a virus research laboratory which would study influenza,
measles, and the common cold. He told Alexander that with a larger lab
he could provide diagnostic services for the entire Pittsburgh community.
Showing him the original hospital blueprints, Salk maintained that the
architect had intended the conference room to be used for laboratories
one day; it already had the wiring and structural arrangements. As soon as
Alexander granted his request for the space, Salk mentioned that his new
laboratory would need additional room for offices.[15] Then he petitioned
the dean for a renovation budget of $35,000, pointing out that a newly
constructed lab cost ten times as much. Furthermore, if he submitted the
work orders within two weeks, the project could be completed in three
months.[16] Before McEllroy could reply, he received yet another note from
Salk acknowledging that it might take the dean a while to obtain the
funds and requesting permission to go ahead and order the furniture so
that it would arrive in a timely manner. Payment wouldn't be due until
thirty days after delivery.[17] He continued to be politely tenacious, and the
dean came through with a grant from the Sarah Mellon Scaife Foundation.

With the dean's endorsement, Salk quickened his pace on the renovation. "He had the first and final and in-between words on everything,"
Donna recalled, "from electric outlets to paint to plumbing to office furniture. He not only knew what was on the floors but was intimately
acquainted with the undersides of the desks."[18] Before long, he notified
McEllroy that the furniture had cost a bit more than originally estimated. That plus some unanticipated plumbing, electrical work, and repair of the floor would cost an additional $10,000. And, he continued, he
still needed an autoclave and a cold room for another $5,000.[19] Some

faculty considered Salk brazen; one called him "a leading example of the genus Rugged Individualis."[20]

Next Salk set out to unshackle himself from Max Lauffer, the director of the Virus Research Program. He told Dean McEllroy that in order to remain at Pittsburgh, he needed autonomy. "All Gaul was divided into three parts," Salk soon wrote his predecessor. "Caesar has meekly stepped down."[21] McEllroy had acceded to his appeal, and now Salk reported directly to the dean. Some colleagues thought Salk took advantage of McEllroy's lax administrative style; many of their arrangements were never documented. "During his meteoric rise at Pitt," a historian wrote, "[Salk] used the confusion to operate as a free agent, almost outside the bounds of university protocol."[22] But if he manipulated McEllroy, the dean did well by it. During his tenure, no other faculty member brought more grant money or fame to the school.

As his research was getting under way, Salk was interrupted by requests to provide diagnostic services for the community—a commitment he had made to Alexander when asking for space. The Pennsylvania Game Commissioner sent him diseased animals for analysis—a rabbit with an abscessed upper jaw, eight dead muskrats, the head of a deer for which they could not determine the cause of death.[23] The director of mammalogy at the Carnegie Museum of Natural History sent him a rabbit carcass from a dog-training area, asking if it had died from a contagious disease. The rabbit had collapsed after running ahead of the dogs for half a mile. Salk sent back a note saying an autopsy revealed a large cyst, which may have contributed to its death. "I might add," he concluded, "that even without such encumbrances, I would probably have suffered the same fate if I had run a half mile."[24]

Salk tried to be a good colleague. He served on the university's Faculty Senate and a number of committees. He taught medical students bacteriology, immunology, preventive medicine, and pediatrics; he gave nursing and public health lectures. Time with Donna and his sons diminished, yet he felt compelled to work harder. He was not progressing on the schedule he had anticipated. "It has been so long since I have had a chance to take hold of... any one thing," he complained to Francis, "and carry it through without one or a thousand distractions."[25] He needed more time not only to conduct his research but also to publish his results. In academia, unpublished work was synonymous with no work; peer-reviewed publications proved research accomplishments. And recognition followed.

Funded by a contract from the Commission on Influenza, Salk continued to conduct vaccine field trials, now at Fort Dix, seventeen miles south of Trenton, New Jersey. The First Army Area Medical Laboratory was responsible for analyzing antibody levels in the blood samples from his study participants, numbering in the thousands. The process did not go smoothly. In November of 1947, Salk inoculated fifteen thousand men with one of two different vaccine formulations—a fruitless endeavor, as no epidemic occurred that winter.[26] The next year, he planned to compare vaccination with Types A, B, and A-prime to vaccination with saline. But with the war over and the threat of an epidemic decimating the armed forces having faded, Salk found the military less cooperative. The relationships he had cultivated over the previous four years became irrelevant as people returned to civilian lives; the name Jonas Salk didn't carry much clout at Fort Dix. Personnel issues plagued him. Supplies were frequently misplaced or lost. Duplication of laboratory numbers and errors in matching numbers with specimens hampered his work. When he asked the Dispensary Unit secretary why she couldn't follow his procedures, her letter of apology, filled with self-deprecation, made Salk regret his reproach. He sent a long conciliatory note.[27] When circumstances didn't improve, he tried to maintain his sense of humor. "Like a bad penny," he wrote another secretary, "I always turn up; and, as usual, I have another request which means additional work for you."[28]

The Army Laboratory staff performed no better. Their seeming indifference generated a substantial backlog. When Salk asked the director to send results to him before passing them through official channels, he replied: "No exceptions are noted which would authorize the transmittal of reports to your office."[29] With no battles to plan, the army seemed to have redirected its energy into bureaucracy. Salk could not keep up with the forms and requirements. All the good work he had done appeared to have been forgotten. Partway through the field trial, he received a letter informing him that in order for the First Army Laboratory to continue to analyze his specimens, he needed to obtain official approval. Salk couldn't even locate proof of authorization to conduct trials at Fort Dix.[30] Added to that, the administrator of the Armed Forces Epidemiological

Board chastised him for presenting a scientific paper without prior permission from the Technical Information Office: "In the future, it is hoped that investigators can adhere to the established Army procedure not only for our sake but theirs."[31] Furthermore, the university bursar notified Salk that the army would not reimburse his trips to scientific meetings because he had not obtained written approval from the Contract Technical Administrator.[32] The man who craved independence felt fettered.

Even the pharmaceutical companies, who were providing vaccine for his Fort Dix trials, were drifting off course. "The curtain goes up on the next act in this comedy of errors," Salk wrote a research associate at Squibb after receiving only one of two cartons of vaccine she insisted she had sent.[33] At one point he became concerned that antibody titers failed to rise to anticipated levels following inoculation. In many cases, the vaccine produced no response at all. Salk told Francis he thought the preparation had been altered; the dose of virus appeared much lower, and he did not know what to make of this "sleight of hand disappearing act."[34] Estimating the viral content to be about one-fifth that of prior vaccines, Salk suspected "somebody's slide rule may have slipped."[35] Months later, Francis sent Salk a letter he received from the Laboratory of Biologics Control at the National Institutes of Health stating that pharmaceutical companies had been instructed to reduce the amount of virus in each vaccine dose to minimize toxicity. Appalled, Salk replied: "This is the first official statement that we have had to support the contention that the content of virus in the vaccines presently being manufactured bears no relationship to the careful work of standardization that was carried out in the Jackson prison studies for this express purpose."[36]

As he would throughout his career, Salk maneuvered around the obstacle to further his own agenda. If the Laboratory of Biologics Control restricted the amount of virus pharmaceutical companies could include in a single dose, he contended that adjuvants should be added to reduce the viral concentration needed in each vaccine. Scientist Jules Freund had reported that adding mineral oil to vaccines held inactivated virus at the injection site for longer and incited antibody-producing cells to accumulate there, thus increasing the response to vaccination. Irritation and abscesses at the injection site, however, had precluded its use in human subjects. Working with a different formulation of mineral oil and method of injection, Salk was able to circumvent these reactions in monkeys. He proceeded to inoculate Pittsburgh medical and nursing students and measured markedly increased antibody titers. "Using the mineral-oil adjuvant," he concluded in the *Bulletin of the New York Academy of Medicine*, "there is considerable latitude for the inclusion of many more strains... to cover the entire antigenic spectrum of both the type A and type B viruses."[37] That had been his original goal—a universal influenza vaccine.

Fred Stimpert, director of biological research at Parke, Davis, agreed to prepare the adjuvant-fortified vaccine for Salk in large amounts. Within just a few months, Salk wrote Stimpert that he had inoculated six thousand people with their mineral oil vaccine with no untoward effects. Antibody levels far exceeded those observed in individuals receiving standard vaccine.[38] Furthermore, he disclosed that the Commission on Influenza had decided to test his mineral oil adjuvant in the next year's field trials. Anticipating widespread adoption of his new vaccine, Salk was startled to receive a letter from a Canadian researcher saying his work had been called into question at an international meeting.[39]

The World Health Organization's Expert Committee on Influenza had just met in Geneva, and, although a member of the group, Salk had been unable to attend. His absence proved unfortunate, as his adjuvant vaccine turned out to be a major topic of discussion. Joseph Bell, a leading epidemiologist at the Public Health Service, reported that he had not observed the same good results with mineral oil adjuvant as Salk had. "It is claimed that use of vaccines containing adjuvants results in greater antibody production," the conference proceedings stated. "These claims require substantiation."[40] The language implied Salk's trials had been flawed and needed a more experienced, reliable investigator to reproduce his results before being accepted. "Although I am by no means infallible," he wrote Bell, having written and discarded several more emotive drafts, "I can assure you that I am severely demanding of myself in regard to what constitutes sound evidence, and I have never yet been guilty and never will be of over publishing or reporting 'claims.'"[41]

To make matters worse, some committee members raised concerns about the potential carcinogenicity of mineral oil. Salk knew coal-tar products could cause cancer, but he had used highly refined mineral oils, and the animals he had inoculated two years earlier showed no evidence of cancer. Nonetheless, several scientists recommended further animal testing before considering use in human subjects. Salk told Stimpert the speculation was just a "red herring." Furthermore, he argued, "When one considers the quantity of mineral oil ingested, the quantities applied to the skin and the face in the form of cold cream, the fact they have been used in medications such as nose drops and as a base for ointments used over long periods, I believe we have much more valuable information from clinical experience than would be derived from doing a rat test."[42]

"New Influenza Vaccine Promises 2-Year Immunity," read the *Providence Evening Bulletin*.[43] "A new influenza vaccine," reported *Newsweek*, "doubles the period of immunity and promises to protect the human body against all known types of flu virus."[44] *Collier's* hailed Salk's results as "phenomenal," describing the vaccine's most remarkable characteristic to be its "roominess."[45] A large number of viral strains could be concentrated into a single shot. "What are we waiting for?" the piece asked. The public was asking the same question.

Just as Lederle Laboratories and Parke, Davis were preparing to manufacture adjuvant vaccine, Salk was notified to proceed to Washington. General DeCoursey of the Armed Forces Institute of Pathology (AFIP) had just learned of two serious problems with the adjuvant. An unnamed scientist had sent DeCoursey microscopic sections from a rabbit injected with Salk's mineral oil emulsion, showing oil droplets in the lungs and kidneys. Who knew what damage this loose oil might inflict in human subjects. Furthermore, a surgeon had warned the general that painful nodules could develop at the vaccination site necessitating surgical removal.[46] At his meeting with DeCoursey, Salk agreed to sacrifice the monkeys he had inoculated with mineral oil adjuvant vaccine two years earlier and send samples of their organs to the AFIP.[47] The pharmaceutical companies suspended vaccine production, awaiting results. Eight months passed before the AFIP issued its report: no abnormalities had been found in any of the monkeys' organs resulting from loose oil.[48] In the meantime, to settle the issue of painful nodules, Salk followed up on eighty children whom he had inoculated with a mineral oil vaccine years earlier. Nine had small nodules at the injection site which, upon removal,

turned out to be scar tissue. "Their occurrence may be a minor evil in relation to the good obtained," Salk rationalized.[49]

The drug companies weren't as sanguine. A prominent cancer researcher at the National Institute of Health predicted that it would take
ten to twenty years to determine the safety of mineral oil adjuvant. If any
injuries resulted, the researcher warned Lederle Laboratories, "the manufacturers of course would be the responsible persons against whom all
claims could and would be legally directed."[50] Consequently, Lederle
withdrew its plans for adjuvant vaccine preparation. Salk tried to hold
on, alleging great progress with a more refined mineral oil, but Parke,
Davis retrenched as well. Years later, Great Britain's Medical Research
Council, which had initially raised the specter of carcinogenicity, reported that their results with adjuvant vaccine confirmed Salk's observations. And the cancer scare later proved to be, just what Salk said it was,
a red herring; eighteen thousand men inoculated with the adjuvant vaccine had no higher incidence of cancer than those given saline. It was too
late; the mineral oil adjuvant vaccine was never patented.

IN THE LATE 1940s, Salk had joined the clique of academic virologists. Although he had helped design and prove the effectiveness of the
influenza vaccine, making a number of important observations along the
way, accumulating publications, and participating in international col-
loquia and virology society meetings, he stood at the edge of this elite
group. In his eagerness to make a universal influenza vaccine, he had
broken a number of their unwritten rules: He did not observe the
expected patterns of behavior for an academician. He was soft-spoken
and polite to the point of appearing ingratiating, yet his contention of
prevailing scientific dogma and dogged adherence to unconventional
approaches irked many. He understood the power of the press and used it
to further his agenda, even reporting results to the public that had not yet
been subjected to peer review. And he seemed too hasty in proceeding to
human application. Salk wanted to be accepted by this cadre of academic
virologists, to enter their inner circle, yet he found the politics of science
stifling. It was reminiscent of his mother's suffocating rules, which had led
him to vow, "Someday I shall grow up and do something in my own way

without anyone telling me how."[51] Now he seemed to be undermined repeatedly by the political maneuverings of senior scientists. In the midst of his thwarted efforts to advance a universal influenza vaccine, Harry Weaver, director of Research for the National Foundation for Infantile Paralysis, came to visit, and Jonas Salk's life changed forever.[52]

Polio

HARRY WEAVER, RESEARCH director of the National Foundation for Infantile Paralysis (NFIP), prided himself on his ability to spot talent, and in thirty-three-year-old Jonas Salk he saw promise. When Weaver came to Pittsburgh in December of 1947 to meet the young investigator, he came straight to the point. He invited Salk to participate in a project, funded by the NFIP, to determine the different types of polioviruses.[1] No one knew how many existed—one, two, or perhaps hundreds? And they couldn't consider making a vaccine until they did. At the time, Salk was still struggling to set up his lab at Pitt, and he immediately recognized the possibilities. "I had no experience in working with polio" he later admitted, "but this...gave me a chance to get funds, to get laboratory facilities, get equipment, and to hire staff."[2] This mundane task—typing poliovirus—could subsidize his primary research endeavor: making a universal influenza vaccine. What began as a financial opportunity evolved into a fascination, then an obsession, with the disease known as polio.

✦

NO ONE KNOWS the exact origin of poliomyelitis.[3] Medical historians have posited that a 1500 BC carving of an Egyptian priest with a withered leg and the twenty-five skeletons from ca. 1400 with deformed limbs found by archeologists in Greenland represent the earliest cases. In 1789, London pediatrician Michael Underwood provided the first clinical description of infantile fever followed by paralysis. A quarter of a century later, Italian surgeon Giovanni Monteggia reported a similar illness in nursing babies. "It begins with two or three days of fever," he observed, "after which one of these extremities is found quite paralyzed, immobile, flabby, and hanging down, and no movement is made when the sole of the foot is tickled. The fever ceases very soon, but the member remains immobile and regains with time only an imperfect degree of strength."[4]

In 1840, German orthopedist Jakob von Heine concluded the malady was an affliction of the spinal cord. Thirty years later, French neurologist Jean-Martin Charcot, examining autopsy material from children stricken with the disease, showed that assumption to be correct. Using a rudimentary microscope, Charcot localized the spinal cord damage to the anterior portion of the grey matter—the central core or marrow of the spinal cord—where motor function is controlled. A contagion or toxin had destroyed the nerve cells, yet he saw no microbes. Based on these pathologic findings, German physician Adolph Kussmaul first used the term "poliomyelitis anterior cuta" from the Greek words *polios* (gray) and *myelos* (marrow).[5]

During the late 1800s, small outbreaks sprung up: four cases in Nottinghamshire, England; ten in Louisiana; forty-four in Stockholm. At the time, physicians had more threatening diseases to worry about than a rare infantile illness. In a single year, twenty thousand in the lower Mississippi River basin succumbed to yellow fever; another year, fifty thousand Americans died from cholera. Then in 1894, Charles Caverly, a Vermont family doctor, reported 132 cases of infantile paralysis in what was the first clear-cut epidemic.

While Caverly rushed around tending patients, he kept detailed notes, and his subsequent publications aroused interest in the medical community. "Early in the summer just passed," he wrote in the *Yale Medical Journal*, "physicians in certain parts of Rutland County, Vermont, noticed that an acute nervous disease, which was almost invariably attended with some paralysis, was epidemic."[6] An astute clinician, Caverly traced the course of poliomyelitis in each patient and reported three distinct patterns. A three-year-old boy (case 2), whom he described as a "sturdy child," typified the most common course.[7] After playing hard on a hot day, his temperature abruptly rose to 104°, accompanied by a headache and restlessness. Three days later, when these symptoms subsided, the boy could no longer move his legs, and merely touching them elicited pain. After six weeks, he could walk holding onto chairs, and in three months, just a slight weakness of his right hip muscles remained. Most with this milder form of the illness went on to full recovery.

Case 88 exemplified the second pattern. This six-year-old girl had similar symptoms of a high fever and headache. On the fourth day, as her fever abated, the muscles in her legs, arms, and side of her face became flaccid. She suffered such excruciating pain that Caverly prescribed morphine for several weeks. After nine months, she only could wiggle her fingers and toes. She never improved. Devastating to patients and their families, permanent paralysis became the hallmark of this disease. Caverly illustrated the most severe form with case 32: A twenty-one-year-old woman, exhausted from nursing her sick child, ran a high fever for a week, after which the muscles of her throat weakened. She could no longer speak or swallow. Agonizing pains in her head and right eye were relieved only by death. With the first frost, Caverly saw no new cases. Of the 132 patients he had attended, thirty remained permanently paralyzed; eighteen had died.

Caverly's accurate clinical descriptions would remain unaltered in the coming decades. In addition, he made several other observations: Overexertion, chilling, or trauma often preceded the onset of disease; in some cases, paralysis involved a recently strained or broken limb. Although earlier cases had been reported mostly in infants and young children—hence its description as "infantile paralysis"—a quarter of Caverly's patients were ages six to twenty-one. And he found that adults had a more severe course with a higher death rate. No longer an infrequent disease of infants, poliomyelitis had become an epidemic disease afflicting all ages.

Like a detective, Caverly searched for clues as to its mode of spread. The epidemic started in early summer and peaked in August, after which it declined, disappearing when cooler weather set in. Most of the cases occurred in Vermont's Otter Creek valley, through which flowed a sluggish stream carrying large amounts of sewage. Yet families living along the stream did not have a higher incidence of poliomyelitis. "That the general sanitary surroundings and methods of living were in anywise responsible for the outbreak is also more than doubtful," he wrote, "since the disease showed no partiality to that class of the population whose habits and surroundings are the most unsanitary."[8] The fever and concentration of cases suggested an infectious origin; however, those living in remote areas seemed more susceptible. "Utterly inexplicable," Caverly remarked, "is the fact that many small, sparsely settled rural townships…were severely visited."[9] At the turn of the twentieth century, pediatrician Ivar Wickman traced contacts during several Swedish epidemics and concluded that polio was highly contagious. Furthermore, he noted that nonparalytic cases outnumbered paralytic ones and suspected they might be responsible for the spread of the disease. Over the next few years, Caverly counted more patients with the nonparalytic form in Vermont. He, too, thought these "abortive cases," undetected and thus not quarantined, served as carriers.[10]

The year 1908 brought the first scientific breakthrough. Searching for the responsible microbe, Viennese pathologist Karl Landsteiner removed spinal cord tissue from a nine-year-old boy who had just died from poliomyelitis. Landsteiner minced the tissue and made a solution which he passed through a filter that retained all microbes except viruses. When he injected two monkeys with the filtered fluid, one developed paralysis; the other died. Under the microscope, the damaged spinal cord tissue from the boy and both monkeys looked identical. Although scientists could not yet see these submicroscopic organisms, Landsteiner had proven that a virus caused this crippling disease.

Three years later, when Sweden suffered the largest epidemic to date, with 3,840 afflicted, researcher Carl Kling isolated the virus not only from patients showing symptoms of the disease but also from healthy children whom he deemed to be carriers. Furthermore, he found virus in intestinal washings, suggesting it was excreted in stool. One of Kling's colleagues noticed that Swedish towns struck by the 1905 epidemic were spared, which he attributed to immunity acquired during that epidemic. Soon thereafter, two French scientists found neutralizing substances (later known to be antibodies) in the blood of humans recovering from poliomyelitis. Continuing to compile Vermont cases, Caverly also observed: "A community visited by an epidemic of this disease has, apparently, comparative immunity thereafter for several years."[11] This poliomyelitis pioneer would likely have contributed even more to the public health field had he not died suddenly in October 1918 from influenza.

No one had anticipated the 1916 poliomyelitis epidemic. The seven thousand deaths in the United States marked poliovirus as a virulent organism. But attention to polio got diverted by the war in Europe and the 1918 influenza epidemic. Poliomyelitis generated only passing interest until one of the country's most charismatic politicians, Franklin D. Roosevelt, contracted the disease.

⬥

ON AUGUST 11, 1921, thirty-nine-year-old Roosevelt became ill.[12] He was exhausted from an intense congressional investigation of the navy's involvement in a Newport, Rhode Island, sex scandal under his watch as assistant secretary. On the way to his summer retreat on Campobello Island off the New Brunswick coast, he had attended a Boy Scout rally, which is where he likely became infected. The evening he reached Campobello he complained of a chill. By the next morning, he couldn't move his right leg; the next day he couldn't stand. Misdiagnosed for days, he was treated with vigorous massage. Finally a specialist was called to the island and diagnosed poliomyelitis. By then, he was paralyzed from the chest down.

Though devastated, Roosevelt had no intention of living as an invalid; he planned to return to politics one day. So Eleanor and his campaign manager, Louis Howe, projected a public image of a strong, vibrant man—a portrayal so successful it was later called FDR's "splendid deception."[13] For the next seven years, Roosevelt tried different therapeutics, always believing he would walk again. He found the most helpful to be the natural thermal spa at Warm Springs, Georgia, a once-fashionable summer resort. There, among other polio victims, he no longer tried to hide his debility, encouraging those in a similar condition. Eventually Roosevelt returned to his law practice, but he still had aspirations for the presidency. A turning point in the history of polio occurred the day Daniel Basil O'Connor, a young New York lawyer, proposed they become partners.

O'Connor was born in Taunton, Massachusetts, on January 8, 1892, the youngest of four children, to second-generation Irish immigrants.[14] His father, working as a tinsmith, never earned more than eighteen dollars a week. At age six, O'Connor peddled newspapers to help support the family, and by ten he was said to have a monopoly on the city's paper routes. Having skipped several grades, he entered Dartmouth College at sixteen, financing his education by playing violin in a dance band. Friends called him "Doc," after the college football coach Doc O'Connor. A slight man at five feet seven, he was a fierce debater, voted most likely to succeed in his Dartmouth class. Initially he planned to teach for two years after graduation to save enough for law school. But Thomas Streeter, a Boston lawyer who judged a debating contest and observed the skillful way in which O'Connor won, offered to loan him money so he could enter Harvard right away. O'Connor took his first job at New York's prestigious and powerful law firm Cravath and Henderson. When the war broke out, ineligible to enlist because of impaired vision, he moved back to Boston to work at Streeter and Holmes while his benefactor served in the armed forces. In 1919, Streeter returned, and O'Connor established his own firm in New York, specializing in oil contracts. Given the large number of Daniel O'Connors in the phonebook, he dropped his first name and became known as Basil O'Connor. That same year he married Elvira Miller, a Catholic of Irish descent from Louisville.

O'Connor had been introduced to Roosevelt at the 1920 Democratic national convention. They met again on October 9, 1922, the day Roosevelt returned to work at a New York finance company. When Roosevelt entered the lobby of the Equitable Building at 120 Broadway, his crutches slipped out from under him on the marble floor. O'Connor, who also had an office at 120 Broadway, saw him fall and helped him up. Shortly thereafter, Roosevelt requested his advice on some legal matters and, finding O'Connor quite helpful, continued to consult him. In 1924, O'Connor proposed they form a joint law practice.[15] He guaranteed Roosevelt ten thousand dollars a year regardless of his client load, which would give him time to pursue his political career and the funds to do so. In deference to Roosevelt's more senior status, he would name the firm Roosevelt and O'Connor.

The two made an unlikely pair. One was born into wealth, imbued with noblesse oblige; the other, who called himself an "Irishman one generation removed from servitude," was hell-bent on making money.[16] One was congenial with a winning smile, the other a no-nonsense man with a sign that read "What are the facts?" over his desk.[17] Nevertheless, the partnership proved mutually advantageous: O'Connor gained Roosevelt's name and contacts; Roosevelt gained a partner who did most of the work. At age thirty-five, with well-tailored suits and a fashionable cigarette holder, O'Connor had a suite at the Waldorf Towers and a gentleman's farm at Westhampton Beach, Long Island. And he and Roosevelt became lifelong friends. "It was that keen, bright spirit, that tremendous humor," O'Connor later said, "which first attracted me to him."[18] He called Roosevelt "Franklin," then "Governor," then "Mr. President." To FDR, O'Connor was always "Doc."

Roosevelt continued to frequent Warm Springs, persuading O'Connor to visit. Once there, he revealed his plans to renovate the dilapidated spa. "I thought he was crazy to want that big goddam four-story firetrap with the squirrels running in and out of the holes in the roof," O'Connor said.[19] Nevertheless, in 1926, Roosevelt purchased the Meriwether Inn, the pool, and 1,200 acres of Warm Springs for $200,000, spending about two-thirds of his fortune. "In 1928," O'Connor recalled, "he ups and becomes Governor of New York and nonchalantly says to me, 'Take over Warm Springs, old fella; you're in.' I tell you, I had no desire to be 'in.' I was never a public do-gooder and had no aspirations of that kind."[20] O'Connor just added managing Warm Springs to the pile of other tasks he had assumed from his partner. To his surprise, he started enjoying it.

The New York governorship provided Roosevelt a stepping stone to the presidency. Although he never allowed himself to be photographed in a wheelchair, FDR came to personify polio, and he used his voice to help others with the same fate. "We have a gospel to preach," he wrote in the Warm Springs *Polio Chronicle*. "We need to make America 'polio conscious.'"[21] He called it a "crusade." It was difficult to raise money for the Warms Springs Foundation, however, and after Roosevelt entered the White House, O'Connor hired a public relations expert, who suggested they raise funds with a series of "President's Birthday Balls." These elegant affairs would be held all over the country on Roosevelt's birthday, with the slogan "Dance so that others might walk."[22] It proved to be sound advice: on January 30, 1934, the President's Birthday Ball Commission raised more than a million dollars for polio treatment, and the balls became an annual event.

With time, the novelty of the Birthday Balls wore off, and Roosevelt's detractors alleged he was using the money for his own agenda. O'Connor concluded they needed a new mechanism to raise money for poliomyelitis, one divorced from the Oval Office. "I could see we were headed for a lot hotter water than Warm Springs," he said, "unless we got going with something much bigger."[23] He conceived of a voluntary health organization, overseen by a bipartisan board composed of laymen, supported by the entire public. This foundation would raise money both to support the cost of caring for polio victims and to supplement the limited federal funds for poliomyelitis research. On September 23, 1937, FDR announced the formation of the National Foundation for Infantile Paralysis, with O'Connor as president.[24] The NFIP would take its place in history as "the most intensive and comprehensive attack on a single disease ever launched by a private agency anywhere in the world."[25]

O'Connor located the foundation headquarters on the eleventh floor of 120 Broadway, down the hall from his law offices. He consulted publicists, who helped design a fundraising campaign which played upon the sympathy and cooperative spirit of the American people. Eddie Cantor of *Ziegfeld Follies* fame was one of the first to volunteer. For the 1938 campaign, he coined the name "The March of Dimes."[26] On his radio show, Cantor expressed its clear and simple message: everyone could help stop polio by sending their dimes to the president. The Lone Ranger made a similar appeal. Two days later the White House mailroom was flooded with dimes.

Perceiving the movie industry to be a major potential source of funds, O'Connor approached Nicholas Schenck, the man who controlled Metro-Goldwyn-Mayer. In the throes of defending himself against charges of violating the Sherman and Clayton antitrust acts, Schenck anticipated earning goodwill by aiding the March of Dimes and volunteered several of his stars to pose with children in braces or wheelchairs, tugging at the national heartstrings. As the CEO of Loews, Inc., which owned two hundred movie houses, Schenck offered his theaters as collection agencies starting in 1941. Before feature films began, a short film ran in which Judy Garland, Mickey Rooney, Robert Young, Jimmy

Stewart, and other Hollywood stars asked their "dear friends in the audience" to give a dime for polio. At its completion, the lights went on, and ushers passed around collection boxes.[27] In its first year, the March of Dimes took in $1,823,000; seven years later, collections totaled more than eighteen million dollars.[28] One-third came from movie theaters.

The unacknowledged element of the NFIP's campaign was the propagation of fear. Its very name—the National Foundation for *Infantile Paralysis*—underscored the most poignant aspect of the disease. In 1947, the NFIP released a short film, *In Daily Battle*, purportedly to stimulate community participation in March of Dimes chapters.[29] No child of that era will ever forget the haunting, eerie music which played as clouds blotted out the sunshine and a shadow of a figure bearing a crutch crept across the countryside, passing over a group of boys swimming in a lake. "My name is Virus Poliomyelitis," said a sinister voice. "I specialize in grotesques, twisting and deforming human bodies. That's why I'm called 'the crippler.'" In the next scene, the shadow swooped down on a farm boy, leading his horse toward the barn. "This is what I've been looking for," the voice intoned, as the boy clutched his stomach and started to fall. The camera then focused on three black children playing outside a tenement. "As you probably know," the voice whispered, "I am very fond of children, especially little children." A well-dressed man with a briefcase left a courthouse and started to get into a limousine when the shadow enveloped him. He clutched his head in pain and collapsed. "I'm quite impartial," the shadow boasted; "I've taken young and old." By then the audience knew what would happen to the towheaded schoolgirl who said goodbye to her mother and headed down the front steps. The shadow fell upon her, and as she tried to run back into the house, her body became limp. "I feel very active today," announced the voice. "I may even start an epidemic."

The public rushed to join the volunteer army to combat polio. The NFIP grew to three thousand local chapters, which became inventive in their fundraising approaches—Halloween trick or treat for dimes instead of candy; collection tins at every checkout counter; scouts, school classrooms, and church groups vying to collect the most money. Before long, Americans could barely look at a dime without thinking about polio. It seemed almost criminal to put the coin into your purse or piggybank.

"For the first time, the average man was given an opportunity to play a personal role in fighting the dread diseases which killed and maimed him and his children," a later NFIP board chairman said. "He became a partner in research. And science was changed, for this new institution called for social accountability by the scientists."[30] Although most academic researchers disdained O'Connor's methods, the NFIP provided funds previously not available in such amounts. Polio researcher John Paul at Yale likened it to "the sudden appearance of a fairy godmother of quite mammoth proportions who thrived on publicity."[31]

The three thousand local chapters were staffed by ninety thousand year-round and two million seasonal volunteers, all supervised by five regional directors who reported to O'Connor. Although the NFIP had an impressive governing board and consensus-building committees, there was no question that Basil O'Connor made all the decisions. Some praised him for his "unique social invention,"[32] calling the NFIP "the apotheosis of organized philanthropy"[33] and O'Connor a "legendary money raiser."[34] Others argued the NFIP exaggerated the threat of poliomyelitis to enhance its coffers. "Often we hear it said," O'Connor rebutted, "that the emphasis on infantile paralysis is disproportionate; that there are other diseases more devastating and of more serious economic consequence on which the Foundation should spend its money. Whether or not infantile paralysis in itself is of particular economic interest to the country, it is all that and much more to the individuals unfortunate enough to become its victims."[35]

By 1938, when the NIFP began its work, much was known about the clinical presentation and course of poliomyelitis, most of which came from observant physicians such as Caverly and Wickman, along with those who had witnessed the 1916 epidemic. Several aspects of the disease still puzzled physicians, however. If sewage provided an obvious means for spread, why did third-world countries experience less paralytic polio? In developed countries, why did the disease attack those in the middle and upper-middle classes, who practiced good hygiene? Once scientists could measure antibodies and determine who had immunity, what they found surprised them: only a small percent of American children from higher socioeconomic groups had antipolio antibodies, whereas almost half of those from lower socioeconomic groups and the majority of children from underdeveloped countries had immunity. Although the introduction of sanitation had reduced the incidence of cholera, dysentery, and typhoid fever, it had enhanced the circulation of poliovirus. Babies from poor hygienic areas were exposed to the virus while they still had protection from their mother's antibodies, transmitted to them in utero. They experienced a mild form of the disease, usually undiagnosed, and acquired lifelong immunity. "Children reared in squalor," concluded a British physician, "grow richer in antibodies than the sheltered children of the well-to-do."[36] Modern hygiene had protected infants from other deadly diseases but left them defenseless against polio. Thus, when poliovirus invaded a community that had good sanitation, it spread relentlessly.

Researchers had made a number of observations that proved to be true, yet misconceptions about the disease abounded. Early on, O'Connor asked Thomas Rivers, director of the Rockefeller Institute Hospital and one of the leading virologists of the day, to serve as his medical advisor and head the Committee on Scientific Research. Rivers fostered the Foundation's credibility within the scientific community, much of which disapproved of the NFIP's publicity stunts.

In 1945, FDR suddenly died of a cerebral hemorrhage. By then O'Connor was immersed in the polio problem. The next year he appointed Harry Weaver as director of research for the NFIP.[37] Weaver had been teaching anatomy at Wayne State University in Detroit when approached. Although his own polio research had not distinguished him, he had attributes that made him well-suited for the position: He was a skilled, exacting administrator who shared O'Connor's penchant for order and efficiency, and he had the insight to predict scientific trends. His academic credentials allowed him to maneuver within the scientific community and connect it to O'Connor's philanthropic world. A scientist himself, Weaver understood how they thought and worked. Yet he had no desire to promote his own research, preferring to foster that of others.

What O'Connor liked best about Weaver was that he had imagination and he thought big. Weaver believed the NFIP could solve the polio problem through a planned, directed research program. "If real progress were to be made," Weaver said, "individual groups of workers would have to sacrifice to some extent their inherent right to 'roam the field'…and concentrate their energies on one or, at most, a few of the objectives."[38] In this, he ran up against Tom Rivers, O'Connor's chief scientific advisor. A short, stocky man from rural Georgia, Rivers "looked and talked more like a redneck cotton farmer than a virologist," science historian Aaron Klein wrote.[39] Paul described him as belligerent when contradicted, "not above the use of pyrotechnics."[40] Rivers believed great discoveries originated in the minds of individuals and decried what he referred to as "gang research."[41] Weaver recalled, "Old Tom Rivers acted as if I were a foreign agent during my first two years around the Foundation. He challenged everything I said."[42] Later, however, Rivers applauded Weaver for initiating round-table discussions whereby NFIP-supported scientists came together to exchange ideas and think through problems, calling him a "catalyst."[43]

At the first NFIP round table in 1947, researchers agreed that before developing a human vaccine, they had to determine the number of different poliovirus types. If polio were like influenza—several viral types—vaccination against one would not protect people from infection with others. If polio were like smallpox—one viral type—the task would be simpler. Until they resolved the issue, they could not move forward. With that as their goal, the group recommended the NFIP support a typing project. Yet no established investigator agreed to undertake the task. "There were a hell of a lot more interesting things to do in polio research," Rivers said, "than to type the various strains of poliovirus that had been gathered by laboratories throughout the years."[44] Besides, many balked at the idea of the NFIP directing their work, even though it had provided them with research funds. "We were beginning to look like a troupe of trained seals," one grantee complained.[45]

It was at this point that Weaver approached Salk about participating in the typing project. Weaver had done enough homework to learn that even though Salk had not engaged in polio research, he had done some first-rate influenza work—and he was ambitious. When he met Salk, Weaver couldn't believe his good luck: here was a gracious young scientist, eager to do his bidding. Salk couldn't believe his good luck either: the NFIP would provide a generous grant to cover the work. Salk's initial interest was in obtaining funds to renovate his lab and hire staff. When

Weaver invited him to the next round table and he read the list of participants, he realized the typing project would permit entry into the privileged domain of polio research.[46] He wanted to be part of that group.
What he didn't realize was that these established scientists weren't quick
to accept suggestions from novices. They touted cooperative spirit but
prized their independence. And although they resented any attempt to
control their own work, they were happy to direct neophytes in the field.

On January 7, 1948, Salk traveled to Washington for his initiation
into the NFIP. The youngest researcher there, he met the key players in
the field. As Weaver made his introductory remarks, Salk couldn't help
but notice how savvy he was in dealing with them. He needed their help
to reach the NFIP's goal of eradicating polio, yet he held the purse
strings. At the time, the National Institutes of Health and other granting
agencies had limited funds. Weaver began with a question: "Do you believe it is important to undertake a program of research to determine the
number, characteristics, and the geographic distribution of the immunogenic types of the virus of poliomyelitis?"[47] The indisputable consensus
was yes. Paul, the senior statesman of the group, suggested that the
group's first task be to adopt a standardized method for typing and decide who would do the work. To that end, two scientists presented their
typing techniques for consideration. They first heard from Albert Sabin.

⁂

SABIN HAD BEEN born Abram Saperstejn to Jewish parents in
Bialystok, a city in the Russian Empire, on August 26, 1906.[48] (The exact
year is in question, since some Jewish parents didn't register the birth of
boys to protect them from conscription into the Russian army.) The
third of five children, Abram got a good education thanks to his mother's insistence. She sent him to a *cheder*, a traditional Jewish school where
subjects were taught in Hebrew and Yiddish, and enlisted a neighbor to
tutor him in Russian. During the World War I German occupation, he
attended public school, where all subjects were taught in German. When
the Bolsheviks invaded the new Polish Republic, he went to a Russian
school. In 1921, Abram's family immigrated to Paterson, New Jersey,
where they lived in near poverty, as his father, a weaver, could barely support them. Two cousins taught Abram enough English and mathematics

to enable him to enter high school. He did so well that his uncle, a dentist, agreed to finance his dental education at New York University. Influenced by Paul de Kruif's *The Microbe Hunters*, a bestseller which dramatized the discovery of microbes, Abram announced plans to switch from dentistry to medicine. His uncle withdrew his support, leaving Abram to finance the rest of his education through scholarships and odd jobs.

In 1930, Abram became a US citizen and changed his name to Albert Bruce Sabin. He received his MD a year later at NYU and began a residency at Bellevue Hospital. That summer, a polio epidemic hit the city, arousing his interest in the disease. After a fellowship in virology at London's Lister Institute, Sabin wrote to Thomas Rivers at the Rockefeller Institute, the launching pad for most academic microbiologists. "Here is a nice young Jewish boy," Rivers told colleague Peter Olitsky, "who is as smart as all outdoors."[49] Olitsky accepted Sabin into his laboratory, even though he had heard rumors about his abrasive personality. "I was warned by several well-meaning persons, I presume, including certain ones in favor with the Lord and with men, that it was a mistake for me to accept him," Olitsky recalled.[50] At the Rockefeller Institute Sabin did prove to be arrogant, acerbic, and condescending to those who did not share his views. Nonetheless, Olitsky found him a brilliant, meticulous scientist. Together the two were able to grow poliovirus in the nervous tissue of human embryos—the first to do so. Four years later, Sabin left Rockefeller to run his own laboratory at the University of Cincinnati.

Salk had first met Sabin in the late 1930s at the Woods Hole Marine Biological Laboratory, where they both were conducting research for the summer. A medical student at the time, Salk looked up to the seasoned Rockefeller investigator. During the war years, both worked for the army's Board for the Investigation of Epidemic Diseases, Salk on influenza, Sabin on viruses that attack nervous tissue. Sabin had distinguished himself by helping to develop vaccines against dengue fever and Japanese encephalitis. Salk later sent Sabin an outline of his technique to inactivate virus, which Sabin called "quite ingenious."[51] But if Salk thought he was establishing a collegiality with this respected virologist, seven years his senior, he was mistaken.

At the 1948 round table, Sabin, dressed in an English tweed jacket and vest, looked older than forty-one with his white-blond hair, pointed nose, and small moustache. His piercing, watchful eyes and sharp features made him resemble a fox, but only in appearance, for he was blunt and outspoken, "irrepressible," Rivers called him. "He just loves to talk. God, he will talk at the drop of a hat. He also just loves to take a poke at the other fellow."[52] Leading scientists may have admired Sabin, but they didn't necessarily like him.

When Sabin presented his typing method, no one dared to interrupt him. His procedure—serum neutralization—entailed immunizing monkeys against a known type of virus and testing to see if their serum protected other monkeys against infection with an unknown type. If it did, one could conclude that the viruses were the same type. If it didn't, they must be different types.

The next speaker was Isabel Morgan, daughter of a Nobel laureate and part of the Johns Hopkins polio research team. Rivers called Morgan a "crackajack experimenter."[53] Nevertheless, as a woman her career opportunities were limited. Before long she married and left the field of polio research.[54] At the roundtable, she presented an alternate typing method—cross immunization. By vaccinating monkeys and testing their resistance to different strains of polio, she could determine if they were the same or a different type. While the group was discussing the pros and cons of the two typing techniques, Salk was struck by the implications of Morgan's methodology. She had used killed, not live, poliovirus to immunize her monkeys. While the group was thinking about typing, Salk was thinking about vaccines.

David Bodian, leader of the Johns Hopkins research team, proposed that with two good typing methods they could proceed. Careful to get consensus, Weaver posed his next question to the group: Did they think it was feasible to conduct a cooperative experiment in which several labs would make the typing of poliovirus their major effort? Yes, the group responded. Bodian and Sabin volunteered to oversee the project. And on January 19, 1948, Salk wrote Weaver that he would be delighted to work on the typing project, assuring him that he could satisfy his requirements.[55] Weaver didn't need assurances; no one had expressed as much enthusiasm for the project as Salk. Although many scientists resented

Weaver's directed approach to research and considered NFIP money a bit tainted, to Salk, Harry Weaver was a savior. The NFIP awarded Salk $148,075 for the first year, the largest grant ever received by any Pittsburgh faculty.[56] Salk had published no papers on poliomyelitis, performed no preliminary research on the virus; he hadn't even attended a polio conference. In short, he had no credentials in this area of investigation. Yet Weaver was willing to bet on him. He had an instinctive feeling that they could expect great things from Jonas Salk.

8

The Chosen

BATTLE PLANS AGAINST polio had been drawn up at Harry Weaver's January 1948 round table. The first charge was to tally the number of different types of poliovirus. Four scientists would be working in the trenches: Louis Gebhardt at the University of Utah, Herbert Wenner from the University of Kansas, John Kessel at the University of Southern California, and Jonas Salk. Albert Sabin, David Bodian, and Thomas Francis agreed to oversee the project. These men constituted the Committee on Typing; this project represented the NFIP's first attempt at directed group research.[1]

Preparations for the typing project took a year, during which time Salk, anticipating March of Dimes funds, expanded his lab and hired staff. As he began to dismantle a conference room, a storeroom, a lounge, he showed consideration for inconvenienced hospital employees. Explaining his laboratory's mission to be the prevention of polio, he made them feel they were playing a part in its defeat. The renovation almost completed, Salk thanked Dean McEllroy profusely, telling him the NFIP considered his lab the finest in the country for polio research, after which he asked for additional space to set up a hospital ward for baby chimpanzees. He thought the female dormitory for housekeepers and nurses' aides ideal and included a sketch, saying he hoped McEllroy would agree to his request to help in "the earliest elimination of the problem of polio-myelitis as a dreaded disease."[2] The dean secured another $20,000 from the Sarah Mellon Scaife Foundation. In the end, Salk's laboratory space—originally forty square feet in the basement—totaled six thousand, spread over three floors of Municipal Hospital.

Salk hired Byron Bennett as his first research assistant.[3] This forty-year-old, self-educated Texan, a former army officer who Salk insisted be addressed as Major Bennett, had been decorated for his work controlling typhus during the war. At Walter Reed Army Hospital, he had demonstrated skill in laboratory organization and field testing, making him well suited to be Salk's chief technician. There was one drawback, however: Bennett drank heavily. Some days he came to work late, some days not at all. Instead of firing him, Salk considered his drinking a medical problem and retained him in his lab, where, as his secretary, Lorraine Friedman, observed, he was appreciated and understood.

Shortly thereafter, Salk hired a senior research associate, twenty-eight-year-old microbiologist Julius Youngner, who had worked on the Manhattan Project and at the National Cancer Institute. From the start, Friedman perceived a bit of reserve in their relationship as Youngner seemed to consider himself the superior scientist. Bacteriologist James Lewis brought experience from the drug-manufacturing world, where he had worked on vaccines. Adding four more research assistants, including Francis Yurochko, who managed the animal quarters, Salk had assembled quite a large team for a relatively young investigator. At this point, he still considered the typing project a means to support his influenza work.

In December of 1948, the Committee on Typing met at New York's Waldorf-Astoria Hotel, where Sabin, Bodian, and Francis dictated how the typing project would be conducted. For years researchers across the country had isolated poliovirus strains from individuals, yet few attempts had been made to classify them into specific groups. Scientists at Johns Hopkins and Yale had determined that their strains fell into at least two distinct immunologic types, meaning they were so closely related that immunization against one strain provided protection against other similar strains. The Committee on Typing didn't know how many strains had been collected in laboratories nationwide—maybe hundreds. They needed to test each one to see if it belonged to one of these two immunologic types.

To begin, the group selected two viruses known to be of different types—Brunhilde strain (Type 1) and Lansing strain (Type 2)—which they called "prototypes." The Brunhilde strain, extracted from the stools of seven Baltimore patients, had been named for the chimpanzee in which it had been isolated. The Lansing strain had been obtained from a deceased polio victim's spinal cord in Lansing, Michigan. The committee agreed that each investigator could choose his typing method: Morgan's cross immunization or Sabin's serum neutralization. Although he considered them equally good, Salk selected the latter. Using Sabin's method, he would immunize monkeys with Brunhilde, the Type 1 virus, and after six weeks collect their serum, which contained antibodies against Type 1. Next he would combine this antiserum and the unknown virus and inject the mixture into the brains of uninfected monkeys. If the monkeys survived, the unknown virus had to be Type 1, as the antibodies for Type 1 had neutralized it. Should the monkeys become paralyzed, it meant that the unknown virus was not Type 1, and the experiment needed to be repeated with the Type 2 Lansing virus. If these monkeys survived, the unknown virus had to be Type 2, as the antibodies made against Type 2 had neutralized it. If these monkeys became paralyzed, Salk could conclude that the unknown virus must be of yet another type.

Salk began contacting polio investigators nationwide to obtain viral samples. Sabin sent him six strains from a 1947 Cincinnati outbreak and three from patients who had died in Akron, Ohio. Strains usually bore the names of the patient from whom they had been isolated or the city in which they had been found, such as "Cincinnati Glenn," "Jacqueline Bean," and "Fofovich Pool." Soon polioviruses were traversing the country: "VIRUS ARRIVED PITTSBURGH TWA FLIGHT 370," read one telegram; "VIRUS LEAVING LOS ANGELES AIR EXPRESS THIS EVENING," read another.[4] Before long, the group had collected 196 strains to type.

Working together, the four investigators developed a camaraderie. Whenever circumstances became tense, Salk's bantering put people at ease. "I envy you for loafing on the job," he wrote Louis Gebhardt, who was waiting for strains so he could begin. "I wish you would send to me in dry ice instructions as to how you do that."[5] Once Gebhardt complained that the container of virus Salk sent had been packaged improperly and arrived with no dry ice, ruining the entire batch. Besides that, the padlock on the container had been removed and replaced with a different one without a key. He maintained he had never had such difficulty with any other lab. Salk wrote back, "I thought that the very next step in the dealings between our laboratories should be the recall of ambassadors and the severance of all diplomatic relations."[6]

In November of 1949, the Pitt team was ready to begin typing the strains they had received. Each week Salk posted assignments: Bennett— receive and catalogue stool and serum specimens from polio patients; Youngner—prepare viral pools for vaccination; Lewis—inoculate monkeys; all staff—rotate examining monkeys for paralysis; Lewis and Youngner—bleed paralyzed animals and conduct autopsies. Before the days of computers and electronic spreadsheets, Salk kept the data on index cards, handwritten in pencil.

Working with monkeys proved problematic; one always seemed to be suffering from vitamin deficiency or dysentery; some arrived infected with tuberculosis, others already dead. Animal caretakers were often scratched or bitten. The typing group needed monkeys in such quantities that the supplier couldn't keep up, causing delays. To obviate these problems, the NFIP established its own monkey conditioning center at Okatie Farms, in Hardeeville, South Carolina. They imported rhesus monkeys from India and cynomolgus monkeys from the Philippines, treated their diseases, and sold them to the investigators. Once, when Weaver got notice of a pending ban on the exportation of rhesus monkeys, he chartered all available space on planes leaving India. Soon Salk's staff was struggling to care for 415 monkeys.[7]

Initially, the four investigators found that all the poliovirus strains fell into one of the two known types. Salk considered this great news with regard to future vaccine preparation. Then John Kessel notified the group about the poliovirus recovered from the brain and spinal cord of L. J. Leon, an eleven-year-old Los Angeles boy who had succumbed to polio.[8] His virus paralyzed monkeys immunized against both Brunhilde and Lansing viruses. Kessel concluded that this strain, which he called "Leon," represented a third type. Now they would have to test all unknown strains against three prototype viruses, which would substantially increase the workload and number of monkeys. Salk's stack of index cards grew.

As expected, the work proved tiresome. "It was scut work," Tom Rivers maintained, "and, for a scientist, almost doing day labor work like digging a ditch, but these boys realized that it was a ditch that had to be dug."[9] If Salk had to dig a ditch, he wanted a better shovel to hasten the work. He turned to the controversial mineral oil adjuvant he had used to bolster the immune response to influenza virus. When he added mineral oil to poliovirus, he found that it amplified the immunizing effect of the virus, facilitating the typing. And mineral oil allowed him to induce antibody formation with only tiny amounts of virus, meaning that the supply of Lansing virus could be diluted one hundred fold. This had major implications for human vaccination.

Salk presented his findings at the January 1950 meeting of the Committee on Typing. "I believe that by a suitable combination of an initial subcutaneous injection with a small dose of . . . virus plus adjuvant," he told the group, "it should be possible to immunize monkeys for your studies more efficiently and more effectively and with less virus in a shorter time."[10] The committee dismissed his idea; no one wanted to change the procedure. Salk proved his point when a physician from the Public Health Service called Weaver requesting urgent typing of several cases. Salk said he could get the answer more quickly by adding adjuvant, and Weaver gave him permission. Unbeknownst to Weaver, Salk had been adding mineral oil for some time. Soon Gebhardt wrote asking for details about the adjuvant, then Kessel, then Wenner. Before long, the committee agreed to add mineral oil adjuvant to the typing process. A year later, Weaver wrote to Salk that he had read with great interest his article "The Use of Adjuvants to Facilitate Studies on the Immunologic Classification of Poliomyelitis Virus."[11] "I might parenthetically add," he admitted, "that after reading this article, I am pleased to forgive you for all your past and even a percentage of your future sins."[12]

At the same committee meeting, Salk offered a more economical method for typing. Currently they used the prototype strain for protection before infecting monkeys with the unknown strain. He suggested they consider the reverse system: if they immunized monkeys with the unknown strain, then tested their antisera, which contained antibodies, against the known prototype, it eliminated several steps, saving weeks of work. According to Tom Rivers, "If you had a thin skin, it was not a good idea to attend these conferences because no one was ever spared. Hell, if you presented a paper or got up to talk, you had to be prepared to be ripped apart. It didn't matter who you were."[13] Nonetheless, Salk proposed his new typing method: Didn't it make more sense to test the ability of an unknown virus to stimulate antibody formation? "Now, Dr. Salk," Sabin replied, "you should know better than to ask a question like that."[14] In a deferential manner, Salk persisted, explaining that he had calculated it required fewer than fifteen monkeys to type each strain compared with forty required by the current technique. After no debate, the group voted to continue the project as planned. "It was like being kicked in the teeth," Salk recalled. "I could feel the resistance and the hostility and the disapproval. I never attended a single one of those meetings afterward without that same feeling."[15]

Salk began to construct a protective shield. He didn't give up on his new typing method and wrote Weaver repeatedly, clarifying why he considered this approach better. Weaver finally relented and told Salk he could attempt to type several strains with his new method; the three other scientists would stay the course. After Salk proceeded to analyze seventy-four strains typed by them, getting the same results in record time, the group agreed to try his technique.

When Harry Weaver first met Salk, the young man's eagerness and ingenuousness had impressed him. He behaved differently from most investigators the Foundation supported—ivory-tower scientists who accepted its money and then disappeared to do their own work, ignoring requests from Weaver. Salk worked tirelessly yet never forgot his manners or patronized those beneath him. He treated an NFIP secretary or telephone operator with the same regard as he did a distinguished researcher. And he had an endearing quality lacking in most scientists. He continued his habit of writing thank-you notes. Partway through the typing project, he wrote Weaver, "Working with you has been a fine experience, and I look forward to an equally satisfying and productive period ahead."[16] Although he was ready to please, Salk also had a tendency to ignore protocol. Weaver had to remind him, like a tardy schoolboy, when grant applications or progress reports were overdue. Salk apologized, although he still attempted to sidestep the rules and regulations. For a while, Weaver held the reins tight. When Salk applied for funds to test gamma globulin to prevent polio, Weaver replied that he must concentrate on the typing project. Salk thanked him, expressed concern about Weaver's recent cold, and mentioned in passing that he planned to try a new tissue culture technique for growing virus.

However exasperating Salk could sometimes be, Weaver could always count on him. He often sent Salk extra specimens to type, such as serum from a surgeon's wife who had contracted polio or samples from a New Jersey hospital where a number of polio deaths had just been reported. If the NFIP wanted one of their grantees to host a foreign scientist in their lab, they asked Salk. When Salk spoke at a fundraiser in Washington, DC, Weaver discovered the young investigator's skill at communicating with the public and his impressive ability to help laymen understand the NFIP's work. Conversant in the arts and current events, he easily mingled with guests, his remarks sprinkled with humor. His earnestness, coupled with his boyishness, charmed donors.

The more Salk did, the more Weaver called upon him. When *Good Housekeeping* was preparing an article on the NFIP's activities, he asked Salk to speak with the writer. Before long a telegram arrived: "Would it be possible for National Foundation photographer to spend day with you taking background pictures on research."[17] Although seven scientists participated in the typing project, it was Salk whom Weaver asked to talk on *Adventures in Science* on CBS radio. In short, Salk was becoming the poster scientist for the March of Dimes. He was a magnet for the press. When Sarah Mellon Scaife of the Scaife Foundation wanted to donate one of Salk's monkeys to the zoo, Salk himself transported little Frances from his laboratory to its new home. A Pittsburgh paper ran a picture of Frances, which helped dispel concerns about use of laboratory animals for research. Such publicity may have put him in good stead with the NFIP, but it was eroding the legitimacy he was striving to build within the scientific community.

For now, however, Salk held one of the biggest caches of polioviruses, which made him indispensable. He received numerous requests for samples, and he was generous. "As possessor of the largest store of anti-polio

sera on this globe," wrote Joseph Melnick of Yale, "will you be able to furnish us with some anti-Brunhilde and anti-Leon sera?"[18] Pierre Lépine of
the Pasteur Institute asked, "Could you bring to New York and give me
the three monkey polio strains?"[19] What had started as a mundane task
had thrust Salk into the center of the polio research world. While providing samples, he developed a cordial correspondence with several
esteemed scientists, such as Harvard's John Enders, moving himself closer
to the collegiality he sought. When Enders wrote to Salk, "Here I am
again begging serum," Salk replied, "Dear John, It is a distinct pleasure to
be able to be helpful."[20] A few months later, Salk received a note from
Enders, vacationing at Camp Harmony Angling Club in New Brunswick,
thanking him for sending a copy of Kahlil Gibran's *The Prophet*. "I shall
always carefully preserve it," Enders wrote. "The sentiment expressed in it
I value deeply although I know I am quite unworthy of it."[21]

Salk also tried to establish a friendship with Albert Sabin. Early on,
Sabin took a gracious stance, acting a bit like a mentor. He signed letters
to Salk, "with all good wishes and kindest personal regards."[22] After a
visit to Cincinnati, Salk thanked him for his kind hospitality at his home
and laboratory. Sabin sent him a birth announcement for his second
daughter, to which Salk replied, "I shall look forward to hearing how the
siblings are doing. 'Siblings' is a technical word derived from the term
sibling-rivalry about which you will no doubt gain first-hand experience."[23] When Salk hosted a meeting for the Committee on Typing in
Pittsburgh, Sabin congratulated him on the fine work he was doing. He
invited Salk to an informal conference on diagnostic tests for polio where,
he said, selected scientists would convene in a leisurely atmosphere, each
bringing his "Pandora's box of unpublished observations, his years of
experience...as well as his critical mind."[24] At meetings, the two often
stayed up talking until after midnight.[25] Sabin appeared to be opening
the door into the polio field's inner sanctum. Yet having once felt Sabin's
sting, Salk accepted these offerings of friendship with caution.

Meanwhile, Salk knew that determining the number of poliovirus
types was only one step toward making a vaccine. In order to supply
large quantities of poliovirus for vaccine production, scientists needed to
be able to propagate virus in a test tube, not just in animals. Viruses can't
survive in culture media alone, however; they must have living cells to

support their replication. In 1949, John Enders, Thomas Weller, and Frederick Robbins had made a major leap in the field when they succeeded in growing poliovirus in cultures from human embryonic tissue. The feat later earned the three a Nobel Prize.

Salk immediately perceived the implications of their accomplishment. He told Weaver he would like to try the tissue culture technique. Weaver replied he could contact Enders if he wanted, but the NFIP would not fund a tissue culture lab at Pitt. Not dissuaded, Salk wrote to Enders. After congratulating him, he said that Weaver thought he might be willing to send him some tissue culture material to study. "I do not want to intrude on anything you yourself might be doing," he wrote. "I would like to offer, however, whatever help we can provide in determining its . . . immunizing capacity in monkeys."[26] Should this interest Enders, he would be happy to plan a joint study. Enders replied he was studying the immunizing effect in their lab already and preferred to have these results in hand before including others. Five months later, when Enders asked for some Leon virus, Salk had an opening. He sent the samples with a note saying he had been thinking of growing virus by Enders's technique and asked again if he might impose upon him for some tissue culture. Enders could not refuse; this eager young scientist who had befriended him would not be deterred. Besides, Enders, a basic research scientist, had no interest in making a vaccine. "I hope something will bring you to Boston during the coming winter," he replied, "as it would be nice to have a chance to sit down and have a talk."[27]

Resolute in his determination to master Enders's tissue culture technique, which he considered the next step in vaccine preparation, Salk appealed to Dean McEllroy for funds, and once again the dean came through with a $7,500 grant from the Spange Foundation. Salk hired a young zoologist, Elsie Ward, who became skilled at tissue culture techniques. A no-nonsense woman with short-chopped hair, Ward had a tireless work ethic and unflagging devotion. Once Weaver realized Salk was setting up a tissue culture lab, and that the Spange Foundation would get the credit, he acquiesced and funded it.

Salk found Enders's technique arduous and set out to simplify the procedure. First, Ward minced monkey testes or kidneys in a Waring blender and cultured the tiny pieces of tissue in a special mixture of nutrients, mixture 199, so called because it had taken Canadian researchers

199 attempts to perfect the combination of sixty-eight ingredients. After several days, long strands of cellular growth could be seen under the microscope. Now Salk had to introduce the poliovirus, which was no easy task. These viruses, which could fell the strongest man, proved impossible to maintain outside a living organism. Instead of growing them in a flask as Enders did, Salk put the tissue culture in test tubes, added poliovirus, and rolled the tubes continually to disperse virus among the cells. When the virus multiplied and infected the cells, their destruction could be detected under the microscope.[28] "There was so much excitement," Ward recalled. "It was such pure joy to come to work in the morning.... To look into the microscope and see what we saw was a great thrill. Dr. Salk was in the lab morning, afternoon, and night. He couldn't wait to see what was going to happen."[29]

Leaders in the field began to take note. "I congratulate you on the fine job that you have managed to do in such a short time," Enders wrote.[30] "Your manuscript has proved considerable help in getting started in the tissue culture work for which we are all so grateful," wrote Bodian.[31] Not everyone was as complimentary. Salk's research assistant Ethel Bailey recalled a visit from Sabin. When she showed him the tissue cultures, he said, "Harrumph, you won't be doing that much longer," assuming Salk's technique would never work.[32]

The NFIP-directed typing project had continued throughout this time, and in 1951 the four investigators completed their work. They found that all the polioviruses fell into three distinct types. Of 196 strains tested, 161 proved to be Type 1, twenty Type 2, and fifteen Type 3.[33] The typing project had required twenty thousand monkeys and cost the Foundation $1.3 million. "I know of no single problem in all of the medical sciences that was more uninteresting to solve," Weaver told the board of trustees. "The solution to this problem necessitated the monotonous repetition of exactly the same technical procedures on virus after virus, seven days a week, fifty-two weeks a year for three solid years. The number of monkeys utilized in this effort is legion. The physical effort expended by the investigators to cope with the struggles, dodges, and antics of this hoard of primates is almost beyond comprehension."[34]

Having spearheaded the project, Salk joined Sabin and Bodian in preparing a series of papers for publication. In the process, several of the traits that would dog him throughout his career became apparent—his unwillingness to conform to the conventional format for scientific manuscripts, his propensity for excessive wordiness, and his need to revise repeatedly, bordering on nitpicking. This should have been Salk's chance to learn how to write clear, concise scientific papers from two of the best. Instead, he told Bodian, "I'm still the non-conformist that I was before we became involved in the cooperative."[35] He did follow Bodian's suggestion regarding authorship. Recalling how disappointed he had been when Francis put himself as first author on papers for which he had done most of the work, Salk added Youngner, Lewis, Bennett, and Ward as coauthors with his own name somewhere in the mix. Bodian told Salk he should be first author on his papers, saying, "You are leaning over backward too far."[36] Salk took his advice, only to be accused later of failing to credit the contributions of others.

Salk was selected to present the results of the typing project in September 1951 at the Second International Poliomyelitis Conference in Copenhagen, marking his debut in the international scientific community. Opened in the presence of the queen of Denmark, the conference was attended by six hundred delegates representing thirty-seven countries.[37] Salk's talk generated a great deal of attention. Identification of the three distinct types of poliovirus paved the way for a vaccine. As well, the typing project represented a milestone in scientific research: a group of investigators in four separate laboratories had collaborated on the project. And it signified a new approach—directed research, whereby a granting agency engaged academic scientists to perform a specific task. "It was a major triumph for the NFIP," wrote Yale virologist John Paul, "to have engineered this cooperative endeavor among a highly individualistic group of research workers, some of whom had hitherto no doubt considered their laboratories to be sacrosanct."[38]

✦

HARRY WEAVER BOOKED Salk to return home aboard the *Queen Mary*. Having traveled to Copenhagen on the *Stockholm*, the smallest North American passenger ship, he now boarded one of the world's grandest ocean liners, unaware that it would provide the backdrop for a significant turning point in his life. Christened in 1934, the *Queen Mary* spanned a thousand feet with twelve decks, holding two thousand passengers as well as a thousand officers and crew. Amenities included two indoor swimming pools, paddle tennis courts, libraries, the Observation Bar and Art Deco Lounge, and kennels. Paneled staterooms with thick carpets and carved furniture bespoke luxury; the Grand Salon, a three-story, columned dining room for the first class, underscored its magnificence.[39]

On board with Salk during the four-day transatlantic crossing was Basil O'Connor.[40] Although they had yet to meet formally, each had undoubtedly sized up the other. Salk admired O'Connor—the son of a tinsmith who had become a successful Wall Street lawyer, who dressed impeccably in tailored pinstriped suits with a white carnation on his lapel. Doubtless Salk had heard from those who worked for O'Connor that he was a bold, blunt, domineering boss who met conflict head-on and did not tolerate buck passers, vacillators, or those who refused to follow orders. And he presented a paradox: he enjoyed a moneyed lifestyle yet took no salary from the March of Dimes. Hell-bent on triumphing over poliomyelitis, he approached it like a complex legal case. "He was fascinating," Salk recalled of his first impressions of O'Connor. "He was different from anybody else in the crowd. He was very much in command of the situation....He had it within his power to cause almost anything to happen."[41]

In Salk, O'Connor saw a nice young man, anxious to please, whom Weaver had plucked from the influenza world to do the Foundation's bidding. And he had done it well. At Typing Committee meetings, O'Connor must have observed how Salk seemed to shy away from conflict. He seldom spoke, except to suggest a novel approach, and he ostensibly deferred to his elders, especially Sabin, when remonstrated. With quiet resolve, however, he maneuvered around barriers. If Weaver or the committee dismissed one of his proposals outright, he did not press his point publicly but waited for the opportunity to demonstrate its validity, letting his results speak for themselves. O'Connor recognized that Salk was not a conventional scientist; he moved quickly, found shortcuts, and did not adhere to the unwritten rules of academic research. He had made a good showing in Copenhagen, enhancing the NFIP's credibility in the scientific community. Added to that, he appeared well groomed for a researcher and met the public with sincerity and humility. It didn't take

O'Connor long to realize how perfect this combination of attributes would be for the March of Dimes' purposes.

Weaver informed O'Connor that two of the NFIP-supported scientists, Enders and Salk, were on board the ship and suggested they join him for dinner. Salk was seated next to O'Connor's eldest daughter, Bettyann Culver, a courageous young woman who not quite a year earlier had called her father and told him, "Daddy, I've got some of your polio."[42] Her entire left side was paralyzed. After lengthy rehabilitation at Warm Springs, away from her family, she had recovered, left only with weak abdominal muscles. Her father had invited her along for relaxation. Watching Salk speak to his daughter with kindness and concern must have touched O'Connor. Perhaps that was when he realized that Salk, whose behavior some construed as obsequious, was indeed ingenuous; and when Salk realized that, far from being dispassionate, O'Connor had a tender side, revealed in his fondness for his daughter.

Salk later recounted the beginning of his relationship with O'Connor: "I stood immersed waist deep in a swimming pool aboard the *Queen Mary* having a philosophical conversation with Basil O'Connor whom I had just met....He made me feel as if I could see more broadly, more clearly, and more deeply than I could when alone or with others....I felt I had found a kindred soul."[43] Almost sixty, O'Connor viewed the world with hard-boiled realism; at thirty-nine, Salk still embodied youthful idealism. Yet both aspired to improve the well-being of mankind—O'Connor in a practical, calculated way, Salk as an almost mystical calling. And both men were prepared to take great risks to achieve their goal—O'Connor as commanding general of the March of Dimes, Salk behind closed doors. Years later, O'Connor recalled his first impressions of Salk: "Jonas is in touch with the world. I don't mean that he's worldly. He's not. In some ways he reminds you of a girl who's never been in a bar before. But he is a human scientist....He sees beyond the microscope....These are the reasons, along with his friendly, modest ways and his unmistakable sense of honor and rectitude, that I liked Jonas. Before that ship landed I knew that he was a young man to keep an eye on."[44]

That day a friendship began that would link the two men for life. Some thought that in Salk, O'Connor had found the son he never had, but that seems oversimplified. Some considered O'Connor to be Salk's patron, though Salk never enjoyed the freedom of creativity such an arrangement implies. Others characterized their alliance as reciprocal manipulation by two opportunists. Salk had found a means to obtain research funding; O'Connor had spotted a good-will ambassador to enhance the March of Dimes' popularity. Self-interest certainly played a part, but that could not have sustained the depth of their friendship, which lasted for twenty years. Whatever the underlying attraction—perhaps simply a mutual admiration—a courtship had begun. Over the next two decades, Salk and O'Connor would help each other realize their dreams and sustain each other through their darkest hours.

Salk left for Copenhagen a young virologist from a mediocre medical school. He returned a rising star in the field. He had stood on the edge of polio's scientific inner circle, and on the trip home aboard the *Queen Mary*, he formed a bond with the power broker for polio research. Before long, those vying for NFIP funds considered Salk "the chosen."[45]

WHILE SALK WAS participating in the typing project, he continued his influenza research in his lab and at Fort Dix, still hoping to make a universal vaccine. Half his correspondence related to influenza, half to polio. "I've been on the go almost continuously for the past six weeks," he wrote a colleague in early 1952.[46] He began to relinquish teaching obligations; his seat at medical school meetings remained empty; memos began, "I'm sorry but . . ." He came home long after the boys had gone to bed. Trying to spend time with his family, he rented Hatch Cottage at Oberlin Beach, where thirteen bungalows sat perched on the cliffs above Lake Erie. The only telephone hung on a pole several cottages away. Donna likely thought she and the boys would have a chance to reclaim Jonas's attention. While they went to the beach, however, he stood at the telephone pole talking.[47] Although Peter saw his father occasionally play Jotto or Scrabble with their neighbor, Bob Tufts, Adlai Stevenson's speech writer, he spent most of his time lying in a hammock, working.

Back home in Pittsburgh, Donna and Jonas did not attend the theater or symphony or movies. Total responsibility for the household fell to Donna. When she wasn't tending to her sons, she read novels or played the piano. She often took the boys to Uncle Herman and Aunt Sylvia's nearby farm, where they romped with their two cousins among the horses, dogs, and assorted animals. At times Salk joined them, although he always seemed preoccupied. Sylvia recalled once when he had asked about her. As she began to talk, his attention seemed to be drifting. "Then I went to the doctor," Sylvia said, testing him, "and the doctor told me that I have only six months to live."[48] Her brother-in-law continued to smile and nod.

Salk needed to find more time. Tired of losing an hour or more each day commuting, he persuaded Donna to give up their country home in Wexford and move into a three-story brick house with pillars on Squirrel Hill, closer to the hospital. That didn't help, however; he still felt overwhelmed. Finally Salk conceded: his workload was simply too great. He could no longer fight on two fronts, conducting research on both polio and influenza. "It has been difficult for me to accept the obvious fact that I must do something about lessening . . . the many responsibilities I have," he wrote to Thomas Francis in early 1954. "I have come to the conclusion that it would be best to take a leave from the influenza program. It has been a difficult decision but one that I know you will understand."[49] Twenty-two years would pass before Salk returned to influenza, a disease he believed he could prevent but for which he had run out of time.

Meanwhile, Salk turned his full attention to polio. Its specter loomed every summer, and Salk didn't want to stand in line behind the cadre of senior scientists, low on the pecking order, waiting to help develop a vaccine on their timeline. He had told Weaver in 1948 that he planned to have a vaccine in five years. Now that he had just jumped two major hurdles, identifying the three types of poliovirus and mastering viral growth in tissue culture, Salk thought he could make that target. "There was nobody like him in those days," Weaver told historian Richard Carter. "His approach was entirely different from that which had dominated the field. . . . He thought big. . . . He was out of phase with the tradition of narrowing research down to one or two details, making progress inch by inch. He wanted to leap, not crawl. His willingness to shoot the works was made to order for us."[50]

Ready to Run

In 1951, THE number of polio cases in the United States was rising—twenty-eight thousand new cases by year's end.[1] No place seemed immune, including Pittsburgh. Diana Ney had just graduated from nursing school when she went to work on Municipal Hospital's polio wards. Aspirating secretions from tracheostomies, passing gastric tubes, trying to manage the patients' excruciating pains with only aspirin, and helping some adjust to a life of dependency, she soon felt drained. A soldier who had survived the war, now to be crippled by polio, asked Ney to play his favorite record over and over: "There's nothing left for me of days that used to be. I live in memory among my souvenirs."[2] A teacher who had just been removed from an iron lung called Ney repeatedly throughout the night shift, annoying the young nurse until she realized the woman was afraid that if she fell asleep she would stop breathing. "One year the ambulances literally lined up outside the place," a senior nurse recalled. "There were 16 or 17 new admissions every day.... To leave the place you had to pass a certain number of rooms and you'd hear a child crying for someone to read his mail to him or for a drink of water.... It was an atmosphere of grief, terror, and helpless rage."[3]

Jonas Salk was now fully engaged with finding ways to prevent poliomyelitis. Several discoveries propelled his work forward: In addition to the
identification of the three poliovirus types and Enders's cultivation of poliovirus in tissue culture, Dorothy Horstmann at Yale and David Bodian at
Johns Hopkins had found that poliovirus was present in the bloodstream
prior to paralysis. Previously scientists thought the virus entered the body
through the nose and traveled along nerves to infect the brain. Now they
knew that not to be the case. Although polio was spread by secretions from
the nose and throat, it now appeared that, once swallowed, poliovirus multiplied in the lymph tissue of the tonsils and intestines, entered the circulation, and from there infected the brain and spinal cord. Horstmann's and
Bodian's discovery had enormous implications. If one could intercept the
virus before it reached the brain, paralysis could be prevented.

The body's best defense against circulating virus is antibodies. These
proteins, produced in response to foreign substances, can attach to and
destroy viruses in the bloodstream. Scientists at the time knew of two
ways to provide antibodies: People could be actively immunized to produce their own through inoculation (with either weakened live or killed
virus). Alternatively, gamma globulin, the fraction of blood serum that
contains antibodies, could be obtained from patients who had already
had polio and injected into healthy people, imparting what was called
"passive immunization." Salk intended to pursue both approaches. He
even considered immunizing cows and hens so the public could acquire
antipolio antibodies from milk and eggs.

"I think that the time has come," he had told Weaver in June of
1950, "for initiating the critical experiments for immunologic prevention, and more than that, the time has come for these experiments to be
carried out in man."[4] Anticipating disparagement from Sabin, Enders,
and other senior scientists, Salk asked Weaver not to subject his proposal
to review by his advisory committee. Weaver consented. The NFIP
granted Salk $184,500, with the stipulation that the money only be used
to develop a vaccine, not to study passive immunization with gamma
globulin, milk, or eggs. Having wisely narrowed Salk's focus, Weaver set
him on an accelerated course in the right direction.

To guide the NFIP in polio prevention, Weaver formed the Committee on Immunization, which included Bodian, Enders, Francis, Paul,

Sabin, Salk, and several other prominent virologists. O'Connor, Rivers, and NFIP medical director Hart Van Riper represented the Foundation, with Weaver as chair. On May 17, 1951, the committee held its first meeting at the Commodore Hotel in New York City.[5] The main topic on the agenda was a proposed human trial of gamma globulin.

William Hammon, one of Salk's colleagues at Pitt, had shown that gamma globulin from infected monkeys, when given to uninfected monkeys, prevented paralytic polio by passive immunization. Its protection, however, was short-lived, making it useful mainly after known exposure or during an epidemic. The public had grown wary waiting for the March of Dimes to do something to protect their children, and Hammon proposed a field trial of gamma globulin. Although the committee concurred with his suggestion, members could not agree on the study's design. As an epidemiologist, Hammon knew that in order to conduct a valid trial, patients needed to be randomized between two groups—a test group who received gamma globulin and a control group who received an injection of placebo. The study should be blinded, such that neither health care workers nor participants knew who received which. Some on the committee argued against this approach, pointing out that children who sustained any type of injury to a limb, including an injection, during a polio epidemic could develop paralysis in that limb. Thus, thousands of children randomized to placebo would be put at increased risk. The group reached an impasse.

Two months later, the committee continued the debate.[6] From the start, the group got bogged down over the smallest details. Salk barely spoke. Then late in the day, he raised his hand and proposed that they let Hammon have the freedom to design the trial as he thought best; they had to trust the experienced researcher. The group paused in its debate. Salk was trying not only to expedite initiation of the trial but also to set a precedent with this powerful committee, so that the principle of scientific freedom would be established when his own turn came. The committee followed his advice.

Hammon chose to start in Provo, Utah, the site of an incipient epidemic, and in September of 1951 he inoculated five thousand children, half with gamma globulin, half with placebo. Each dose required a painful injection of up to ten milliliters of fluid into the buttocks. On December 4, he reported to the Committee on Immunization that the results looked promising: the number of paralytic polio cases in the treatment group was one-quarter of the number in the group who had received placebo. And he found no indication that any child developed paralysis in a limb as a consequence of the injection.[7] Even so, the trial was too small to withstand the scrutiny of statisticians. To prove its efficacy beyond a doubt, Hammon conducted two major studies in the summer of 1952. As polio struck Houston, thirty-three thousand children were enrolled in another randomized study. By now the public knew the potential benefit of gamma globulin, and parents pressured their doctors to obtain doses for their children on the black market, confounding results. At the same time, sixteen thousand children entered a trial in Iowa and Nebraska, where an epidemic was threatening. Combining data from these three studies, totaling fifty-four thousand subjects, Hammon confirmed that gamma globulin conferred significant protection against polio.[8]

Gamma globulin would not solve the polio problem, however, as Hammon and the NFIP knew full well. The antibodies in gamma globulin were eliminated from the body gradually, providing protection for only two to five weeks. Furthermore, in order to get high levels of antibodies to all three types of poliovirus, the Red Cross had to pool serum from tens of thousands of adult volunteers, making it inordinately expensive. To inoculate children in New York City alone would cost millions of dollars. Even worse, gamma globulin could be contaminated with other viruses, such as hepatitis. Nevertheless, it was the only protection the public had. "O'Connor wasn't the type to stand idly by while children were needlessly paralyzed," NFIP official Gabriel Stickle recalled, "even if gamma globulin was only marginally effective."[9] He set out to corner the world's supply, committing eighteen million dollars from the March of Dimes. "35,000 TO GET POLIO SHOTS IN ELMIRA AREA," announced the *Chicago Daily Tribune* in June of 1953. "Health authorities rushed crews into two polio stricken counties today to set up the biggest mass anti-polio inoculation in history," the article reported about an outbreak in south-central New York which had reached epidemic proportions.[10] O'Connor knew gamma globulin could never provide worldwide prevention. He called it a "stopgap" until they had a vaccine.[11]

⁂

BACK IN 1951, when Salk began to talk about active immunization to the Committee on Immunization, it brought back painful memories of the 1934 attempts.[12] The outcome had been disastrous. That year, William Park, director of the New York City Health Department's research laboratory, announced that his assistant, Maurice Brodie, had prepared a polio vaccine using virus extracted from the spinal cord of infected monkeys, presumably inactivated by formalin. Six volunteers, including Brodie and Park, received the vaccine. "There is no danger," Park told the press.[13] At the same time, John Kolmer of Philadelphia's Institute of Cutaneous Research made a vaccine using a live virus weakened by chemicals. Having inoculated forty-two monkeys, his two children, and himself, he publicized his success two days following Park's announcement. A deadly polio outbreak had just devastated Los Angeles. The public was pressing for protection. The two researchers raced to see whose vaccine would be first to rid the world of polio—Brodie's inactivated virus or Kolmer's attenuated live virus.

Before the scientific community had time to review their data, both hastened to conduct field trials involving over ten thousand children. Ten suffered paralysis. Kolmer and Brodie speculated that the children had become infected prior to immunization. More cases followed. Tom Rivers of the Rockefeller Institute tested both vaccines in monkeys and found neither prevented polio. Worse yet, several became paralyzed. At an American Public Health Association meeting in November of 1935, Rivers chastised the two scientists, saying they had rushed into human experimentation without proper animal work and safety tests. "Gentlemen," Kolmer replied, "this is one time I wish the floor would open up and swallow me."[14] Brodie's career plummeted; a few years later, he died suddenly from a suspected suicide. Investigators in the field became leery, constraining further vaccine work.

Years had passed with almost no progress toward a polio vaccine. Then in March of 1951, three investigators presented their work at an NFIP round table. Isabel Morgan of Johns Hopkins reported that she had prevented paralysis in monkeys using multiple inoculations of a chemically inactivated poliovirus extracted from the nervous tissue of infected monkeys. She remained cautious, saying her results could not be translated into human use. Her colleague Howard Howe, after testing his inactivated-virus vaccine in chimpanzees, had inoculated six mentally disabled individuals at Rosewood Training School in Owings Mills, Maryland.[15] Although he measured elevated antibodies in each, no one wanted to give his vaccine to millions of healthy children. Researchers had found a virus could be inactive in one species and cause paralysis in another. Even more worrisome, these vaccines had been prepared from monkey spinal cord, and injected nervous tissue could cause inflammation so severe that it destroyed the human brain.

Next to speak at the NFIP round table, virologist Hilary Koprowski surprised the group with the announcement that he had made a live virus vaccine. A graduate of both Warsaw Conservatory of Music and Warsaw University, where he studied medicine, Koprowski was fluent in several languages and stood out in the group with his cosmopolitan charm and striking good looks.[16] Two years younger than Salk, Koprowski had already made his mark in the virology field through his research on rabies and yellow fever. Now he was tackling polio. He had grown poliovirus in the cotton rat and passed it through several generations, called "serial passages," until the virus became weak enough to stimulate antibody formation without generating polio. One afternoon in 1948, he and his assistant had ground up rat brain and spinal cord, teeming with the live attenuated poliovirus, and drunk the gray, oily mixture, thus vaccinating themselves.[17]

At the 1951 round table, Koprowski disclosed that he had administered his rodent-adapted poliovirus to twenty volunteers. All developed antipoliovirus antibodies with no ill effects; most excreted virus in the stool. "How dare you," Albert Sabin yelled. "Why did you do it? Why? Why?" Koprowski, who rivaled Sabin in brazenness and imperiousness, rejoined that someone had to do it, to which Sabin retorted, "You may have caused an epidemic."[18] As a scientist at Lederle Pharmaceutical Labs, Koprowski had the funds and freedom to move ahead with his work on a live-virus vaccine outside O'Connor's sphere of control, which would later cost him.

The work of Morgan, Howe, and Koprowski supported Salk's belief that polio could be prevented. Yet they had made their vaccines before the three types of poliovirus had been identified, before the virus could be grown in tissue culture instead of rat brains or other nervous tissue, and before antibodies could be accurately measured. Thanks to the work of Enders, Salk now had the requisite tools. His influenza research had trained him in the preparation of vaccines and the conduct of clinical trials. He had NFIP funding and a smooth-functioning laboratory. If left alone to do his work, Salk knew he could be successful in a brief period.

At this point in the history of polio, most virologists, including Sabin, Enders, and Koprowski, favored a live-virus vaccine. Epidemiologist Alex Langmuir said there was "an almost religious fervor on the part of many in the scientific community that killed vaccines are incomplete."[19] They believed that only live viruses could provide lifetime protection by inducing a low-grade, almost imperceptible infection. Salk believed that a killed virus, although it had lost its ability to cause infection, could still retain its "antigenicity," the ability to stimulate production of antibodies. He and Thomas Francis had shown that to be the case with the influenza vaccine. Salk held fast to his conviction and set out to make a killed-virus vaccine to prevent polio.

⁂

WITH HIS 1952 NFIP grant, amounting to $196,920, Salk made several important additions to his team: Donald Wegemer, a Pitt graduate student and laboratory jack-of-all-trades; German physician Ulrich Krech, who developed their vaccine safety tests; and Percival Bazeley, an Australian physician, who had mastered techniques to mass-produce penicillin during World War II, making Australia the first country to supply the life-saving antibiotic to its troops. Bazeley provided Salk with the expertise he lacked in large-scale drug manufacturing, a crucial skill when they undertook widespread vaccination.[20]

In the lab, Salk's team had to be inventive. They didn't have hoods to protect tissue cultures from infection. Working on open lab tables, they used towels soaked in mercuric chloride to prevent air currents from contaminating the cultures. Nothing protected the researchers themselves. On one occasion, lab assistant Ethel Bailey was carrying 152 tissue culture tubes into an incubator the size of a walk-in refrigerator when she tripped. Several tubes containing live virus shattered. "We just cleaned it up with Lysol," she said.[21] Reporter John Troan recalled the time he was visiting the lab, and Jonas spilled some tubes of virus. "I broke the 110-yard dash [record] getting out," he said.[22] Salk wiped it up himself.

The team worked around the clock, as some experiments required testing samples every two hours for forty-eight hours. Despite the pace, their boss seemed relaxed. His optimism and excitement permeated the lab, now spread over the basement and first two floors of Municipal Hospital. Polio patients were housed on the three floors above them. "If you want inspiration," Salk told his staff, "look to heaven, and take your views of the third, fourth, and fifth floors."[23] They soon found themselves working harder than they ever had, though none harder than Salk.

To begin the process of creating a vaccine, they needed to choose three viral strains, one of each immunologic type, that could induce high durable antibody titers. For Type 1, Salk picked the Mahoney strain, isolated by Thomas Francis from a patient in Ohio. For Type 2, he chose the so-called MEF-1 strain, isolated by Rockefeller scientists in 1943 from spinal cord tissue of a British soldier who had died from polio while serving in the Middle East Forces.[24] For Type 3, he selected the Saukett strain, isolated in his own laboratory from the stool of a ten-year-old who had been hospitalized at Municipal Hospital with paralytic polio. (The boy's name was actually Jimmy Sarkett; it had been misspelled by a clerk.)[25] Salk's assistant Elsie Ward grew the three types of poliovirus in cultures of monkey kidney tissue.

Next Salk needed to devise a method to inactivate virus completely. As Isabel Morgan had done, he used a solution of formaldehyde called formalin to inhibit the virus's infectivity but not its antigenicity, the ability to stimulate antibodies. To determine if any live virus remained in the batches of vaccine, he placed minced monkey kidney tissue in a test tube and under the microscope looked at the long strands of cells growing from the tissue. If he introduced live virus into the test tube, the cells were destroyed. If he added virus that had been inactivated by formalin, the strands of cells continued to expand. This method was cumbersome, however. Salk and his research associate Julius Youngner devised a simpler method, using phenol red, a color indicator that turned yellow when mixed in an acidic solution.[26] They added phenol red to the tissue-culture system. If the kidney cells grew normally in the culture, the solution became acidic, turning yellow. If they added live virus, which killed the kidney cells, the solution stayed red. Thus, yellow meant the virus had been inactivated; red indicated the presence of live virus. This ingenious method greatly facilitated vaccine preparation. (Although he said nothing at the time, Youngner later alleged that his boss had taken credit for his idea.)[27]

After that the team investigated the optimal formalin exposure time, temperature, and dose required to inactivate each of the three strains. They assayed each batch for the presence of live virus using the color test, and if a trace remained they discarded it. To double check, they injected inactivated virus directly into the brains of a dozen monkeys and after twenty-eight days sacrificed the animals to search for live poliovirus in their brain tissues. Finding not a single live virus, Salk concluded complete inactivation had occurred; the vaccine preparation was safe. Finally, based on his experience with the influenza vaccine, he added mineral oil adjuvant to enhance the effect. Ready to test the preparation's ability to stimulate anti-polio antibodies, his staff inoculated monkeys with vaccine and several weeks later injected a paralyzing dose of virus into the bloodstream. The vaccine prevented paralytic poliomyelitis in every case. The entire procedure of making a vaccine took Salk and his team only three months.[28]

Salk was poised to prevent polio. He had the skills, a modern laboratory, a committed staff, ample funding, and a good relationship with the pharmaceutical companies who could produce large amounts of vaccine. Above all he had passion. He was like a racehorse ready to run, not because he wanted to outpace the other horses but because there was a finish line he wanted to reach. He longed to be let out of the gate. But two forces were holding him back—his growing fame and the politics of science.

Salk was beginning to find the press burdensome. He did not want to raise expectations for a polio vaccine prematurely, and he did not want to become a public figure. As he began to gain renown, however, people wanted to know more about this potential knight in shining armor. Yet the more reporters asked about his private life, the more he shied away. Eventually, he made one exception. When John Troan of the *Pittsburgh Press*, whose beat included the medical school, first approached him, Salk declined an interview. Troan assured him he had an interest in "factualism," not "sensationalism," and gradually gained Salk's trust.[29] Still, as a reporter, Troan had a job to do. Soon after Salk had confided in him that human tests were imminent, headlines in the *Pittsburgh Press* read: "PITT TO TEST POLIO SERUM ON HUMANS."[30] As a result, reporters besieged Salk with requests for interviews. He avoided most, though he agreed to *Life* magazine's request for a brief photo shoot, at Troan's insistence. When the photographer remained until late into the afternoon, Salk told Troan, "It's a damn good thing this is Leap Year. I can make up the lost day."[31] The two were sometimes seen having lunch together in a local Chinese restaurant. Rumor spread among Pitt faculty that they had made a deal: if Troan promoted Salk in the press, Salk would see to it that Troan became the medical editor for the Scripps-Howard newspapers.[32]

As the public became more aware of his work, Salk's volume of mail increased. He never learned to dodge these intrusions. He told Lorraine they must respond to each letter; he had great regard for the public and thought each voice should be acknowledged. No other scientist would have answered the Toronto, Ohio, housewife who said she thought cats caused polio. "It is very kind of you to share this idea with me," he wrote.[33] When S. H. Tyler of Raymond, Minnesota, suggested that anxiety predisposed people to paralytic polio, he replied, "Your suggestions are interesting."[34]

It wasn't just the general public that made demands on Salk's time; Weaver didn't hesitate to make requests either, knowing that Jonas would oblige him. When a Saint Louis scientist wrote that Weaver had suggested he visit Salk's laboratory for two or three days to learn his techniques, Salk replied he would have to wait until later in the month, as he already had visitors the entire first part of the month. On another occasion, Weaver wrote that he was coming to Pittsburgh with a photographer and hoped to do a picture story on tissue cultures. Weaver never would have asked the same of Enders.

Salk's second major impediment was the NFIP Committee on Immunization. At its December 4, 1951, meeting, Salk presented preliminary data demonstrating that antibodies in monkeys vaccinated with inactivated vaccine plus adjuvant were equivalent to levels following natural infection in man. Rivers interrupted his presentation, saying, "I think we will all admit that there is no test to be sure this stuff is inactive. Why not just accept that?" Sabin, too, chastised Salk: "Human experimentation with vaccines which cannot be assayed and compared in a definite way are useless."[35] Talk of the 1934 Brodie disaster followed.

Sabin went on to propose the committee's next steps. Not all NFIP-funded investigators should be working on the same thing, he argued.

They had a large enough army of researchers to divide into regiments, each of which could tackle different aspects of the problem. One regiment would determine the optimal three polio virus strains to include in a vaccine. Another would work on weakening live virus to be used in an oral vaccine. Yet another would feed live virus to volunteers. Salk felt himself being demoted to noncommissioned-officer status under General Sabin. He did not want to be constrained by Sabin's or anyone else's timeline. And he did not want to be told what to do. Ready to initiate a human trial himself, Salk did not reveal his intentions.

Research Sub Rosa

EPIDEMIOLOGISTS FORECAST THAT 1952 would be a record year for poliomyelitis. "Eight in One Family Stricken," announced the *Chicago Daily Tribune* on September 12.[1] "Fifth Polio Case on North Carolina Campus Strikes Freshman Guard on Football Squad," read a *New York Times* headline on October 4.[2] The press was full of harrowing tales of innocent people being maimed or dying, such as twenty-three-year-old Philip Thorpe. Three days before he was to receive his US Air Force flight wings at William Field in Chandler, Arizona, he got a flat tire. When he tried to lift the spare tire out of his trunk, he found he couldn't. Then his legs gave out. He was rushed to Phoenix Memorial Hospital. The young man never walked again.[3] Twenty-two-year-old Lawrence Lubin had just come back from a Cape Cod vacation when he became so weak he couldn't even scratch his nose; then he couldn't swallow. "Bulbar polio," he heard a doctor tell his wife from the iron lung in which he had been entombed. "Be prepared for somebody who is going to be pretty useless his whole life."[4]

In early 1952, Jonas Salk told Harry Weaver the time had come to test his vaccine in human subjects. Both knew the Committee on Immunization would block such a study and agreed Salk should conduct it sub rosa. In his first trial, he planned to determine the levels of antibodies induced by vaccination. He thought it best to start with children who had already survived a bout with polio, since he wasn't trying to demonstrate prevention, rather the safety and antigenicity of an inactivated virus vaccine. It was a dangerous step, one he would be taking alone.

On June 6, Salk contacted Dr. Jessie Wright, Director of the D. T. Watson Home for Crippled Children, located in Leetsdale, Pennsylvania, eighteen miles northwest of Pittsburgh. He had chosen this potential test site carefully, at a safe distance from reporters and colleagues. Wright had an interest in polio research, having already made her mark by adapting a rocking bed, which used gravity to enhance respirations. This simple device allowed a number of patients to leave the iron lung and return home. Lucile Cochran, administrator of the Watson Home, recalled Salk's first visit: "He was charming and gentle, and obviously he was not just a scientist on an experiment but a man deeply concerned about the human importance of the experiment."[5] Wright agreed to his proposal, and Cochran contacted parents to obtain written consent:

> I have been informed that Dr. Jonas E. Salk...with the financial support of the National Foundation for Infantile Paralysis, Inc., has inaugurated in the D. T. Watson Home...a project for test purposes in connection with a study of infantile paralysis, its causes, remedies, and prevention....It is proposed to inject into children a poliomyelitis vaccine that has previously been injected into animals without subsequent harm....The vaccine will contain several ingredients consisting of the vaccine itself and a vehicle that will result in different rates of absorption. It is proposed to test small samples of blood to determine level of immunity before and at intervals after treatment. To assist in this project I hereby consent that the preparations above mentioned may be injected into my child.[6]

Salk had one firm proviso: no one could talk about the trial until its completion. He did not want the press hovering, photographing children or predicting results. And he did not want scientists sniping at him before he began. "For many months we have been bursting with the desire to tell our friends," a participant later wrote for the *Sunny Hill World*, the

Watson Home's school paper, "but we and our families were sworn to secrecy."[7]

Before inoculating the patients with his vaccine, Salk measured the levels of antipolio antibodies in their blood. Lorraine Friedman accompanied him to keep records. She observed how much the children liked Dr. Salk; he was tender and playful, yet firm. He remembered each child's name and where they lived, recalling things they talked about on his last visit. Among the patients was Jimmy Sarkett, whose poliovirus had been used to make the vaccine. (After Salk left Pittsburgh, he often took Sarkett and his wife to dinner when he was in town.) The staff became enamored of Salk as well. If the cook knew he was coming, she baked a strawberry pie.

Back in his lab, Salk and his staff determined that almost every patient who had had paralytic polio still had measurable antibodies against one type of polio, mostly Type 1. He hoped his vaccine could induce the production of antibodies against all three subtypes. Soon he would find out.

On July 2, 1952, Salk addressed the patients and staff assembled in the Watson Home auditorium. "This is it!" he announced, holding up a small vial.[8] Sixteen-year-old Bill Kirkpatrick volunteered to go first. A year earlier, he had been preparing to play high school football when he contracted polio. His symptoms began on the way home from his grandmother's house, where the family had spent Labor Day. He had been running laps and throwing a football. "I thought I had overdone it," Kirkpatrick recalled. "My neck felt stiff. My skin felt chapped." That night he had a fever, the next morning excruciating pains. "It was just like someone taking a sledgehammer and beating it against your spine. I could feel my legs get soft like jelly, and all of a sudden I couldn't move them."[9] His breathing became shallow; he felt like he was suffocating. A spinal tap confirmed the diagnosis of poliomyelitis.

As he was wheeled to the isolation ward, down halls lined with iron lungs, Kirkpatrick felt overcome by fear. His parents were not allowed to visit. His only solace from the masked attendants and crying children was a nurse who came back to his bedside after finishing her shift to hold his hand and comfort him. Once the immediate crisis had passed, he was transferred to the Watson Home, where he was relearning to walk. A metal frame held him upright; ropes extended from his legs to above his head. "I was like a puppet, he recalled."[10]

Even though Kirkpatrick's parents had been reluctant to give their consent to his participation, the sixteen-year-old insisted on it, thinking of Peggy, a pretty redheaded teen admitted to the hospital with acute poliomyelitis just before him. She had sent him a rose, which he kept under his pillow. When he was able to write, he sent a thank-you note. It was returned, marked "DECEASED."[11] And he thought of his older brother's children. He'd do anything to help protect them from polio. So when the first group of volunteers in wheelchairs and on stretchers gathered in the auditorium, Bill Kirkpatrick was among them. One glimpse at the long table on which bottles of alcohol, cotton swabs, and hypodermic needles were arranged was enough to frighten the other kids, Kirkpatrick recalled. "So I stepped up to bat first."[12]

Initially Salk inoculated fifty-two subjects, giving every shot himself. Although confident of the vaccine's safety, he later confided in reporter John Troan, "When you inoculate children with a polio vaccine for the first time, you don't sleep well for two or three weeks."[13] He returned that night to check up on them; no one suffered any ill effects from the shots, just some redness at the injection site. He gave a second injection six weeks later and measured antibody levels five weeks after that. In the first twenty-seven children vaccinated, he found increased levels of antibodies to the Type-2 virus; they were still measurable four months later. Although Salk had demonstrated the vaccine's safety, those children already had low levels of antibodies from a previous infection. Now he needed to confirm its safety in subjects who had never had poliomyelitis. This was a dangerous move, as uninfected children had no natural protection. If any live virus remained in the vaccine, it could infect and even kill a child.

For this trial, Cochran identified patients at the Watson Home who had been crippled by conditions other than polio, such as congenital abnormalities. Salk inoculated twenty-seven children. Then he waited. "He phoned frequently," Cochran recalled, "and returned frequently in that old rattletrap car of his."[14] Salk was relieved that not one child showed symptoms of poliomyelitis. His formalin technique had inactivated the virus in the vaccine; it was safe. Now he needed to determine if the vaccine had done its job. He took blood samples from the children two weeks following vaccination, returned to his lab, and mixed their serum with Types 1, 2, and 3 polioviruses. Then he inoculated cultures of monkey kidney cells with the mixtures. Instead of dying from infection, the kidney cells thrived. His vaccine worked.[15]

Years later, Salk told John Troan that he considered this to be the most remarkable moment in the entire polio saga, for it was then that he knew he could prevent poliomyelitis. "It was the thrill of my life. Compared to the feeling I got seeing these results under the microscope, everything that followed was anticlimactic."[16] That evening, his sister-in-law recounted, he came bursting into his house and cried, "I've got it!"[17]

In a few weeks, Salk again measured antibody titers against all three types of poliovirus in the same group of children. The levels proved to be as high as those from a natural infection. Although Salk's trial had been successful, the number of subjects was small. To confirm his results, he needed to vaccinate a larger group of children who had never had polio. For that, he looked to the Polk State School.

Situated on twenty-one acres an hour west of Pittsburgh, the Polk School compound included residences, a modern hospital, a dairy, and acres of crops and orchards. There 3,400 mentally disabled individuals were being trained for activities of daily living.[18] Salk chose this site because it provided a controlled environment, accurate records, and long-term observation. He contacted Gale Walker, superintendent of the school, who agreed to volunteer his charges. Salk soon became a familiar face at the Polk School. The expense account submitted to the NFIP included lunch for Dr. Walker and lollipops for patients. He and Walker shared the same sense of humor. "I hadn't realized what a good doctor you were until I read one of your letters long-hand," Walker wrote Salk. "They say you can tell a doctor's ability by the illegibility.... At first I could not figure out who was writing me."[19]

The children trusted the kindly Dr. Salk. On November 11, 1952, he inoculated the first of sixty-three. Again he measured a rise in antipolio-virus antibodies. Again no one contracted polio from the vaccine. When he had completed the trial, Salk sent Walker a letter to be printed in the Polk School newsletter, thanking the children and staff: "I can only admire the spirit that prompted you to give me the opportunity you did."[20]

Salk now had data demonstrating the vaccine's safety and its ability to induce antipolio antibodies, supporting his hypothesis that one could inactivate a virus, destroying its infectivity while retaining its antigenicity. Up to this point, Weaver and Salk had kept the Watson Home and Polk School trials from the public eye as well as from other scientists. As 1952 drew to a close, Weaver decided the time had come for Salk to reveal his work to the Committee on Immunization. Although O'Connor had suffered a heart attack that summer, he had recovered sufficiently to attend what he must have known would be a contentious meeting.

⁜

ON JANUARY 23, 1953, the Committee on Immunization met in Hershey, Pennsylvania, "the sweetest place on earth." The luxuriously appointed Hotel Hershey's old-world charm, with its mosaic tiles and archways, villa-style balconies overlooking formal gardens, and cigar lounge, didn't seem to pacify the quarrelsome committee members. Weaver began the meeting by introducing two new members. "This is always an informal, free-wheeling group," he told them, "and although it may not seem so at times, it is really quite a friendly group."[21]

First on the agenda, guest scientist Jerome Syverton presented a new method for growing polioviruses on HeLa cells, a line of cells derived from a patient with cervical cancer. This highly effective process for growing large quantities of virus would be advantageous when the time came to produce massive amounts of vaccine. A spirited discussion followed. John Enders said he would be hesitant to inject viruses grown on cancer cells into humans. Others contended the public would never accept a vaccine linked to cancer. David Bodian said the group should try to reach consensus "without slaughtering each other."[22] Nevertheless, he didn't think they should attempt it at that meeting. "Our experience indicates that it would take a good week of hammering and beating each other's brains out to get it done."

They then turned to the second agenda item, listed as "A presentation by Jonas Salk of some recent work," giving no hint of the full content. The night before, Sabin had dined at Salk's home, and they rode the train from Pittsburgh to Hershey together.[23] Salk said not one word about the Watson Home or Polk School. Now he faced a formidable group of scientists who believed that only a live virus could provide immunity, who thought they were years away from a safe vaccine, and who were quick to condemn anyone who rushed to early human experimentation. Tom

Rivers recalled some "ding-dong fights" over scientific matters as no one on the committee vacillated or tempered his opinion.[24] Joe Smadel had humiliated Salk back when he was just an intern giving his first scientific presentation. Albert Sabin had slashed many fellow scientists with his rapier-sharp tongue.

Salk began by acknowledging that Isabel Morgan already had accomplished vaccination with inactivated poliovirus in monkeys, giving her credit that scientists later would say he didn't. He proceeded to describe what he called a "preparation," avoiding the word "vaccine," composed of three poliovirus strains (Mahoney Type 1, MEF-1 Type 2, and Saukett Type 3) grown in monkey kidney cell culture.[25] To inactivate the viruses, Salk explained, he and his team had treated the preparation with formalin for thirteen days at 1° C, the temperature of melting ice. When Smadel asked, "Why did you pick melting ice?" Salk replied that the electricity in the cold room had gone off one day, and the ice started to melt, which he thought had ruined one of the experiments. Instead, he found the temperature of melting ice ideal for inactivating the virus. To be certain that the preparation contained no live virus, he had injected monkeys with the most virulent strain. Whether injected into their bloodstream or directly into their brains, the formalin-treated poliovirus had infected not a single one. "The margin of safety is great," he concluded.[26] He proceeded to show the group data demonstrating a relationship between the amount of virus injected into monkeys and the antibody levels eight weeks later. The addition of mineral oil adjuvant, he stated, induced a greater and more lasting effect.

Committee members were about to critique Salk's approach when he made an unexpected disclosure: he had inoculated fifty-two children at the D. T. Watson Home for Crippled Children with his preparation. Calling his results "preliminary," he demonstrated a fourfold or greater rise in antibody titers to the Type 2 virus in children who had had paralytic polio. Smadel interrupted him, stating that such findings appeared to be a booster effect in children who already had antibodies. The real question was whether the vaccine could stimulate antibody formation safely in children who had never had polio. Salk did not yet disclose that he was in the midst of conducting such an experiment. A few technical questions followed. Sabin remained silent.

After lunch, Weaver began the afternoon session in a light-hearted manner, saying they had just passed a motion directing Sabin to talk more. Then he asked Salk to continue. Salk presented his next set of experiments, explaining they had been designed to test a preparation that contained all three strains of poliovirus incorporated into one preparation, mixed with mineral oil adjuvant. He had inoculated ninety previously uninfected children at the Watson Home and Polk School, observing no side effects from the injection. And no child contracted polio. Data on the first fifteen showed measurable antibodies against all three types. The group sat speechless. He proceeded to present detailed data that answered many anticipated questions: He compared antibody levels with and without mineral oil adjuvant, and levels based on the method of injection—into the muscle or into the skin. He demonstrated how the antibody levels following inoculation with this preparation appeared to be as high as those from a natural infection. "I am not holding anything back, Albert," he said, inundating them with data.[27] "Thank you," Sabin replied. Everyone laughed. After several hours, Salk concluded, "That is all I have to say."

The interrogation began slowly, then gained momentum. Most of the committee doubted the level of antibody from an inactivated virus vaccine could ever be as high as that from natural infection. They expressed concern about using mineral oil adjuvant. They worried that material derived from monkey kidneys would cause organ damage. "They examined Jonas closely," Rivers recalled. "That's not surprising—these boys would have questioned their own mothers if they were foolhardy enough to give a paper at a conference."[28]

Sabin conceded that Salk had produced some antibodies against poliovirus with a killed vaccine. The real issue, he said, was the quantity of antibody. Likely, Salk's preparation just boosted the antibody already present in children at low levels. When Salk posed a possible alternative explanation, Sabin snapped, "If you had the data, you can discuss it. You can't discuss it without the data." With this, the arguments intensified, and Weaver intervened: "Why don't we have a good sleep on this first and all of us kind of mull this over a little bit?"[29]

Weaver had shown his usual wisdom, for on the morning of the second day Sabin began on a positive note. "As I was lying in bed last night thinking about this, it occurred to me that even if it turns out this is primarily a booster phenomena...this is really, I think, truly a new discovery that none of us could predict—that in an individual who has one type of antibody the administration of such a small amount can give rise to antibody at dose levels of the other types."[30] Salk must have felt heartened, until Sabin began to dissect his work. Salk had not searched extensively to determine the best viral strains for widespread use, Sabin argued, implying that he had selected three that he happened to have on hand. Regarding mineral oil adjuvant, the Biologics Control Laboratory would not approve a vaccine containing the agent. "I hope Dr. Salk doesn't mind if I tell you some other things he told me," Sabin continued. "Go ahead," Salk replied. Sabin went on to say that Salk had expressed concern before giving the influenza vaccine with adjuvant because of the carcinogenic potential. Bit by bit, he discounted much of Salk's work.

Salk found Sabin's comments demeaning. "His interpretations made my work seem incredible, of no meaning or significance," he later told Richard Carter. "We hadn't done this and we hadn't done that and this was premature and that was unsubstantiated."[31] As Sabin continued to try and undermine Salk's efforts, Weaver broke in and said that while he didn't think anyone disagreed with Albert's concerns, they shouldn't hold up production of vaccine. Others disagreed. Thomas Turner, chairman of the Department of Bacteriology at Johns Hopkins, said he worried about an allergic reaction and organ damage. Bodian thought the Mahoney virus was the worst they could select because of its high rate of paralysis. Smadel suggested they test it in two hundred monkeys to settle the issue of safety. The committee seemed to be resetting the clock, sending Salk back to the laboratory for years.

Then, in the middle of this interchange, Smadel suddenly reversed the discussion and asked when they wanted to conduct a field trial. "We are playing for high stakes....If a preliminary trial is not done this year, it means waiting another year."[32] In the meantime, polio would strike thousands more children. Turner proposed the NFIP initiate one in the spring, given that in Salk's judgment he had a vaccine which met rigorous safety criteria. With that, the debate shifted from antibody levels and viral strains to trial design: Should it be a safety test or a controlled trial to determine whether the vaccine could prevent paralytic polio?

Turner and Norman Topping, vice president of medical affairs at the University of Pennsylvania, favored the latter. Enders thought a large field trial was premature: "It would mean that we could go off half-cocked." There were still too many unknowns: the most suitable strains of poliovirus, the optimal route of vaccination, and whether adjuvant should be used. "I would suggest more experimentation along the same lines that [Dr. Salk] is doing so admirably at the moment," Enders said, "and not enter into a large experiment which will inevitably be connected with a lot of publicity and may jeopardize the whole program."[33]

Turner concurred they should show caution. "On the other hand," he argued, "there comes a time when a thing is so in your grasp that you have to push ahead as rapidly as possible. I think the foundation is in that situation, so that a summer does mean a great deal."[34] He suggested they set up another meeting at which Salk would present his plans for a field trial. The committee members had taken sides: those in favor of a field trial—Smadel, Turner, Topping, and Weaver; those against—Enders and Sabin, with Bodian neutral. Salk remained quiet during the discussion. Finally, he was asked what he would like to do. "I would like to continue the work as we have been doing it, and enlarge the scope of the studies just as rapidly as possible," he replied. "I can assure you that I will be the one that will be the fall guy if a mistake is made, and no decision by this group or any administrative body is going to force me into doing anything before I am ready." Embarrassed by his seeming defiance, Salk apologized to Weaver. "I am sorry, Harry," he said. "It's just because we know each other so well and love each other that I said that."[35]

Sabin said the safety tests should be postponed until they decided upon the preparation they would use in large studies. "I agree with you, Albert," Salk replied, "and I think that safety tests should be done on batches of material that should be sufficient for 20,000 to 25,000 people."[36] Sabin retorted, "I didn't mean that." He believed that the committee should select the optimal strains and method of preparation, postponing a large clinical trial until they reached consensus on a vaccine preparation that could be used year after year. "Do not rush in," he cautioned.

Weaver's impatience started to show. "We have confidence in what has been done," he said. "We would like to see it pushed forward as rapidly and intelligently as it can be."[37] Sabin replied, "Let's be practical about this. We don't think that he has presented us with a lot of stuff that he never got. That is not at issue. There is no use taking a vote 'Are we for good work and intelligently pushing forward as fast as possible?'" Trying to avoid further derailment by Sabin, Weaver concluded the meeting.

At no time during the two-day exchange did Salk champion his vaccine. He, too, considered a large trial premature. "There was no vaccine, no product to try out in hundreds of thousands of people. All we had was a flicker of light," he later recounted. "The talk by some about hurrying into field trials was as disheartening as the wearisome reviews by others of all the facts we had not yet established.... The sense of being caught between two lines of fire made me ache to retreat to Pittsburgh and continue my work in my own way."[38]

Harry Weaver and Basil O'Connor felt otherwise. Two days after the Hershey meeting, Weaver met with the board of trustees to report that one of their investigators had produced a poliomyelitis vaccine that appeared safe and effective. It may be time to consider a field trial, he told the board, but he could not yet reveal the specifics or the investigator's name. Despite his insistence on confidentiality, someone leaked his statements to the press. A friend at the NFIP told Troan to come to New York, where Weaver was about to break some big news to the board. Troan took the night train and arrived at the Foundation headquarters the next morning. Before the board even met, Troan learned enough to send the following story to the *Pittsburgh Press*:

> A vaccine that may make polio as extinct as smallpox is due to get its baptism this summer.... The news that science may be so close to total victory over polio broke here today with dramatic suddenness. From all indications, the promising vaccine was developed by a team of University of Pittsburgh scientists working under Jonas E. Salk.... If it holds up in the field as well as it has in the laboratory, the vaccine could spell final doom for polio.[39]

Troan had put consideration for his own journalistic career above the interests of Salk. That same day, Broadway columnist Earl Wilson's headline read: "New Polio Vaccine—Big Hopes Seen."[40] These articles turned the spotlight directly on Salk, resulting in a barrage of letters, phone calls, and interview requests. Worse yet, they would soon force him to take an action that would create disfavor in the scientific world.

Weaver, Rivers, and O'Connor agreed they were nearing the time for a large national trial to prove the vaccine could prevent polio—the crowning glory, the raison d'être for the NFIP. The annual polio statistics had just revealed a record 57,879 in 1952.[41] They still had reasons to be cautious: a field trial of a polio vaccine would constitute one of the largest national trials ever conducted, and it would involve human experimentation with subjects who had almost no say over their participation, namely, children. They didn't know how the public would view this. A year before, Pope Pius XII had publicly stated the Catholic Church's stance on the moral limits of human subjects research. Three federal prisoners had recently died from hepatitis following experiments with blood products. And now they were talking about experimenting with children. If any child suffered harm from the vaccine, it would be disastrous for the NFIP, to whom the American public had given their dimes and their trust.

Weaver, ever the tactician, knew they needed the backing of influential public figures. To that end, he invited a group of such people to meet at New York's Waldorf-Astoria Hotel on February 26, 1953. Attendees included the president of the American Medical Association, the assistant surgeon general, esteemed members of the Rockefeller Foundation, the chancellor of the University of Pittsburgh, and the editor of *Ladies' Home Journal*. O'Connor began the gathering by thanking attendees and saying the NFIP sought their advice. Rivers gave an overview of the issues; then Salk presented a summary of his work to date. "Dr. Salk is a very cautious man," Rivers told the group. "Some people want to go much faster than he wants to go. Some want to throw all he has got out the window and try something else." Once the public becomes aware of Salk's results, Rivers continued, "everybody and his brother is going to want vaccine."[42] Serious pressure would be put on Salk and the Foundation. "There is always the danger of going too fast," he warned. At the same time, there was also the danger of going too slow. "That is the problem before the group this morning," he concluded. Those in attendance asked questions and debated the various courses of action. At the end of the day, they gave Salk their blessing to increase the number of children vaccinated until he felt satisfied with its safety.

The press continued to incite the public; exaggerated and inaccurate reports created unreasonable expectations. Feeling compelled to reach out to the American people, Salk told O'Connor he thought if he explained his results and cautioned against premature conclusions, he could stem the frenzy created by the media. O'Connor agreed and arranged for Salk to appear on a special CBS television program, *The Scientist Speaks for Himself.* On the evening of March 26, millions turned on their televisions expecting to hear that polio would soon be eradicated. O'Connor addressed viewers first: "Never before in history have scientist and citizen worked together so effectively toward this great goal. You, the American people, have characteristically made yourselves active partners—stockholders, if you will—in this cooperative enterprise which seeks to attain better health for the peoples of the world."[43] Then he introduced Salk.

For the first time, the American public heard from the young scientist on whom they pinned their hopes. If they had expected a knight in shining armor, instead they saw an unassuming man of medium height with thinning hair and black-rimmed glasses. He seemed too young to carry the weight of polio prevention on his shoulders. Salk began by saying that a preliminary report of his studies on vaccination against polio would appear in the March 28 issue of the *Journal of the American Medical Association.* "This topic has, in recent months, been featured prominently in the news, and there has been much speculation varying from cautious optimism to definite conclusion."[44] He welcomed the opportunity to clarify the situation, he told viewers. After describing earlier vaccine attempts, he outlined recent advances, giving credit to several scientists. Then he turned to what the public was waiting for—results of his human trials.

These trials, Salk stressed, were still "in progress" and "incomplete."[45] He explained that he had vaccinated a group of children at the Watson Home and Polk School who had never had polio and measured antibody levels similar to those following a natural infection. "The results of these studies," he said, "provide justification for optimism." Although he noted that progress had been more rapid than expected, he was careful to temper public expectations: there would be no vaccine available for the next polio season. "I am certain that you will understand that the actual accomplishment of our purpose cannot be achieved in a day," he cautioned. "Certain things cannot be hastened." Wanting to end on a positive note, he concluded, "With this new enlightenment, we can now move forward more rapidly and with more confidence."

For the NFIP, Salk's appearance on national television proved a great success. He came across as a modest, concerned, and articulate scientist, supported by the March of Dimes, and he gave the public the hero they craved. For Salk, however, it proved disastrous. He had hoped his comments would calm the hysteria; instead they enhanced the frenzy. And he had done something considered taboo in the medical world: he had revealed his results to the public before physicians and scientists had a chance to review his work and draw their own conclusions. Patients would soon be clamoring for this vaccine while physicians only knew as much about it as they did from the television program.

Many in the scientific community were annoyed by Salk's television appearance. Some thought him a grandstander, looking to the public rather than to fellow investigators, to judge his work. Salk wanted acceptance by his colleagues, but he had unintentionally hurt his chances. And when the article on his work did appear in the *Journal of the American Medical Association*, it did not further his cause. Published quickly, Salk's manuscript had undergone minimal editing which was unusual for a journal of such repute. The long, wordy article skipped back and forth between animal and human data, mixing methods, results, and conclusions, at times resembling a stream-of-consciousness piece. Even the authorship seemed a bit unconventional, listing Salk as the sole author "with the collaboration of Bennett, Lewis, Ward, and Youngner."[46] Scientists and statisticians who thought his data intriguing likely found his irregular style of presentation irksome.

The press read his manuscript with a less critical eye, glossing over his acknowledgment of those scientists whose work had preceded his, misrepresenting the conclusions he described as tentative. Troan's takeaway—that this young scientist had developed a vaccine that could prevent poliomyelitis—stood. Salk did not welcome such attention: "I wanted to avoid the hue and cry of publicity so that I could get on with my work undisturbed," he told a reporter. "It was nothing I did to become public property.... [I was] a scientist, working in the public interest, working with funds provided by the public, doing a public service. I was neither a politician nor a performer."[47]

Jonas Salk had become a household name. No longer could he conduct research without intense public scrutiny. And to many, his assertion that he didn't expect such a reaction rang false. "What adult would be naïve enough to think he could go on radio and television to talk about a polio vaccine he was making and expect to be allowed to retreat to his cloister afterward?" Carter reported an unnamed critic as saying. "Naïve, my foot. Whether he believes it or not, Jonas went on the air that night to take a box and become a public hero. And that's what he became."[48]

Out of His Hands

In June of 1953, when Salk read in the newspaper that the NFIP was planning a field trial to begin in the fall, he was stunned. "I had no inklings of these conferences and plans," he later complained. "Weaver and Rivers had been meeting for weeks... planning field trials of a product that did not exist and planning my duties for me as if I were a staff technician."[1] He insisted upon talking with O'Connor in person and took a train to NFIP headquarters in New York. Weaver had usurped clinical assessment of his vaccine, Salk told O'Connor, a vaccine which was not yet ready for widespread use. Added to that, a newly appointed group, the Vaccine Advisory Committee, from which he had been excluded, had been given control over the details of its testing. As much as O'Connor wanted to see a field trial go forward, he did not want to agitate his star scientist. He told Salk not to worry. "Nobody is breathing down your neck. It's your work and nothing will be done with it that you don't want done. You have my word on it."[2] Salk returned to Pittsburgh secure in O'Connor's promise.

But Harry Weaver made no such promise. He was moving ahead with plans to coordinate the NFIP trial himself. "[Salk] could not be the architect, carpenter, and building inspector—or judge, jury, prosecutor, and defense attorney all at once," he reasoned. If Salk tested his own vaccine, the results would be suspect. Weaver did understand his reaction, however. "Jonas... felt that his baby... was being torn from his arms," he explained. "Yet it couldn't be any other way."[3] As far as Weaver was concerned, Salk had played his part: he had prepared and tested a polio vaccine. Now he was hesitating, talking about continuing to study dose and sequence of inoculations with the tacit understanding that the NFIP supported his time schedule. Weaver and Rivers had a different agenda.

In mid-May, just three weeks after Salk had revealed his vaccine work to the public, Weaver had prepared a confidential memorandum for O'Connor, outlining plans for a field trial to be initiated on November 15, a mere six months away.[4] Anticipating an outcry from the Committee on Immunization, whose members were split in their opinions regarding almost every aspect of polio prevention, Weaver and Rivers had conceived of an ingenious plan. They recommended that O'Connor bypass the group and appoint an advisory committee to determine the specifics of the poliomyelitis vaccination program. Although Weaver said publicly that this new group had been created to broaden the base of responsibility, later on he privately acknowledged, "We formed the Vaccine Advisory Committee to break a logjam."[5]

For his Vaccine Advisory Committee, O'Connor had selected forward-looking men, all with extensive public health experience, who were willing to make decisions rapidly: David Price, the assistant surgeon general; Thomas Murdock, a trustee of the American Medical Association; Ernest Stebbins, director of Johns Hopkins School of Hygiene and Public Health; bacteriologist Thomas Turner, dean of Johns Hopkins Medical School; Norman Topping, vice president of medical affairs at the University of Pennsylvania; and Joseph Smadel and Tom Rivers. Notably absent were Enders, Bodian, Sabin, and Salk. All the members had one thing in common—they favored initiating a field trial before the 1954 polio season began.

On May 25, 1953, Rivers had convened the first meeting of the advisory committee.[6] Although asked to report on his work, Salk had been excluded from its deliberations, so he didn't know that one of its first recommendations concerned the field trial design. Salk had assumed the NFIP would conduct a trial in which a defined group would receive vaccine on a voluntary basis, and the incidence of polio among them would be compared with another group who received no injection—an observed control group. Weaver, Rivers, and O'Connor favored the same plan. The Vaccine Advisory Committee preferred one whereby children would be randomized to receive the vaccine or placebo, stressing its more scientifically sound design. Salk first learned about the recommendation from the press.

Salk wasn't the only one disturbed by Weaver's tactics; they infuriated the NFIP medical director, Hart Van Riper. A Florida pediatrician, Van Riper had moved to New York to join the NFIP when his wife became paralyzed with polio. Tall, articulate, and urbane, he represented the Foundation well at congressional hearings and medical society meetings. He had preceded Weaver at the NFIP, and Weaver supposedly reported to him. This was a mismatch from the start. Van Riper adhered to administrative protocol, whereas Weaver sought the quickest path, circumventing rules and regulations. Increasingly Weaver spoke directly to O'Connor, bypassing Van Riper. Now he appeared to be reorganizing Van Riper's department, holding meetings without his knowledge. They regularly clashed: Van Riper accused Weaver of usurping his role; Weaver complained Van Riper was impeding his trial. "Van Riper felt that Harry Weaver was too big for his britches," recalled NFIP regional director Charles Massey, "that Harry Weaver had not only sold O'Connor on Jonas Salk but had sold him on the idea of the field trial all without consulting with him."[7] They had reached an impasse; Weaver threatened to leave. O'Connor was torn: Weaver and Van Riper were equally valuable. So he left for Europe, telling Van Riper to settle the problem.

On August 29, Weaver resigned. "This action was taken," he wrote to Salk, "following the realization that I could no longer discharge my responsibilities in an effective manner within the administrative framework in which I had to work. It was not easy to write this letter to you— sorry but it had to be."[8] Weaver had given Salk a major opportunity when he engaged him in the typing project. He had provided funding to build his laboratory and launched his career in the polio field. Nevertheless, once Weaver could taste victory, he had taken over, unwittingly making Salk feel like a hired hand. "I must tell you quite honestly that I was a very unhappy person for many months," Salk wrote to

O'Connor after Weaver left, "and regretted that I could not talk to you alone rather than through Dr. Weaver or in his presence."[9] O'Connor knew Jonas felt ambivalent about Weaver's departure and sent him a telegram: "All will be much better."[10]

But it wasn't. With Weaver out of the way, Van Riper appointed Joseph Bell, chief of the NIH Epidemiology Unit, as scientific director of the field trial. A physician with a PhD in public health, Bell had substantial experience in vaccine assessment. With this expertise, however, came a tendency for inflexibility and top-down decision-making, which wouldn't sit well with O'Connor. At the onset, Bell agreed with the Vaccine Advisory Committee: a randomized, placebo-controlled trial had become the gold standard for proving efficacy of a new vaccine. In addition, he refused to test any vaccine that contained mineral oil adjuvant; they would use an aqueous (water-based) vaccine for the field trial. And he intended to get his way.

Bell's pronouncement sent Salk back to his laboratory to repeat his experiments with an aqueous vaccine. In monkeys, he found the best response occurred when two doses were administered a week apart followed a month later by a third dose, which he called a "booster." Because human responses did not always parallel those in monkeys, he needed to study a new group of subjects. Salk contacted Pittsburgh's Industrial Home for Crippled Children and the Sewickley Academy, a prep school located just north of the city. Parents readily volunteered their children as Salk set out to answer a number of questions: Could aqueous vaccine, devoid of adjuvant, produce an adequate antibody level? What were the optimal dose, number, and timing of inoculations? No matter how hard he worked, Salk worried that he couldn't answer them in time to start a field trial in November.

The field trial design posed a bigger quandary.[11] Initially O'Connor had supported Salk's scheme: children in the second grade would receive vaccine on a voluntary basis, and the rate of polio would be compared with that of first and third graders in the same community who did not receive vaccine—an observed control group. This was the fastest, easiest, and least expensive trial to run, and parents would know whether or not their child received vaccine. O'Connor had already informed health officials in thirty-three states that this was the NFIP's plan. The Vaccine

Advisory Committee continued to resist this design, emphasizing its pitfalls. Those likely to volunteer would come from upper socioeconomic groups, the ones most susceptible to polio. Thus, children with a lower chance of contracting polio would be in the control group. The committee stressed that randomization, whereby children would be assigned by chance to inoculation with either vaccine or placebo, represented the most reliable statistical method.

Bell proposed yet a different design. He, too, favored a randomized trial, but instead of a placebo such as saline, the control group would receive influenza vaccine. He thought it was unethical to inoculate children with a solution of no value. Some committee members accused him of trying to piggyback an influenza field test onto the poliomyelitis trial. Salk was opposed to both plans, the committee's and Bell's. He still favored a nonrandomized trial in which second graders would be vaccinated and first and third graders would serve as observed controls. He pressed his design at every opportunity. "For arguing this as often as I did," Salk recounted, "I earned scorn as an eccentric nuisance."[12]

Additionally, Bell insisted the trial be double-blinded, such that neither the treating nurse, physician, and patient nor the NFIP would know who received which inoculate. Everyone would be coded, and the code would be broken only at the end of the trial. That way, no favoritism could be shown, and physicians, in making a diagnosis of polio, wouldn't be biased by knowing whether or not the patient had received vaccine. Double-blind trials had the most scientific credibility. The Vaccine Advisory Committee agreed with him on this point, yet they continued to debate whether the control group would receive an influenza vaccine or placebo. Salk still resisted using a randomized trial altogether. Each felt passionate about his position, and the altercation made good copy. The *Pittsburgh Press* reported that the NFIP planned to inoculate more than a million children with either the new polio vaccine or a placebo. "This means they are to be given an injection of something which will look like the milky-white Pitt vaccine but actually will be only sugar water.... Dr. Salk is known to be opposed to giving any youngster 'blanks,' however, and may object to this proposal."[13]

The dispute ran throughout September, and the start date for the trial was delayed until March of 1954. "It was never a tea party argument," Tom

Rivers recalled, "and the fur flew more than once."[14] During all this, O'Connor remained calm, trying to keep a broader perspective. Melvin Glasser, administrative director for the field trial, recalled one particular exchange when O'Connor quietly scribbled numbers on a yellow pad while the advisory committee and Bell were arguing. Suddenly he inter-rupted: "I have just figured out that during this coming summer thirty or forty thousand children will get polio. About fifteen thousand of them will be paralyzed and more than a thousand will die." Caught up in their dispute over control groups and placebos, they inadvertently might delay vaccinations until after the next year's outbreaks had begun. "Let me re-mind you," he continued, "that we are supported by the people, and it is our duty to save lives."[15] With that, the debate ended. When Bell realized the Vaccine Advisory Committee would not budge from its position, he resigned.

Salk did not yield. He sent O'Connor an eleven-page letter pleading for a trial with observed controls: "I would feel that every child who is injected with a placebo and becomes paralyzed, will do so at my hands." Those demanding a placebo-controlled trial, he argued, took that posi-tion in order to reach some statistical endpoint because of "values in which the worship of science involves the sacrifice of humanitarian prin-ciples on the altar of rigid methodology." Such a trial would make Hippocrates "turn over in his grave."[16] But the decision had been made.

"Many Thousands to Get Polio Vaccine Next Year," ran headlines on October 9. Starting in March of 1954, hundreds of thousands of children would be getting shots—half with a vaccine against all three known types of poliovirus, half with salt solution. "When the 1954 polio season has come and gone, scientists will count noses to see how many in each group got polio."[17] O'Connor's public announcement provoked a groundswell of opposition among scientists, beginning with members of the Committee on Immunization who had been excluded from decision-making for the past nine months. How did they feel when news of the field trial screamed from every headline? The NFIP would soon find out. Henry Kumm, who had replaced Weaver as director of research, convened a meeting of the group on October 24 in Detroit where he intended to bring them up to date on the immunization program and invite their collaboration. The evening before the meeting, Salk told John Paul that he was concerned about how members of the committee would react when they learned how far along the NFIP had moved toward the trial.

Salk's unease was well founded. The next day, when a committee member asked if they had a choice as to the kind of vaccine, O'Connor replied, "That's not the function of this Committee."[18] Following the advice of the Vaccine Advisory Committee, the NFIP had already decided on the inactivated-virus vaccine. The Foundation had kept these deliberations from its own scientific advisers. "Decks had been cleared for action on a vaccine," Paul said, "and if in the process some individuals had been hurt and some wrong decisions had been made, that was just too bad."[19] Sabin and Paul tried to convince the NFIP to postpone the trial, calling the Mahoney strain too virulent to use in the vaccine. Their concerns were brushed aside. The breach that resulted, Paul recounted, "remained for some members of the Immunization Committee an open and sore wound."[20] Since O'Connor wouldn't listen to them, the disgruntled scientists targeted Salk. Sabin and Paul urged him to block the field trial, telling him he was being controlled by O'Connor and that it would ruin his reputation in the scientific community. Salk did not belong to the Vaccine Advisory Committee and had been ostracized by the Committee on Immunization. The former was moving too fast; the latter was suggesting he retreat. He felt like a pariah. "I'd walk down a corridor," he said, "and people would stop talking as I approached."[21]

Remarkably, the relationship between Salk and O'Connor remained as strong as ever despite this turmoil. "Jonas was the nicest, sincerest young man you ever met," O'Connor told science reporter Victor Cohn. "There wasn't a mean or selfish bone in his body."[22] On October 28, he sent Salk a telegram on his thirty-ninth birthday: "Twenty years from now this will be Interesting But Good History.... Best wishes from one who knows."[23] During the months that followed, as tensions rose, they grew even closer.

Although members of the Committee on Immunization had left Detroit frustrated and angry, no one resigned from the committee. Many still received considerable research funding from the NFIP and did not contest O'Connor's decisions publicly, except Sabin. At the American Medical Association convention in New York the prior June, Sabin had informed its forty thousand members that the Mahoney strain was highly infectious and just a small amount of live virus left in the vaccine could cause paralysis. At a congressional hearing in November, he contended that Salk's vaccine provided weak protection and that the safety of a killed-virus vaccine had not been confirmed by others. He opposed inoculating hundreds of thousands of children based on the work of one investigator. Sabin did not address the concern that waiting for him to develop a live vaccine would leave the public unprotected for several more years. "He could not suppress his own desire to be recognized," NFIP official Charles Massey related. "He kept using the idea that Jonas was rushing too fast and that this would be risky and people might die. But, in my judgment, he was doing that to protect his own ego, rather than to be concerned about humanity."[24]

The press began to portray Sabin and Salk as adversaries, racing to see who would make medical history. John Troan capitalized on this presumed contest. "Dr. Sabin," he wrote, "is the first top-level scientist to cast a jaundiced eye on the vaccine developed at the University of Pittsburgh."[25] In this alleged rivalry, Sabin was often depicted as the villain who tried to block Salk at every turn, who repeatedly maligned him behind his back. Letters between them suggest otherwise. Following the Hershey meeting earlier that year, Sabin had written to Salk, warning him not to be pushed "to make liters of stuff for Harry Weaver's field test." He said he felt confident Jonas would do the best possible job, "regardless of what is said by others," signing his note "All good wishes and affectionate regard."[26] When he wrote to a prominent pediatrician critiquing Salk's vaccine, he sent him a copy, penciling at the top: "This is for your information so you'll know what I am saying behind your back.... Love and kisses are being saved up. Albert."[27] No one close to Salk ever heard him make a derogatory comment about Sabin. "The race was a myth," his research assistant Don Wegemer said.[28] Each stuck firmly to his belief regarding the principles that guided immunization— live or killed virus. Thus, at that point in time, a rivalry was brewing between two scientific principles, not between two scientists.

While Sabin was campaigning against an inactivated-virus vaccine, other scientists began to question Salk's results too. "Polio vaccine researchers got into a hassle last week," *Time* magazine reported on November 23.[29] Chicago physician Albert Milzer had presented a paper at the eighty-first meeting of the American Public Health Association, stating that his group had followed Salk's published directions faithfully, and formalin had failed to kill all the poliovirus. In response, Salk sent a letter to the editor of the *American Journal of Public Health*. "The implication that our methods have been followed, but our findings were not repeatable, is rather serious." Milzer seemed to lack an understanding of the formalin inactivation process. "These investigators have, without justification, impugned experiments that were carefully conducted, and they have aroused fear and doubt by their irresponsible remarks in a scientific paper in which evidence, rather than opinion, should stand out."[30] Nevertheless, the damage had been done; the Illinois state health director banned vaccine studies until they had adequate evidence of its safety.

Then, four days after the *Time* article, C. Henry Kempe, a junior pediatrics professor at the University of California, San Francisco, started a conflagration when he wrote to Aims McGuinness, a leader in the American Academy of Pediatrics, objecting to the Academy's endorsement of the upcoming field trial. He and a number of others had three substantial concerns: First, they thought the formalin-inactivated vaccine had not been tested sufficiently to assure its safety. Second, Salk grew poliovirus in a monkey kidney culture, and a reaction against this foreign protein might damage a child's kidney. Third, Salk's published work was based on a vaccine mixed with mineral oil adjuvant, yet an aqueous vaccine was to be used in the field trial. "It seems remarkable," Kempe wrote, "that there seems to be a general unwillingness on the part of the virologists to go on record in public against the plans of the National Foundation for Infantile Paralysis."[31] McGuinness sent Kempe's letter to a large number of scientists, including Salk, seeking their comments.

Before Salk could compose his reply, Sabin wrote to McGuinness attacking Salk's work as well, stating that most leading virologists held similar views.[32] Thomas Francis, Jr., lambasted McGuinness, saying the statements about Salk's vaccine appeared to be founded on "an accumulation of rumors." He chastised him for not contacting Salk directly before spreading Kempe's letter widely: "I count it neither valorous or virtuous to attack an individual by indirection in such a way as to cast doubt on his scientific integrity when the very doubts are neither documented nor affirmed."[33]

Weeks later, Salk finally responded himself. Fully aware of the blistering letters going back and forth among leaders in the field, he wrote several long drafts, the first full of emotion, each subsequent draft less so, until he finally sent McGuinness a brief note: "I can only say that Dr. Kempe's statement is replete with inaccuracies."[34] McGuinness sheepishly responded that in a field moving as fast as polio vaccine development, it was impossible to keep abreast of the latest information. Emboldened by the apology, Salk wrote back:

> I am unaware of anything that I have done in the past that should merit the degree of distrust that is implied by the great concern that so many people have.... What right does one go forth casting aspersions and for these aspersions to parade as facts without what one might call the accused being faced by his accuser.... Science has come to a pretty pass when relationships between scientists have been so debased.[35]

In response to the concerns raised by Kempe and Milzer, the Vaccine Advisory Committee asked Salk to test a sufficient number of children to detect any resultant kidney damage prior to commencing the field trial. This time-consuming task would require drawing blood and collecting gallons of urine from hundreds of children. With regards to the aqueous vaccine, Salk was already testing it; Smadel insisted the number of subjects be increased to five thousand.

The NFIP had bigger problems to resolve than Kempe's letter. Salk had prepared an effective, safe inactivated-virus vaccine in his lab; however, he couldn't produce enough vaccine for the nation, let alone the world. That was a job for pharmaceutical manufacturers. And once it was out of his hands, Salk couldn't attest to the vaccine's reliability or safety. So he insisted that vaccine produced by drug companies pass safety tests not only in their own labs and the NIH Laboratory of Biologics Control but also in his laboratory. He knew this triple testing might delay the trial, yet he was firm. "While we can shorten the time between the taking of each step," he warned those leading the field trial, "I do not think we can skip any without running the risk of tripping... [and] that would open us to criticism on the part of those who are only too ready and eager to destroy that which has been constructed thus far."[36]

In early November, NFIP executives met with ten pharmaceutical companies to discuss their potential participation. Although O'Connor told them the Foundation prohibited patents for work performed under its research grants, five more companies asked to participate. By this point, Salk and his group had honed their technique for vaccine production: Monkey kidneys were minced in a blender and incubated in test tubes along with nutrient 199 for six days. Each of the three strains of live virus was added to separate tubes of kidney cells and allowed to proliferate for four days. Debris from the minced kidney was filtered out, after which the viral suspension was put into refrigerated tanks. Over the next six weeks, the fluid was tested repeatedly for possible contamination with bacteria or tuberculosis (TB). The solution was then heated to 96.8 degrees and deposited in roller tubes with formalin. At three days and again at nine it was tested for live virus. If none remained, the solution was inactivated for three more days and analyzed again for residual live virus. If negative, sodium bisulfate was added to neutralize the formalin. The viral suspensions of all three strains were then combined to form the vaccine. That was just the halfway point. Over the next twenty-eight days, Salk's team checked and double-checked for live virus in tissue cultures, mice, and monkeys. If a lot proved clear, they bottled it. Each production cycle could take up to four months. And it was already November.

Once production left Salk's hands, there was always the possibility for error, serious error that could result in an ineffective product or a vaccine tainted with live virus. In order to prevent this, instructions had to be spelled out in detail in a document entitled "Minimum Requirements." For this the Vaccine Advisory Committee turned to Salk. "I was not an industrial engineer," he said years later. "Specifications for large scale manufacture could not be my responsibility."[37] Yet only he knew all the particulars. With his many competing tasks—continuing his laboratory investigations, inoculating thousands of Pittsburgh school children, answering hundreds of calls and letters—he didn't complete the first draft of the "Minimum Requirements" until December. Even then it had to be edited extensively. That completed, he was assigned the onerous task of reviewing the procedures of each company and answering their numerous questions.

The NFIP selected Parke, Davis and Company to lead off vaccine production. At first, its scientists could not get the vaccine to induce antibodies, and Salk was called upon to investigate the problem. He started at Connaught Laboratories, a Toronto group with which NFIP had contracted to cultivate virus for the field trial. Salk found no issues; they were sending frozen virus to Parke, Davis. Next he traveled to Parke, Davis's lab in Detroit and discovered the problem lay in the way in which the technicians were thawing the virus. Just as that issue was solved, Parke, Davis scientists reported live virus in their inactivated vaccine. Again Salk visited their lab and found the incubator to be unreliable, varying the temperature from what Salk had specified. Although Parke, Davis blamed Salk for writing vague manufacturing directions, he was beginning to suspect they wanted to produce vaccine their own way. "The entire program is being jeopardized by the attitude that prevails," he wrote O'Connor, "and I would urge very strongly that we waste as little time as possible attempting to bring them into line."[38] It seemed unlikely they could make enough vaccine by March. "We all believed that the Foundation had to put on a field trial in the spring of 1954," Rivers recalled. "If it didn't, the lid would be off and the following year everybody and his aunt would be trying out their own vaccine."[39] Swedish scientist Sven Gard was preparing a vaccine already.

It didn't take Salk long to comprehend that drug manufacturers were entrepreneurs, not academic scientists; they occasionally ignored the "Minimum Requirements" and made cost-saving decisions. When Cutter Labs, located in Berkeley, sent Salk their production manual, he could already spot instances where some specific details of his instructions had been omitted. He sent a list of corrections, acknowledging that they would make the process more time-consuming. "Every batch of vaccine is a damned research project," a Cutter scientist complained.[40] When Salk found another company had omitted Type 2 virus and just added extra Type 3, his confidence was shaken. Reluctantly, the NFIP announced the field trial would be delayed until April 2.

O'Connor sensed Salk's growing frustration with the pharmaceutical companies and hired G. Foard McGinnes, a former medical director of the Red Cross, to oversee vaccine procurement and distribution. O'Connor chose well. McGinnes had a strong background in product management as well as the collaborative style required to achieve team-work between the pharmaceutical laboratories and Salk. In the end, only Parke, Davis and Eli Lilly would be ready to supply vaccine for the field trial.

Meanwhile Salk was trying to continue some much needed labora-tory work. His group, now consisting of nine research professors and fellows as well as fifteen staff, worked long hours, leaving only when they completed experiments, not when the clock struck five. Many experi-ments ran on a twenty-four-hour basis. "Salk liked to do multiple tests on everything," Wegemer recalled. "He duplicated, duplicated, and redu-plicated to make sure everything was right."[41] When a *New York Times* reporter asked about his "punishing load," Salk replied, "An investigator who develops a new vaccine assumes responsibility for its safety."[42]

Initially his research group had a great deal of camaraderie. Salk had shown sensitivity and concern for every member. Now things had changed. The lab could not function like a usual academic laboratory with regular meetings, proper training of postdoctoral fellows, and seminars; they were too busy. Each morning Salk passed out slips of paper listing the tasks to be accomplished that day. He returned late at night to review the results. This angered some members of his team, in particular Julius Youngner, who considered the many daily tasks to be menial chores, not creative science. But these were extraordinary times; the lives of thou-sands of children were at stake. Salk held no one captive; any technician, trainee, or research professor could go elsewhere, yet no one left, not even Youngner. Although he later carped that Salk had more time for reporters than for his research team, Youngner did admit: "You had at your fingertips the prevention of a terrible disease, an epidemic disease. I can't describe to you the kind of excitement this generated."[43]

Salk was spending up to eighteen hours a day in his lab, eating most of his meals there when he wasn't traveling to NFIP headquarters, the NIH, or the pharmaceutical labs. His grueling schedule left no time for nine-year-old Peter, six-year-old Darrell, three-year-old Jonathan, or his wife. Donna must have been amused when she read in the *New York Times*: "Busy as he is, Dr. Salk makes time for his three sons who range in age from three to nine. On Sundays he usually takes them out riding or walking in the country... and he tells them about the magical life

processes of the plants and animals around them."[44] Donna never talked
to the children about polio or their father's work, and she never showed
them pictures of Jonas, which now appeared with regularity in newspapers and magazines. While her husband was doing something with
enormous global potential, she made sure her children lived ordinary
lives. If Donna appeared to tolerate the situation with sangfroid, it was
because she understood her husband's aspirations. Reflecting back on
their conversations the summer they met in Woods Hole, she said, "Jonas
had the idea from a time when he was quite young, that he wanted to do
something that would make a difference to humanity."[45] If she thought
that once he had accomplished his goal of preventing polio she and the
boys would recapture his attention, she was wrong.

⸻

As 1953 CAME to an end, the 35,968 reported polio cases marked the
third-highest incidence in US history. A survey of public fears ranked
polio second, just behind the atomic bomb. Everybody awaited a preventive vaccine, and their hopes were directed toward the NFIP. The field
trial would be a costly endeavor, one solely supported through the March
of Dimes. O'Connor set seventy-five million dollars as his fundraising
goal for 1954. To accomplish this, three million volunteers from the 3,100
National Foundation chapters across America joined forces. The NFIP
needed widespread publicity, and its public relations department sent the
press human interest stories to encourage donations—like the "tipping
from a waitress" anecdote out of Portland, Oregon.[46] A group of volunteers had gathered at a local restaurant to plan their fundraising activities. At the end of dinner, as they started to leave, their waitress, Evelyn
Higgenbottom, called them back and gave them their first contribution—the three dollars in tips they had left for her.

   No one, however, sold magazines and newspapers as well as Salk. He
had come to personify the fight against polio. In his white coat and over-
sized, clear-rimmed glasses, he imparted the impression of the archetypal physician-scientist; yet two things helped the press create a congenial
image—his humility and his engaging smile. The public wanted to hear
about this man who had risen from Harlem to free them from the fear
of polio. His image was burnished by the press and the NFIP. A *New*

York Times reporter wrote that without him "not a public health official, not a physician would move. The whole vast network of medical personnel and volunteer aids the National Foundation is erecting for the test—the largest medical test in history—would not get off the ground."[47] A friend from Syracuse wrote Salk that he had pushed the Korean conflict off the front page. "With the conquest of polio in sight," wrote a *Life* reporter, "the currently lively topic in the medical world is who will get the Nobel Prize?"[48] Troan, who professed to be Salk's friend, was among the most egregious practitioners of sensationalism. "He's the Man Who May Lick Both Polio and Flu," Troan wrote for the *World Telegram*. "Don't miss this absorbing article about a man who may be on the verge of making miracle contributions to humanity!"[49]

Salk remained uncomfortable with such publicity. When *Life*, *Time*, and *Newsweek* asked for his personal story, Salk gave them no details of his life outside the laboratory. He considered his private life irrelevant. "Why do they all want to know what I eat for breakfast?" he asked Troan.[50] On the one hand, he frustrated newsmen by talking in general principles, not specifics, and answering questions with questions. On the other hand, they liked him; he was polite and well-spoken and made science accessible to the public. Limited facts didn't keep reporters from speculating, however, based on the tidbits they had gathered. An old acquaintance sent him an article from the *Jewish Daily Forward* that revealed his dreams of being a rabbi. "The figment of someone's imagination," Salk replied.[51] Interruptions by the press, many of which the NFIP had instigated, increasingly annoyed Salk. He told Tom Rivers, "I hope the intensity with which the spotlight has been focused on us will be turned off before we are burned to a crisp."[52]

One of the things that embarrassed Salk most was that the press referred to his preparation as the "Salk vaccine," an improper appellation in scientific circles. No one called Pasteur's rabies vaccine the Pasteur vaccine or Jenner's smallpox vaccine the Jenner vaccine. Salk knew he did not deserve such credit and feared scientific colleagues would think it a form of self-aggrandizement. Many did. He tried referring to it as the "Pitt vaccine," but that name never stuck. When Salk asked Troan why the press insisted on calling it the "Salk vaccine," he explained, "It fits in a headline."[53] Besides, naming it after their hero-in-waiting distinguished the vaccine. Many in the scientific community considered Salk's protestations disingenuous. They thought he courted the press out of self-interest. When a picture of Salk vaccinating his three sons appeared in the news, some thought it another publicity stunt, lending proof to their contention that Salk was a celebrity-seeking NFIP puppet.

◈

READY TO INITIATE a field trial of historic proportions, the NFIP still had not selected the person to conduct the all-important data collection and analysis after Bell resigned. Although Salk would have readily accepted the charge, the Vaccine Advisory Committee recommended the trial be analyzed by a scientist outside the NFIP. That way detractors couldn't claim bias in the vaccine's assessment. Van Riper, O'Connor, and Rivers concluded that Thomas Francis, Jr., had the capability, integrity, and credibility they were seeking. Van Riper contacted Francis, who was on sabbatical leave in Europe. He replied that he would not consider the task unless they agreed to his stipulations: First, the NFIP must provide him with funds to set up an evaluation center at the University of Michigan where he would have complete control over all data with no interference from the Foundation. Second, results of the trial would be released when he deemed them ready. Finally, regarding the trial design, Francis insisted that it be a randomized, double-blind trial with one group receiving vaccine and a control group receiving placebo. He understood that O'Connor had already promised some communities that they could participate in a nonrandomized study giving all second graders vaccines, with first and third graders serving as observed controls. He would honor that pledge. The primary trial, however, would be a randomized trail conducted in first, second, and third graders. Van Riper agreed to all Francis's stipulations, and on January 25, 1954, Francis accepted his offer to evaluate what he knew would be history's most closely watched clinical trial.

Before the field trial could commence, Salk needed to complete assessment of his aqueous vaccine, after which he would test commercially prepared vaccine in 2,500 Pittsburgh children, observing them for twenty-one days for toxicity and response. The work was proceeding at a rate that would allow the trial to begin on April 2, in advance of the summer outbreaks. It was at this point that the federal government stepped in.

Although O'Connor planned to bear the entire expense of the field trial, the NIH Laboratory of Biologics Control, under William Workman, eventually would be responsible for licensing the vaccine. Workman knew that if something went wrong during the trial, Congress would investigate why his bureau had not protected the public. So he began to get involved. He agreed that each commercial lot would be tested for potency, safety, and sterility in the pharmaceutical laboratories, in Salk's lab, and at the Laboratory of Biologics Control. Then he mandated that the antiseptic Merthiolate be added to all vials of vaccine. He reasoned that after the vaccine was bottled, bacteria or fungus might grow and contaminate the vaccine before its use. Salk countered that he had never observed this problem, and vaccine would be used promptly. Besides, he didn't know if Merthiolate would interfere with the vaccine's activity, and he didn't have much time to find out. Workman remained adamant—no Merthiolate, no trial. Salk had no option but to submit to his directive.

On March 21, Salk notified Van Riper that he had completed the inoculation of four thousand children with aqueous vaccine to address the concerns raised by Kempe. It had proved effective and produced no ill effects, including kidney damage. He was ready to assess commercially prepared vaccine in 2,500 children when Fred Stimpert called with disturbing news: at Parke, Davis, guinea pigs injected with the vaccine tested positive for TB. The NFIP dispatched a tuberculosis specialist to the Parke, Davis laboratory to examine the guinea pigs. He found no infection. Merthiolate, the antiseptic Workman had insisted be added to the vaccine to prevent contamination, had caused false positive TB tests.

While Salk was trying to meet the April deadline, enormous pressure was being exerted from all sides. The public stood by in anxious anticipation, incited by the press. Salk's picture appeared on the cover of *Time*; "Polio Fighter Salk: Is This the Year?" it asked.[54] *Life, Collier's, Consumer Reports, Popular Mechanics*, and *U.S. News and World Report* all ran feature articles on the vaccine. The *New York Times Magazine* portrayed Salk as the star in an article entitled "A Stirring Medical Drama."[55] *Time, Newsweek*, and *Science News Letter* gave weekly updates. On the other side stood the vaccine opponents from the legitimate to the psychopathic. "Several States Balk at Tests of Polio Vaccine," read a headline in the *Chicago Daily News*, with the subheading "Health Officers Call Plan Hasty, Doubt Safety of Mass Inoculation."[56] The World Health Organization issued a statement that read, "Mass immunization should not be generally adopted until such times as scientific data are available on the innocuity and efficacy of the vaccine."[57] Opening his talk before the Michigan State Medical Society in mid-March, Sabin quipped, "I felt certain that after you all had read the *Life* magazine story of the conquest of polio, no one would be here." He called the field trial premature: "Let us not confuse optimism with achievement."[58] Among the most vitriolic was D. H. Miller, self-proclaimed president of Polio Prevention, Inc., in Coral Gables, Florida, who sent Salk a number of his articles, which he had circulated nationwide. One, entitled "Little White Coffins," began, "Only God above will know how many thousands of little white coffins will be used to bury the victims of Salk's heinous, fraudulent vaccine."[59]

At the end of March, Workman approved the first batch of Parke, Davis vaccine, and O'Connor was inoculated with it. The following day, Salk had just returned from Colfax Elementary School, where he had begun vaccinating children with commercial vaccine, when he received an urgent message from Workman: safety tests performed on commercial vaccine in the Biologics Control Laboratory had revealed that Parke, Davis lots 501–506 and Eli Lilly lot E-2178 were causing polio in monkeys. Workman was calling a halt to the field trial. McGinnes asked Workman for seventy-two hours to solve the problem. He and Salk found that the companies had not followed the specifications for inactivation exactly as written. Parke, Davis had shortened the exposure time to formalin, allowing virus to survive. Eli Lilly had not filtered the viral suspension properly, leaving cellular debris that could interfere with inactivation.

On March 25, Rivers and O'Connor met with NIH Director William Sebrell and his assistant James Shannon to review the situation. Rivers pointed out that these mistakes had been caught in the safety tests, and contaminated vaccine never would have been released to the public. Shannon said their statistician had calculated that in order to validate the data, they should test samples of each lot in 350 monkeys instead of 54, the current number. O'Connor pointed out that would make the cost of vaccine prohibitive and would delay the trial to a date past polio season. "I've been making vaccines all my life," Rivers told Shannon, his temper rising. "As far as I'm concerned, you can take your pencil and paper and shove them up your ass."[60] O'Connor sent Rivers back to New York to cool off. That night he called the other members of the Vaccine Advisory Committee. "This is General O'Connor speaking," he said. "I have been attacked from all sides and need reinforcements. Can you be here tomorrow morning?"[61]

Over the next three days, the NIH and NFIP reached a compromise. They would continue triple testing every lot with the same number of monkeys. Each company, however, would have to produce eleven consecutive lots that tested safe before the first lot could be released. If one lot tested positive for virus, they all had to be destroyed. Someone leaked the story to the press, and on April 4 Walter Winchell in his Sunday night radio program shocked the American public when he announced: "In a few moments I will report on a new polio vaccine. It may be a killer!"[62]

This popular newsman for ABC, who specialized in sensationalism and scandals, threw the public into a tailspin. Some reacted with fear, others with outrage. "The public is entitled to accuracy in journalistic reporting," a Pittsburgh judge wrote to ABC, "not tips on horse races or the stock market nor statements made in reckless disregard of their accuracy."[63] The University of Pittsburgh sent a notice to parents telling them there was no live virus in the vaccine their children had received. When Troan asked Salk if he wanted to make a statement, he said, "Winchell should stick to propaganda or rumors and not dabble in medicine."[64] Even Sabin called Winchell's broadcast "irresponsible."[65] Nonetheless, the harm had been done. The NFIP estimated that approximately 150,000 children were kept from participating in the field trial by frightened parents.[66] The state of Minnesota withdrew from the trial. Then, one week before the trial was to open, workers at the only factory that could provide the two million needles required for the trial called for a strike.[67]

On April 24, O'Connor and the Vaccine Advisory Committee returned to the NIH. The time had come for a decision about the field trial: it was either now or a year's postponement. Salk reviewed his data— 7,500 vaccinated with no toxicity. The commercial vaccine was now free of virus. Then, Workman told the committee that a group of mice recently inoculated with vaccine had become paralyzed. They called in David Bodian—the world's expert on poliomyelitis in animals. It was no secret Bodian originally had not favored the inactivated vaccine. Now the decision to go forward rested on his opinion. Workman showed Bodian a tape of the mice swaggering around in their last days of life. The problem started with a subtle change in gait, followed by dragging of their hind legs, falling, and eventually death. Workman expected Bodian would need several days to determine if the mice had polio. "I don't know," Bodian said almost immediately. "But I know it's not polio."[68]

The Vaccine Advisory Committee met the next morning at the Hotel Carlton to vote.[69] Many reported a sleepless night. A no vote guaranteed thousands would die from polio in the coming season. With a yes vote, they accepted responsibility for harm done to any child by the vaccine. Dorothy Ducas, the public relations director for the Foundation, stood by for the news release. She found Salk sitting alone on a bench outside the meeting room. When she asked why he was there, he replied he thought he might be called in for last-minute questions. Although Salk had vaccinated thousands at that point, he was not included in the proceedings. "It's not my decision to make," he told Ducas.[70]

Inside, the Vaccine Advisory Committee passed a unanimous resolution to start the polio vaccine field trial. The US Public Health Service issued a statement declaring the decision sound. At 9:35 a.m. on April 26, 1954, the biggest clinical trial in the history of medicine began when six-year-old Randy Kerr of McLean, Virginia, received the first vaccination at the Franklin Sherman Elementary School.

⁂

THE PERIOD BETWEEN January of 1953, when Salk first presented his work to the Committee on Immunization, and April of 1954, when the polio vaccine field trial began, was among the most trying in his life. He felt responsible for the health of the nation. Salk knew his vaccine was both effective and safe. How to demonstrate this to the satisfaction of the federal government, practicing physicians, and his scientific colleagues while answering to his own conscience, formed the crux of a major dilemma.

Salk stood by almost helplessly as the NFIP, through the actions of Weaver and Rivers, took over what he thought should have been his trial, giving him little say as to design, excluding him from the national evaluation of his vaccine. They contended that he couldn't take responsibility for the definitive assessment of his own discovery. No large organization had wrested the smallpox vaccine from Jenner's hands, calling it improper for him to test his own vaccine. The vaccines for yellow fever, diphtheria, and rabies had been tested by the scientists themselves, not a foundation or a government agency. And Salk and Francis had not only developed the influenza vaccine but also tested it on military recruits. The conduct of clinical trials had changed, however, and in the long run insistence on a randomized trial, evaluated by a nonbiased investigator with strict statistical oversight, would validate what was certain to be a controversial study. To make matters worse, Salk had watched his carefully prepared and tested vaccine be adulterated when the pharmaceutical companies began large-scale preparation, taking shortcuts which reduced its safety. The removal of the mineral oil adjuvant and addition of Merthiolate by the Biologics Control Laboratory added to his discontent.

In the meantime, the public, the overzealous NFIP, and Basil O'Connor, whom Salk revered, pulled at him from one side, while scientists he respected and a group of vocal physicians pulled from the other. The press stood by, reporting every move, every dispute, stretching the facts whenever necessary to make a good story and keep Jonas Salk in the headlines. Even so, his wife, Donna, maintained, "No external pressure could possibly match the internal pressure under which Jonas operated. He had decided that there ought to be a polio vaccine and that's what he was going to do."[71] During that year Salk had heard leaders in the field, men he aspired to emulate, criticize him at every turn. When asked later in life whether that criticism had hurt his feelings, he replied, "Hurt? That's one thing. Being deterred is another. I just plowed on."[72] Engulfed in conflict, this man who avoided confrontation reacted with equanimity. "When other people might have caved in, he didn't," his son Peter said. "It was just not his nature; he never caved in."[73] Some interpreted his conviction as arrogance.

While trying to complete his work with utmost speed, Salk was bombarded with hundreds of letters from parents begging for vaccine and heart-rending requests from people afflicted with polio. The sanctuary of his laboratory was invaded by researchers coming to learn his techniques and by the press hoping to get a glimpse of this man who was rapidly rising to saintly status. Always a private man, Salk had few friends in whom he could confide. He couldn't trust colleagues in the field. His mentor, Thomas Francis, had long since distanced himself. Although he had a close relationship with O'Connor, it became clear that the NFIP was O'Connor's favored son. And he did not seek sympathy from Donna. He rarely made it home, and when he did, it was to sleep a few hours or change his shirt. Her focus had to be her three sons, whom for the most part she was raising alone while coping with her husband's growing celebrity.

The polio vaccine saga, one of the most controversial in medical history, was being played out on a grand scale, with the health of the public at stake. During that year Salk had to draw upon all the inner strength he had stored up since childhood when he dreamed of helping humanity, of making a difference. "I desire to so conduct the affairs of this administration," his childhood hero, Abraham Lincoln, had said, "that if, at the end, when I come to lay down the reins of power, I have lost every other friend on earth, I shall at least have one friend left, and that friend shall be down inside of me."[74] Jonas Salk persevered because, in the end, he believed, he had to answer only to himself.

The World's Largest
Clinical Trial

ON APRIL 26, 1954, the National Foundation's polio vaccine trial commenced. Children around the country, from Kingsport, Tennessee, to Laramie, Wyoming, rolled up their sleeves and gritted their teeth. Never before and never again in the history of medicine would there be a trial this monumental in size, conducted solely on children, financed and run by volunteers.

From an operations standpoint, the trial involved substantial logistical issues. In his studies leading up to the field trial, Salk, his staff, and a handful of physicians and nurses had done everything themselves—identify the subjects, obtain consents, inoculate children, and collect and analyze the data. The number of subjects, however, totaled about 7,500, and they all lived within an hour of Pittsburgh. Now a voluntary organization of laymen, not a scientific research team, was embarking on a study of almost two million, spanning the entire United States.[1]

Basil O'Connor had selected NFIP medical director Hart Van Riper and operational director Melvin Glasser to lead the trial, adhering to the research plan agreed upon by the Vaccine Advisory Committee. For sites, they chose rural, suburban, and urban counties of approximately fifty thousand to two hundred thousand in population, big enough to include different socioeconomic groups yet still manageable. They picked areas that had had high rates of polio in 1952 and 1953 and those whose health departments seemed capable of carrying out the trial. They eliminated Minnesota, whose health officials had not authorized the trial in time; Maryland, Arizona, and the District of Columbia, where the school year would end before the series of three shots could be given; and Georgia, where poliomyelitis outbreaks had been reported already. The final group comprised 211 study areas in forty-four states, as well as a few in Canada and Finland.

The field trial consisted of two concurrent studies. The primary trial—a randomized placebo-control study—would involve approximately 750,000 first, second, and third graders, the group known to have the highest incidence of polio. It would be run through elementary schools, where students in each classroom would be assigned by random draw to receive either vaccine or placebo. Coding assured that no one, neither the child, parent, nurse, nor the NFIP, knew who received which injection until the code was broken. At the end of December, Thomas Francis and his statisticians would compare the number of cases between the two groups. In the second, parallel trial—the observed-control study—four hundred thousand second graders in selected areas would be offered vaccine on a voluntary basis. The rate of polio among this group would be compared to approximately 725,000 first and third graders in the same community, who would receive no injections, serving as the observed controls.

Parke, Davis and Eli Lilly, the only pharmaceutical companies whose lots passed stringent safety testing in time for the trial, supplied all the vaccine, produced according to Salk's specifications with three strains of formalin-inactivated virus plus Merthiolate. Children would receive the first two doses a week apart, followed by a third dose, a booster, a month later, all injected into the upper arm muscle. In a subset of forty thousand children, blood samples were to be drawn before and shortly after inoculation, as well as six months later, to measure antibody levels. This would allow Francis to estimate how many had antipolio antibodies prior to vaccination and compare potency and protective effect of different vaccine lots.

Orchestration of such a trial posed huge challenges. The Foundation needed to educate and obtain permission from more than a million parents.

Although teachers would give children consent forms to take home, someone had to be certain they didn't get left on the playground or in book bags. Once signed, consents had to be collected, the list of subjects prepared, and basic demographic information entered onto forms. Health officials had to receive cartons of vaccine and placebo, along with needles and syringes, and distribute them to trial sites; others needed to set up inoculation stations in school gymnasiums and auditoriums. As children lined up, their assigned number had to match the one coded on the vial so that each child received the proper inoculate. Volunteers needed to be on hand to comfort children and pass out lollipops, others to make sure the children returned for their second and third inoculations. For those forty thousand subjects designated to have blood taken for antibody levels, samples had be drawn at the right time from the right child, labeled, processed, and mailed to special laboratories. Any child who developed a reaction to the shot or any illness throughout the trial period had to be examined by a physician. Every death required an in-depth investigation. And data on every child, including the demographics, lots used, specimens, and illnesses, had to be recorded and coded as precisely as if done by an academic research laboratory.

Although the mechanics would have daunted the most seasoned investigators, Melvin Glasser seemed unfazed. He had served as chief of field operations for the International Red Cross during World War II. Even his title, operational director of the Field Trial Unit, evoked the image of a military campaign. To carry out such an undertaking, Glasser needed an army. That's exactly what the NFIP provided—an army of volunteers. Many had been preparing to go to war against polio since 1938, the year the National Foundation had been founded. When the *National Foundation News* announced it was looking for volunteers, three thousand Foundation chapters around the country responded.[2] Other organizations joined them: the National Congress of Parents and Teachers; the National Councils of Jewish Women, of Negro Women, and of Catholic Women; and men from the Rotary Club, the Kiwanis Club, and the Chamber of Commerce. Housewives constituted the highest percentage of volunteers. Actress Helen Hayes, whose only daughter had died from polio, served as chairwoman for the National Mothers March on Polio. "It was a prayer that led me into the fight against polio," she told *American Weekly*. When she felt unable to face the future after her daughter's death, Hayes said, "Providently, God led me to a consciousness that in the crusade against polio, I might find surcease from pain."[3]

Next Glasser faced the task of training those who would execute the trial: 20,000 physicians and public health officials, 40,000 nurses, 14,000 elementary school principals, 50,000 teachers, and 220,000 volunteers. When someone at the Foundation suggested hiring trained personnel to do a task, O'Connor refused. He insisted the trial be conducted by those who had demonstrated loyalty to the March of Dimes. "It was O'Connor's sense of the vitality and power of his voluntary movement," Glasser recalled, "that kept the project going."[4] They trained the volunteers during two-day workshops held at each of the 211 sites. A fifty-eight-page "Manual of Suggested Procedures" assisted local health officials, as well as those staffing the vaccination clinics, in completing each step in the proper manner. Instructions for the placebo-control trial were printed on yellow paper, those for the observed-control on blue. A purple kit provided instructions on what to do in case of an accident. A booklet entitled "Operational Memoranda" contained seventeen sets of detailed directions for different tasks. Eighteen bulletins, issued along the way, clarified processes such as "Notification of Deaths and Untoward Reactions."

Once the volunteers were ready, the NFIP needed to encourage parental consent. Each child brought home a note from O'Connor that began, "This is one of the most important projects in medical history. Its success depends on the cooperation of parents. We feel sure you will want your child to take part."[5] Walter Winchell's warning about the vaccine, "It may be a killer," still rang in the ears of many parents. Winchell had quoted medical writer Paul de Kruif as saying, "If a batch can bring down monkeys, it is capable of bringing down children." The popular newscaster pointed out that the New York Health Department required parents to sign an agreement that released them from liability. "In short," Winchell scoffed, "they assure you that the vaccine is completely safe. But you cannot sue them if it isn't."[6] *Time* quoted a researcher as saying, "This year's mass trials are the greatest gamble in medical history";[7] *Newsweek* referred to children as "guinea pigs."[8] Despite these warnings, most of the public believed in a savior named Jonas Salk and enrolled their children in the trial.

Above all, the Foundation needed to engage the subjects of the trial—the children. Dave Preston, a science writer for the NFIP, coined the term "Polio Pioneers" to give them special attention. After completing all three injections, a child received an official card from the NFIP with his or her name on it and the coveted Polio Pioneer button. Teachers impressed upon their classes the importance of the historical event in which they were about to take part. The smiling face of Randy Kerr, America's first Polio Pioneer, beamed from magazines and pamphlets along with his quote, "I could hardly feel it."[9] A group of towheaded children from Provo, Utah, posed in a line, holding their right hands over their left upper arms in a kind of Polio Pioneer salute. Television, newsreels, magazines, church and school bulletins depicted a nation united in an attempt to eradicate the disease that had instilled fear in its citizens for the past forty years.

In the meantime, Francis set up the Poliomyelitis Vaccine Evaluation Center at the University of Michigan's old maternity hospital. A sign on this inconspicuous brick structure read "Special Projects Research Building." The *Michigan Alumnus* described rooms crammed with desks, typewriters, filing cabinets, and IBM machines, "nothing to suggest a medical experiment." One visitor remarked that it looked like "the head office of a mail order company."[10] On the wall in the anteroom hung a large map of the United States dotted with brightly colored pushpins, each denoting the status of the trial in that area—270 pins stuck in forty-four states where more than fourteen thousand schools were taking part. Francis's job was to design the forms, collect and process all records, and tabulate the final data with assistance from a group of statisticians, epidemiologists, and clerks.

If Francis thought he could sequester himself in the Vaccine Evaluation Center, analyze the data, and write the final report, he was mistaken. For an entire year, it seemed, his phone did not stop ringing, the list of problems never-ending. A child got two injections on the same day; should they skip his second dose a week later? A child moved to another county in the middle of the trial; should she be registered as a participant from the first or second county? His previous trials, many conducted in the military, had been under his complete control. With a group of laymen running the vaccine trial, mistakes were certain to happen. In Denver, the city that boasted the highest participation rate, all the registration forms had been filled out incorrectly. The pharmaceutical companies had done such a good job making the vaccine and placebo look identical that several volunteers mixed up the vials, and it was unclear who got what. In Schenectady, New York, nurses reused syringes without cleaning them between subjects, thus combining small amounts of vaccine and placebo. Physicians in Guilford County, North Carolina, took home study vaccine to inoculate their own families. As serious as some of these problems were, considering the size of the trial, they occurred with relative infrequency.

A bigger concern was tracking the potential side effects from the vaccine and documenting cases of poliomyelitis. Since the number of children contracting polio in the vaccinated and control groups constituted the endpoint of the trial, every illness, as minor as diarrhea or a cold, had to be reported and reviewed. If the physician considered polio a possible diagnosis, a complete neurological exam needed to be performed, with blood and stool samples collected and sent to special labs. Each death had to be thoroughly investigated and an autopsy performed. When a seven-year-old from Jackson, Mississippi, died suddenly, Francis learned that the body had been embalmed before blood samples and tissue from the spinal cord could be obtained. They had to be precise. By the trial's completion, the Evaluation Center had received more than 144 million pieces of data that were entered onto IBM punch cards for analysis.

True to their agreement, the NFIP did not press Francis for preliminary results. Citizens, the press, and O'Connor remained patient—for a while. Before long, however, the public became curious about this scientist whom reporters described only as "impeccably dressed, looking younger than his fifty-four years." Unlike Salk, Francis refused to charm or even oblige them, and soon the press began to use less complimentary portrayals, calling him "phlegmatic on first acquaintance" and "a man no one can push around." When a reporter told Francis that the three-quarters of a million dollars he was getting paid for the evaluation meant "the integrity of the conclusions might be open to question," Francis told him to inform the editors of his newspaper that "the Center's integrity was at least the equal of their own."[11]

Frustrated with his behavior and inaccessibility, public relations director Dorothy Ducas sent someone from the NFIP to tell Francis his report would be better received if the public knew more about him. Francis practically threw the man out of his office. Moreover, his job was made more difficult by the public's belief in Salk's vaccine, leaving Francis to play the possible role, in the words of the *Michigan Alumnus*, of a "wet blanket."[12] To add to the strain, Francis's wife, Dorothy, was seriously injured in an automobile accident and remained hospitalized for six months. Francis's chronic ulcers began acting up.[13]

In June of 1954, the pharmaceutical companies working on the vaccine raised the question of whether they should continue production in anticipation of the next year. If the field trial demonstrated that the vaccine was beneficial in preventing polio, millions around the world would be clamoring for it. If it proved ineffective, they wanted to shut down the costly production facilities and move on to other drugs. They turned to Van Riper for the answer. He replied that he had not been able to extract even the slightest hint from Francis. Van Riper, in turn, looked to Salk, hoping he had more sway with his former colleague. Salk knew Francis well enough to understand that when he had stipulated no outside interference, he meant it. In July, Francis told Van Riper he would not complete evaluating the data until early spring of 1955.

O'Connor faced a dilemma. On the one hand, he could not ask the pharmaceutical firms to place their facilities on standby, ready to gear up production at a moment's notice. On the other, he could never tell the American public that although the vaccine had worked, none would be available for the coming polio season. Pushed to make a decision six months before he knew the outcome of the trial, O'Connor gambled, ordering twenty-seven million doses of vaccine at the price of nine million dollars.[14] Since he had spent more than twenty-five million dollars already on the vaccine trial and the research leading up to it, this decision put the NFIP finances in a precarious state.

✦

THE VACCINE TRIAL under way, Salk anticipated a quiet year. In June, he wrote Danish virologist Herdis von Magnus that he was sitting in the backyard in the sun, dictating letters. Soon he would be leaving for a month's vacation at their cottage on Lake Erie and then on to Rome for the International Poliomyelitis Conference. When von Magnus wrote back that she hoped he was relaxing and didn't miss the excitement, he replied, "I do miss it but with great pleasure. You know what it is like when you take off a tight shoe—it feels so good."[15] What should have been a relatively peaceful year would turn out to be an exasperating one instead, stretching his equanimity to its limits.

Salk felt certain the vaccine would prove to be effective, but he recognized two modifications which might preclude its protection in every child. The first was timing of inoculations. For this he took full responsibility. He knew that the third dose should be given no earlier than seven weeks after the first to allow the immune system to mount a booster response. Because the trial had started later than planned, seven weeks would place the third dose in the fall, after the polio season had ended. So they administered it five weeks after the first dose instead, knowing full well that might be too soon. The second alteration, the addition of Merthiolate, had been thrust upon Salk, against his advice. He had never seen the need to add an antiseptic to the vaccine; the Laboratory of Biologics Control had mandated it. Salk worried that Merthiolate had weakened the vaccine's potency, and he had not had time to test it fully.

During that year, the number of people begging Salk for vaccine increased as polio spread from one community to another. "As a father of three," he told Mrs. L. Meltzer of Brooklyn, "I think I know what you . . . are experiencing, and if it were within my power to ease your anxiety, I would do so."[16] Even harder was denying requests from friends and colleagues. "If I had departed from this position even once," he informed one, "my life would have been extremely difficult."[17] Neither the rich nor the famous could move him from this position. He replied to Marlene Dietrich that he could not provide vaccine for her grandchildren. "I find it very difficult and unpleasant indeed to admit my limitations in being unable to do more."[18]

Meanwhile he received many questions from physicians regarding the vaccine, the answers to which they could have found in his reports, had they been accepted for publication. He had submitted two papers on vaccine preparation to the *Journal of the American Medical Association* (*JAMA*), the most widely circulated medical journal. Both had been rejected as too "technical." Eventually they were published in specialty journals not usually read by practicing physicians. As the number of inquiries increased, so did his irritation with the American Medical Association. When its president complimented Salk on a television interview, calling the manner in which he had explained complicated immunological material "a masterpiece in health education," Salk took the opportunity to express the resentment that had been festering for months.[19] "I have not been unmindful of the great need for education, not only of the public but of our profession as well," he wrote back, It was for that reason he had submitted two articles to the editor of *JAMA* written with the practicing physician in mind. "Both were intended to answer for him the questions that I thought were uppermost in his mind." The rejection of both, he wrote, "increased the burden upon me enormously. Many inquiries came to me that would not have come otherwise. Much doubt, and in some cases indignation, was aroused which could have been avoided if usual channels of communication had been available." He did not take it personally, he maintained, but felt "it was unfortunate for those who may have advised the editors or allowed their personal feelings to cloud their objectivity in decisions that concern not themselves but all of our colleagues who are desirous of being kept abreast of moving frontiers."[20]

In early September 1954, Salk boarded the SS *Independence* in New York, headed for the Third International Poliomyelitis Conference in Rome.[21] Photographers snapped pictures of him on deck in a casual pose; fruit baskets and flowers filled his stateroom. "May this journey afford you the rest and relaxation you so richly deserve," read a telegram from a friend.[22] In 1951, Salk had made his debut as an up-and-coming polio researcher at the Second International Poliomyelitis Conference in Copenhagen. Now, just three years later, he returned a celebrity, his picture on the cover of every major American magazine and newspaper.

Held at the University of Rome starting September 6, the five-day conference attracted more than one thousand physicians and scientists from forty-nine countries. Speakers from London, Madrid, Copenhagen, Milan, and the United States discussed the social aspects of polio, physiotherapy, orthopedic management, respirators, tissue culture techniques, and gamma globulin. Many came to hear Salk update them on his inactivated-virus vaccine. Some came to this meeting determined to topple him. Chief among this group were the live-virus vaccine advocates, led by Sabin.

Considering this debate to be one of the highlights of the conference, the organizers scheduled both Salk and Sabin to speak in the same session. Salk began by acknowledging that investigators in the field were divided between the two approaches to polio immunization. Many believed that live-virus vaccines provided the only satisfactory means for protection. Yet he had found that antibody levels following the third (booster) shot of killed-virus vaccine resembled those from a natural infection. By manipulation of dose and intervals between inoculations, it should be possible to provide long-term immunity. Then he turned to the issue of the vaccine's safety. Plotting data on infectivity against hours of exposure to formalin, he showed graphs from thirty-three commercially prepared lots. In each one, all the points fell on a straight line, showing that at three days, no live virus could be measured. Thus, if they continued inactivation for six days, he predicted the amount of residual virus to be infinitesimal. "The ultimate objective is not merely a reduction in the amount of crippling and death from poliomyelitis," he said in conclusion, "but rather elimination of these as a cause of fear."[23] An unusual way to end a scientific presentation, this statement sounded more like a press release.

Sabin followed. In chimpanzees he had been able to attenuate strains of all three poliovirus types so that they could induce antibody formation while causing no overt infection. He should have avirulent viral strains ready for oral vaccines in the next few years. His data on a live-virus vaccine looked promising in monkeys. Even Rivers, who had pushed for the killed vaccine trial, called his work "exciting," stating it should be continued "vigorously but with caution."[24]

Francis moderated a discussion of the two papers. First to speak, Swedish scientist Sven Gard said he could not reproduce Salk's data showing that viral inactivation occurred in a straight line.[25] Salk suggested Gard had used the wrong temperature or too much formalin. Wendell Stanley agreed with Gard. Some began to joke about Salk's "elusive straight line."[26] Even stronger condemnation came from the Harvard group. Thomas Weller, Enders's colleague and a soon-to-be

Nobel laureate, contended that Salk's technique for detecting residual traces of live virus was faulty. Prior to the conference, he told Gard he was upset by "the moral and ethical aspects of the manner in which the whole vaccine program has been handled." Pressure had been exerted on public officials as well as scientists in order to fit the NFIP "party line."[27]

Sabin again brought up the potential for allergic kidney disease since Salk grew his virus in monkey kidney cells. Salk said he considered the issue no longer germane, as he had shown no damage in children who had received three inoculations. Sabin countered that he could not dismiss his concern for kidney damage so blithely, since immunity from the inactivated vaccine lasted just one year at most, necessitating repeated inoculations throughout life. David Bodian rebutted, saying that Salk's vaccine appeared to confer long-lasting immunity, making repeated inoculations unnecessary; Sabin argued that this was impossible to predict. The discussion began to resemble a free-for-all. Throughout, everyone ignored the proverbial elephant in the auditorium: by then, almost a million children had been inoculated with the vaccine under attack. In seven months, they would know whether it was as impotent and dangerous as Sabin, Gard, Weller, and Winchell asserted.

Salk came to realize that even if the field trial demonstrated the inactivated-virus vaccine to be beneficial, the majority of polio experts considered it a stopgap while they waited for the live-virus vaccine. He could feel attendees pulled toward the live-virus camp. Koprowski, a master in debate, had the last word. "We are living in the era of live-virus vaccine. What we want is to elicit as nearly as possible all the latent capacities of human talent to apply principles established by Jenner."[28] Salk had left for Rome amidst cheers of "Bon voyage"; he returned exhausted.

⁂

MEANWHILE, THE ISSUE of Merthiolate still had not been settled. Salk needed to persuade Workman to lift his mandate that the antiseptic must be added to all vials of vaccine. With the success of the vaccine at stake, Salk arranged a meeting among all six vaccine manufacturers, as well as Workman, Van Riper, Rivers, and O'Connor, on November 2. He came armed with compelling data regarding the harm done by Merthiolate.

Workman stood firm: since the field trial had tested vaccine with Merthiolate, that was the only formulation the Laboratory of Biologics Control would license in the event of a positive trial. Rivers said he was "sore as hell," yet this time Salk fought his own battle.[29] "Would it be improper for me to ask for the basis upon which the decisions concerning the poliomyelitis vaccine are being made?" he asked Workman. "It seems to me that factions have developed in relation to a problem that has a single goal. This is not only inappropriate but unfortunate." He felt, as he thought Workman did, too, that decisions should be based on facts acquired by experimentation. "In this way we approximate the truth and reduce dependence upon opinions." He went on to quote the medieval English philosopher Roger Bacon's list of impediments to the acquisition of truth, ending with "concealment of ignorance by ostentation of seeming wisdom."[30]

It is not clear what political maneuvering followed, but eventually the NFIP, NIH, and commercial firms reached a compromise. Workman agreed to consider licensing vaccine without Merthiolate if Salk inoculated five thousand children with commercial vaccine to establish its safety.[31] Salk agreed. With regard to the field trial, there was nothing he could do. He felt certain that some children had received lots spoiled by Merthiolate. This was not his trial, however. All he could do was report his concern to Francis and hope he took that into account in his final evaluation.

Salk's usual optimism was flagging. So when O'Connor, attempting to appease the disenfranchised Committee on Immunization, announced a joint meeting with the Vaccine Advisory Committee on December 18, Salk declined to attend. "I will not subject myself nor my work nor my principles," he wrote O'Connor, "to a combine such as the so-called committees on vaccine and immunization."[32] O'Connor had witnessed the beating Salk had taken in Rome. He knew how disapproval from scientific colleagues affected him and that this underlay his refusal to attend the meeting. He sent Salk a 1772 quote from Benjamin Franklin: "We must not in the Course of Public life expect immediate Approbation and immediate grateful Acknowledgment of our Service—But let us persevere thro' Abuse and even Injury. The internal Satisfaction of a good Conscience is always present, and Time will do us Justice in the Minds of the People, even of those at present the most prejudiced against us."[33] As he always did with O'Connor, Salk relented.

On the first day of the meeting, the two groups again debated the merits of live versus killed virus vaccines. Sabin announced he was set to test his vaccine on volunteers at the federal prison in Chillicothe, Ohio. Salk had not attended that day, saying he had scheduled booster shots at the Watson Home. He arrived the second day to witness a contentious discussion regarding the authority of the two committees. Members of the Committee on Immunization still smarted from being excluded from decisions regarding the field trial. John Paul suggested they proceed as they had with the typing project and enlist researchers for work agreed upon and supervised by an expert committee. Salk thought Paul was implying that he had ignored the advice of the Committee on Immunization when he prepared a vaccine on his own. Pretending to have misunderstood Paul's remarks, Rivers suggested Salk could use some help, having shouldered the burden of the vaccine alone. When he turned to Salk and said, "I don't know how you feel about it though, Jonas," Salk could contain himself no longer.[34]

"What I have done," Salk said to the group, "has been by default, by virtue of the fact that this is something that needed to be done." At no time along the way, he insisted, had he objected to anyone else working on the problem. "I have carried an enormous burden, an unjustifiable one, one that continues to be unjustified." His composure shattered, he continued: "I don't know why I should be the one that should have to stand and hold the fort against the NIH and against the pharmaceutical houses. These are unreasonable things for one individual to have to do, and I say right here and now that I am perfectly prepared at this point to withdraw completely because I think I have done enough....I am tired."[35] The group must have sat dumbfounded—Paul shocked by Salk's emotional outburst, Sabin smug in gaining the upper hand, Rivers pleased with his "give it to them with both barrels" reply, and O'Connor sad it had come to this.

Salk returned to Pittsburgh frazzled. Once again scientists he revered and from whom he wanted acceptance had demeaned his research and him. "I don't think those aspersions touched where he lived as a scientist," his wife, Donna, said, years later. He had confidence in himself and

his work. But "they touched where he lived as a human being, because...
approval was certainly important to him."[36]

The stress was starting to take a toll on Salk. He began to lash out at
innocent bystanders. "Bill Kirkpatrick," he wrote an NFIP assistant
about his first volunteer at the Watson Home, "is a very nice boy; his
mother is a very nice woman; his father is a bore. More than that, he has
a great passion for publicity.... If you detect any cynicism in these
remarks, please be assured that it is not accidental."[37] A filmmaker, producing a documentary on inequity in medical school admissions, asked
Salk about discrimination he had endured as a Jew. "You say that as a
result of these 'vicious and frivolous religious barriers the community
may well have been deprived of the talents of other Doctor Salks,'" he
replied. "This is merely conjecture and the fact of the matter is that Salk
did get into medical school. I might say that I had far fewer difficulties
of a religious discriminatory nature than I have had of a scientific discriminatory nature."[38]

The director of special events for ABC complained to O'Connor
that he had recently attended a meeting summoned by the NFIP for
radio, television, and the press to receive an important announcement
from Salk. To his surprise, Salk would not permit recording of his
remarks, and he refused to read the Foundation's summary of his paper,
as was the usual procedure at such news conferences. Salk later apologized to O'Connor, making a feeble excuse, but his unusual behavior
continued.[39] He even took on public relations director Dorothy Ducas,
saying he found her fundraising approach objectionable. He suggested
that they extol the volunteers who contributed their dimes to develop
the vaccine rather than focus on him. "This, it would seem to me, would
have more effect upon the average person than to eulogize Salk as the
'Polio Man of the Year.'"[40]

Frustrated that some virologists still doubted his findings, frustrated
in his dealings with the press, frustrated that his time and identity had
been taken from him, Salk decided to decline all interview requests.[41]
But he couldn't resist Edward R. Murrow. In February of 1955, he agreed
to appear on *See It Now*, joining the ranks of such distinguished guests
as Carl Sandburg, Robert Oppenheimer, and Jawaharlal Nehru. The interview started on the right note when Salk emphasized, "This is not the

Salk vaccine. This is a poliomyelitis vaccine." He credited the scientists upon whose work his was based, especially John Enders, a recent Nobel laureate. "Enders threw a long forward pass," he told Murrow, "and we happened to be at the place where the ball could be caught."[42] So far, so good. Then Salk proceeded to demonstrate how they made the vaccine, showing television audiences how he minced monkey kidneys in a Waring blender. In ending, he warned listeners that the vaccine used in the trial might not prevent every case of polio and explained why. Salk said he went on *See It Now* to enlighten the public; his critics considered this yet more evidence that he was a star-struck fame-seeker.

WHEN THE NFIP reported that 1954, with 38,741 new polio cases, had surpassed 1953 to mark the third highest incidence of polio in US history, neither the press nor the public could sit by idly, waiting for results of the field trial.[43] Francis was besieged. Parents called to find out if their child had received the placebo or the real vaccine, as the start of the next polio season would soon be upon them. Leaders of the US Armed Forces wanted to know whether they should prepare for mass inoculations. Francis divulged nothing. The press tried to pry answers out of him using some old tricks. On March 30, 1955, the *New York World Telegram* announced it had just heard from "an unimpeachable source" that the vaccine had proved 100 percent effective. Reporters began to call Francis's office for verification. "I have absolutely nothing to say," he replied. "I advise you to go back to that unimpeachable source from whence the rumor originally... came."[44]

Francis anticipated that reporters might try to obtain tips from his staff at the Evaluation Center. To avert a security breach, he had divided up the data among different groups of statisticians. Reporters attempted to take a straw poll among local health officers involved in the field trial, but Francis had put a ban on any form of advance release. When O'Connor heard rumors of the poll, he asked Francis what he was going to do. "Nothing" he replied. "The health officers won't talk."[45] Most upheld the vow of silence. Not all. A South Carolina official revealed that of the twenty-seven polio cases in his area, none had occurred in children who had received vaccine. Rumors originated from Salk's lab as well. In late March, Troan got a call from James Lewis informing him that Workman had come from Washington to see Salk. When Troan asked who Workman was, Lewis told him he was the head of the Division of Biologic Standards at the NIH. "They license vaccines," Lewis said. "He's in the room with Jonas, and they're going over the protocols."[46] Troan called the pharmaceutical firms to confirm this lead and began writing an article about the vaccine's success. Lewis's tip turned out to be misleading; they were talking about Merthiolate. Even the AMA tried to get a preview of Francis's results. When they approached him about allowing an AMA committee to review his findings so they could be published immediately in *JAMA*, Francis replied, "No peep shows."[47]

Finally, Francis informed O'Connor that results would be ready by mid-April. They agreed the findings should be presented at a national meeting. The American Medical Association, the most appropriate venue, didn't hold its annual conference until June. They considered a special forum, and Salk suggested the National Academy of Sciences in Washington, DC. This society of elite scientists included Francis and Enders; no doubt Salk hoped to be nominated for membership someday himself. When the Academy declined, public relations for the University of Pittsburgh put forward their medical center. According to John Paul, "Gradually the forces of publicity and sensationalism took over, and since the Poliomyelitis Vaccine Evaluation Center had been established at the University of Michigan, it seemed that this university had the right to capitalize on the project."[48] Francis agreed but insisted upon a scientific presentation, not a public relations event or press conference. The NFIP Public Relations Department advised that a Tuesday was the best day for an announcement and offered Francis two dates in March and two in April. He chose the latest, April 12, which happened to be the tenth anniversary of Franklin D. Roosevelt's death. Although critics of the NFIP and Salk called this another publicity stunt, Francis rejected the charge: "The choice was made by my staff and me with no knowledge that any political significance attached to the date."[49]

On April 8, Francis finished the draft of a 563-page report: "An Evaluation of the 1954 Poliomyelitis Vaccine Trials." In the end, what he would present in Ann Arbor were the results not just of a trial but of a tour de force. The NFIP, under the direction of O'Connor, had stimulated a cooperative effort among a diverse group of investigators to solve a practical problem and had persuaded the public to fund that work. Although the vaccine's development represented the culmination of creative work by a number of esteemed scientists and hours of drudgery by the Pittsburgh laboratory group; although Francis had collected and analyzed millions of pieces of data to make a coherent report; although the public in large part funded and executed the trial; and although the NFIP, led by O'Connor, was the powerhouse behind it all, Jonas Salk became the symbol for the prevention of polio. On April 12, 1955, the entire world's attention would focus on him.

Relief from Fear

ON APRIL 11, 1955, when Jonas Salk boarded a plane for Ann Arbor, he didn't yet know the outcome of the field trial.[1] Although the trial had been conducted to evaluate the vaccine he had developed, culminating seven years of work, he had been excluded from its design and execution. He had not seen the data, or a summary, or conclusions—not a word, not even a hint from Thomas Francis. Salk would hear the results at the same time Francis announced them to the rest of the waiting world. And while Salk was confident about his vaccine's efficacy and safety, he still did not know how much the addition of Merthiolate or the early booster shot had reduced its potency. He was scheduled nonetheless to address the audience at the University of Michigan right after Francis, putting him in an awkward position. If Francis reported that the vaccine prevented polio, it would be hard to top that; his comments might sound like an afterthought. If Francis reported no difference in the rate of polio between those had who received the vaccine and the controls, he would face a disappointed audience and a disheartened public, a failure. Any explanation he offered would seem a feeble excuse.

Salk had suggested that Donna and the boys accompany him to Ann Arbor. Their sons would have their first plane ride; Peter and Darrell could see the city in which they were born. Their Uncle Lee would join them. Donna thought they would hear the report, catch up with some old friends, and come home the next day. She packed for a two-day stay. University officials had arranged for the Salks to stay at the Inglis House, a guest residence owned by the university. Up a long driveway, behind great stone walls, stood a gracious mansion with a slate roof and wisteria surrounding the entrance. French doors led to a terrace and formal gardens, graced by a fountain with four bronze turtles. These accommodations, along with engraved invitations sent to five hundred guests, should have indicated this was not going to be a typical scientific forum.

The NFIP expected heavy press coverage. "If Tommy were to announce his findings in a men's room," O'Connor said, "the reporters and cameramen would be there."[2] Presenting a paper under the bright lights of television cameras would be a new experience for Francis. KTTV in Los Angeles was planning to broadcast the entire symposium live. *Voice of America* was preparing to transmit the talks throughout Europe. Eli Lilly was sponsoring a closed-circuit telecast to fifty-four thousand practicing physicians in sixty-one cities, costing the company a quarter of a million dollars. The Ann Arbor event was looking more like an international press conference.

On April 12, Salk awoke to a bleak, cloudy day. At 8:30 he had breakfast at the Inglis House with O'Connor, Van Riper, Rivers, and Alan Gregg, vice president of the Rockefeller Foundation, who would moderate the symposium. When Francis joined them, he finally divulged the results of the trial: they were positive; the vaccine was safe and effective. The four men could barely contain their excitement or relief, but they had to keep the news to themselves until after his presentation. Since it was too early for champagne, they shook hands and left for Rackham Hall.

As Salk greeted guests and prepared to take his seat, he may not have noticed the setting, which was magnificent. Built in the late thirties, the Horace H. Rackham Building was an award-winning showplace for the university, a tasteful blend of classical and art deco styles.[3] The main entrance hall, painted Pompeian red, opened to a marble staircase with bronze railings. An Italian sculptor had provided lavish wall decorations, using both interior and exterior bas-reliefs. Bowl-shaped chandeliers and Chippendale furniture added to its elegance. The building's focal point, Rackham Hall, was of classical Greek style, terra cotta in color, with 1,200 plush seats arranged in a semicircular pattern; fluted columns abutted the stage. Recessed lighting and art deco detailing made the ceiling resemble a starry sky. On the stage, a gold-and-blue University of Michigan seal adorned the front of the lectern behind which the dignitaries would sit. An eight-foot-wide platform, erected over the last two rows of seats, supported sixteen television and newsreel cameras, radio microphones, and a tangle of cables.

Jonas's brother Lee and Donna sat a few rows from the front with the three boys. Although she tried to concentrate on what was happening, Donna was busy quieting five-year-old Jonathan, answering eleven-year-old Peter's questions, and separating him from eight-year-old Darrie. "It was an important day," Peter recalled, "because it was the first day of baseball season."[4] A staunch Brooklyn Dodgers fan, he wanted to listen to the game. As a consolation, his mother gave Peter a miniature marble bowling game to keep him occupied.

As guests gathered in the auditorium, few were aware of the commotion going on upstairs. In the large third-floor library with its stained-glass windows and ornate paneling, forty-one telephones, fifteen typewriters, and six Western Union teletype machines had been set up on the mahogany library tables. The clickety-clack of typewriters, clouds of smoke, and scattered paper cups, half-filled with cold coffee, transformed the dignified sanctum into a noisy pressroom. An estimated 150 reporters had gathered from as far away as Denmark, France, and Israel.

The plan for distributing the report to newsmen had been prearranged. Each was to receive several packets that contained the entire report, an abstract, a press release prepared by the University of Michigan science reporter Lou Graff, and the speakers' talks. A gentleman's agreement had been struck: In order to give them time to absorb the material, reporters would receive the packets at 9:15 a.m. In return, they would instruct their newspapers, television, and radio stations not to release the news until after 10:20, the time Francis was scheduled to speak. To maintain security, the university hired an Ann Arbor policeman to guard the packets. In theory it was a sound plan, but almost immediately it went awry.

At 8:30, while Francis was giving the good news to Salk and O'Connor at the Inglis House, Robert Voight, the chief of statistical operations; Graff; and the guard loaded the packets onto a truck and drove to the back entrance of the Rackham Building. Stacking the reports onto a dolly took longer than expected. Upstairs the reporters were pacing. Graff had planned to place separate piles of material on the tables. When they reached the third floor and the elevator door opened, reporters mobbed them and started grabbing copies. Graff climbed up on a table and threw packets to the reporters, who shoved and jumped over tables to catch them. One glance at the material told them what they needed to know. "It works! It works!" they yelled as they ran for the phones and typewriters.[5] Dave Garroway of NBC's *Today* was the first to violate the gentleman's agreement when he announced the vaccine's success on live television at 9:30. Garroway later admitted that when "The Vaccine Works" came over the wire, the news was just "too good to keep."[6] Thus before Francis said a word, everyone watching *Today* knew the vaccine had been a success.

In contrast to the celebratory atmosphere above them, Rackham Hall was sedate. Hart Van Riper opened the meeting, thanking President Harlan Hatcher for hosting them, followed by comments by Alan Gregg, who acknowledged polio victims everywhere and thanked the children who had participated in the trial.[7] Hatcher spoke next, extolling the university and the chosen master of ceremonies who had become indisposed. If the public wondered how Salk was reacting at this pivotal moment in history, they couldn't tell. Although he sat on stage, he was positioned behind the podium, not visible to the audience or television cameras. Rivers, however, could be seen fidgeting and rubbing his eyes. The group moved to the first row for Francis's presentation.

Dressed in a black suit, white shirt, and striped tie, Francis looked dignified as he approached the lectern. He put on his glasses and for the next hour and a half presented an objective, detailed report, complete with technical slides. In a monotone, he read his typed lecture, occasionally glancing up. Using standard scientific language, not the lingo of the popular press, he stumbled over some phrases and stopped for sips of water, offering no dramatics for radio and television audiences.

Francis said that in the fall of 1953, the National Foundation had announced its intent to conduct a large field trial in order to test the efficacy of the formalin-inactivated poliomyelitis vaccine. The study design comprised two concurrent trials: In the placebo-control study, the main trial, they randomized first, second, and third graders to receive placebo or vaccine in a double-blind fashion. In the observed-control study, they offered vaccine to all children in the second grade, with those in the first and third grades serving as observation controls. Although this design could pose problems of unintentional bias, it was the initial NFIP plan, and several states had agreed to participate on this basis. The main population Francis analyzed totaled 1,080,680, although they followed another 1.8 million children in the study areas. The vaccination period ran from April 26 to June 15, 1954. More than three hundred thousand physicians, epidemiologists, health officials, nurses, schoolteachers, administrators, local volunteers, and clerks had assisted in the program.[8]

Before giving the results, Francis reviewed the side effects from the vaccine. The Evaluation Center received reports of thirty-two major reactions: paralysis or muscular weakness (15), nephritis and kidney infections (7), shock (4), high fever (3), and hives (3). At least half had occurred in children receiving placebo. They found no evidence of kidney damage. In those vaccinated children who developed polio, the time between vaccination and infection was too long to implicate the vaccine as the source. They felt confident in concluding that the vaccine had not caused poliomyelitis in a single child.

Francis had been speaking for fifty minutes. Finally, he turned to the section everyone, including Salk, was anticipating—the effect of vaccine on the incidence of poliomyelitis. He showed slides packed with numbers before he reached the crux of the trial—the prevention of paralytic polio. Among the 749,000 children in the placebo-control study, 33 from the vaccinated group developed paralytic polio compared to 110 in the placebo group, making the rate among controls 3.3 times that of the vaccinated—a significant difference, according to statistical analysis. Addressing the observation study, they found the incidence of paralytic polio to be 2.7 times greater in the control group, with 331 cases among 725,000 children compared with 38 cases among the 222,000 who had been vaccinated—also a significant difference. Overall, Francis said, the vaccine was 80–90 percent effective against paralytic poliomyelitis. Analyzing the data by poliovirus strain, he found the vaccine to be 90 percent effective against Types 2 and 3, and 60–70 percent effective against Type 1. In closing, Francis stated: "Properly prepared vaccine of the Salk variety is safe, antigenically potent and has a high degree of effectiveness in the prevention of paralytic poliomyelitis."[9]

Although Francis had just presented one of the finest clinical trials ever conducted, this was Jonas Salk's day. As he walked to the lectern, the audience rose in a standing ovation. He began by complimenting Francis, whom he called "one of the great masters."[10] He then thanked a long list of those responsible for the trial's success. Starting with the NFIP, he singled out Harry Weaver for his "energetic devotion and foresight." He thanked Connaught Laboratories, which had prepared the virus, and the pharmaceutical manufacturers who had performed a "Herculean task in an unbelievably short time." He talked about the role of Rivers and the Vaccine Advisory Committee, who, he said, "pulled the switch." He thanked community volunteers. And finally, he praised Basil O'Connor, without whom the entire project would not have been possible.

Salk then reflected on his first study at the D. T. Watson Home for Crippled Children, conducted in those already afflicted with polio. The parents and children had come forward even though they had little to gain themselves, Salk told the audience, and Dr. Jessie Wright had agreed to keep the work secret lest it create false hopes. He called Lucile Cochran, the Watson Home's administrator, another Florence Nightingale and explained how, with the gracious help of Dr. Gale Walker, they had extended their studies to the Polk State School. He recognized the University of Pittsburgh, including Chancellor Fitzgerald, Dean McEllroy, and the trustees, who provided him with academic freedom. Finally, Salk thanked his own staff: "This opportunity would have no meaning if it were not for the devotion with which each of the … group that comprises our laboratory contributed and shared in that which needed to be done."[11]

Salk then turned to the scientific portion of his talk. "During the course of our work," he began, "it has become quite clear that commonly accepted opinions that are not founded on quantitative observations cannot be supported for long."[12] In other words, he said in his moment of triumph over the disbelievers, they had shown that exposure to a live virus is not the only way to provide protection against polio. Then he explained why the vaccine used in the field trial had not been completely protective, presenting data obtained after the trial had begun that indicated Merthiolate had diminished its potency. He showed how delaying the booster shot for several months produced higher antibody levels. "We might say," he continued, "that the study conducted in the field in the spring and summer of 1954 was a test of the question as to whether or not primary vaccination alone could prevent paralytic poliomyelitis," even though the vaccine was flawed.[13] The new 1955 vaccine, he proclaimed, "may lead to 100 percent protection from paralysis."[14]

When the enthusiastic applause at long last started to wane, Rivers took his turn. Few in the audience knew that this elder statesman for the NFIP had brokered a number of crucial deals that had allowed the trial to go forward. He praised the thoroughness with which Francis completed the trial and talked about the long road that led to the vaccine's development, highlighting the typing project and the work of Enders, who was conspicuously absent. Finally, O'Connor came to the podium wearing his trademark boutonnière, smiling broadly. He praised the public for their participation and underscored how there had never been such a cooperative and coordinated effort between scientists, doctors, and laymen in the history of medicine. On this glorious day, his thoughts turned to Franklin D. Roosevelt. "The soul of the man who had that dream and who inspired this movement must be rejoicing with us."[15] William Workman, director of the Laboratory of Biologics Control, ended the meeting by saying the vaccine warranted careful consideration for licensure, leaving them with the anticipation that the vaccine would soon be made available to the general public. The formal program ended at 2:00 p.m.

⁂

CHURCH BELLS TOLLED, horns honked, and sirens rang out as the nation rejoiced. Some cheered; some cried. In department stores, loudspeakers blared out the good news. Storekeepers painted "Thank You Dr. Salk" on their windows. Public address systems in schools, courtrooms, and factories called for a moment of silence. Churches and synagogues held impromptu prayer meetings. And the presses started rolling. Upstairs in the Rackham Building newsmen dispatched their headlines: "POLIO IS CONQUERED," announced the *Pittsburgh Press*.[16] "VICTORY OVER

Polio! Polio Vaccine Works!" blazoned the *Chicago Daily News.*[17] Hong Kong's *South China Morning Post* proclaimed Salk's "Triumph over Polio."[18] Downstairs, reporters rushed to get comments from Salk and Francis; hundreds of cameras were flashing. Everyone seemed to be speaking at once. "It was a madhouse all over the place," Rivers remembered, "created by newspaper people and photographers. God, it was just a madhouse, it really was!"[19]

The University of Michigan and NIH had scripted the remainder of the day. After posing for pictures, the speakers adjourned to a press conference upstairs. As they waded through the crowd, hundreds reached to shake hands or slap them on the back. Meanwhile, a panel of experts met with Workman to advise him on licensing the vaccine. This panel had two hours to review Francis's hundred-page document, production protocols from five pharmaceutical firms, and safety data on lots tested by the Laboratory of Biologics Control. Workman told the group that as soon as they made their decision he would telephone Surgeon General Leonard Scheele, who would make a recommendation to the secretary of the Department of Health, Education, and Welfare (HEW), Oveta Hobby. A signing ceremony and press conference had been scheduled for 4:00 p.m., and Hobby had already prepared her remarks. Approval seemed inevitable.

Most on the expert panel were members of the quarrelsome Committee on Immunization, a group that resented any attempt to use them as a rubber stamp. Sabin immediately proposed replacing the Mahoney strain. Others expressed concern about Salk's inactivation methods. What was not adequately discussed was the crucial point that, once licensed, vaccine production would be in the hands of the pharmaceutical companies, meaning that new lots of vaccine would no longer undergo the triple safety check.

The panel was running late, and word came that the HEW secretary was waiting. The attractive wife of a Texas governor, as well as the daughter of a Texas state legislator, Oveta Culp Hobby was prepared for her shining moment. Workman called Scheele to apologize; they would have to cancel Mrs. Hobby's press conference. "Indeed in the atmosphere of triumph which prevailed," Paul wrote later, "it is doubtful whether the committee could have viewed the results of the field trial dispassionately. And it is doubtful whether any group would have had the fortitude to hold out for long against the tremendous pressure to release the vaccine for general use."[20] Everyone on the panel, including Sabin, voted to license the vaccine. At 5:15, Mrs. Hobby signed the official documents. For the second time that day church bells tolled, horns honked, and sirens rang out as the nation rejoiced. "City May Get Its Supply in Forty-Eight Hours" announced the *Pittsburgh Press*.[21]

At six o'clock Francis and Salk made a live presentation to physicians nationwide via closed-circuit television. Salk had arranged for his parents to view the program at the Waldorf-Astoria Hotel along with two thousand New York physicians. The presentation ended at seven in the evening, after which the stars of the day rushed through a formal dinner in order to prepare for *See It Now*, to be shot in the conference room of the Vaccine Evaluation Center.

Promptly at ten-thirty, Edward R. Murrow began. "The sun was warm, the earth coming alive; there was hope and promise in the air. The occasion called for banners in the breeze and trumpets in the distance." After a commercial break, he praised the children and adults who had taken part in the polio field trial. "Today," he continued, "a great profession made a giant step forward, and the news that came out of this room lifted a sense of fear from the homes of millions of Americans."[22] When Murrow introduced Francis, many saw for the first time the man who had determined the vaccine's fate. Exhausted by the long day and uneasy in front of a television camera, Francis came across as a somewhat stuffy scientist, using phrases such as "a protective effect of no insignificant level."

Salk, on the other hand, appeared refreshed and at ease, instinctively knowing how to speak to the camera and what language to use. The *National Jewish Monthly* described him as a "deep-voiced and attractive young man...whose chief characteristic seemed to be modesty."[23] He told Murrow that no one man could take sole credit for most scientific advances, and that in preparing the vaccine, he, too, had built upon the work of others. Salk smiled a lot; he was charming, the people's scientist. And if the public didn't love him enough already, when Murrow asked who owned the patent on the vaccine, Salk answered with a statement that would be quoted often: "Well, the people, I would say. There is no patent. Could you patent the sun?"[24]

A reception followed at the Inglis House. At midnight, the phone was still ringing with congratulatory messages. "People were milling around the room," Salk recalled, "arguing about my future as if I...had just swum the English Channel or something. It all seemed unreal, the sort of thing that would surely end and be forgotten as suddenly as it had begun."[25] Edward R. Murrow knew better. Putting his arm around Jonas's shoulders, he said, "Young man, a great tragedy has just befallen you."

"What's that?" Salk asked.

"You have just lost your anonymity," Murrow replied.[26]

⁂

SALK PLANNED TO stay in Ann Arbor one more day, relaxing with Donna and the children, before they returned to Pittsburgh. An old friend from Francis's lab, Elva Minuse, was coming to visit. Since the formal events had ended, the boys could take off their suits. Francis departed for Boston to visit his daughter; O'Connor and the NFIP staff returned to New York City; and Lorraine Friedman left that morning for a vacation. Salk told Tom Coleman, the University of Pittsburgh public relations person, he could return to Pittsburgh. If he needed anything, he would call. "Jonas was slow to catch on to what was happening," Coleman recollected. "He was behaving as if the situation would blow over in a few hours."[27]

When the sun came up, the phone started ringing. Magazine editors were calling for photo shoots, newsmen for private interviews. The mayor of New York invited Salk to a ticker-tape parade; the governor of California wanted to hire him as a consultant. A public relations firm guaranteed him a million dollars if he would sign an exclusive contract. Someone wanted to erect a statue of him. When Coleman arrived at the Pittsburgh airport, he was paged by a distraught and overwhelmed Salk. He turned around and flew back to Ann Arbor to take over the phones, but he soon became hoarse and had to call for assistance. Murrow was right; Salk had lost his anonymity. "I actually thought I'd go to that meeting, hear the report, read a paper of my own, talk to a few newsmen, and return to Pittsburgh and my laboratory the next day," he said a few years later. "I was totally unprepared for what happened at Ann Arbor."[28]

Donna, too, was taken aback. Reporters swarmed around her. Because her husband had become a folk hero overnight, she also had been conferred celebrity status. She attempted to remain calm and make sure the boys looked presentable and didn't misbehave. "We just had to take things as they came—interview after interview after interview, and photograph after photograph."[29] Even so, Peter recalled overhearing his mother complain about being "in the eye of the hurricane."[30] And it was not just hard on Donna. Although Darrie delighted in the throng of newsmen and movie cameras, all the attention upset Peter. "I remember the discomfort of having to dress in these stupid jackets and ties and Bermuda shorts," he said, "and having to pose for photographers in these set-up family shots."[31] The boys gathered around their father holding a kite they never flew; they sat in a large easy chair looking at a copy of *Life* magazine they never read. The photographs were supposed to show the happy family relaxing together following the vaccine's success. Yet they were hardly relaxed. The boys were restless; Peter grumbled about missing the start of the baseball season. Donna and Jonas tried to keep a sense of humor. When Coleman took a call from a West Coast hospital that was being renamed the Jonas E. Salk Memorial Hospital, Salk quipped, "Memorials are for dead people. I'm only half dead at this time."[32] And when someone asked Donna about her plans for the future, she replied, "The first thing I'm going to do is change my name to Smith."[33]

Though they attempted to maintain appearances in the face of public scrutiny, the Salk family had suffered from Jonas's single-minded focus. The American public got a glimpse of the tension in Jonas and Donna's marriage during a live television interview. Salk sat with his arms folded across his chest while Donna related how she and the children were probably the least excited of anyone, rather than stating, as many expected, how proud she was of her husband. When Salk said, "The question that keeps being asked most frequently is 'What am I going to do now?' I think that the answer should be implicit in all that you've heard—...." Donna interrupted.

"From my experience," she said, rolling her eyes, sounding piqued, "what is implicit is that whatever you do it is something that will keep you busy."[34]

Elva Minuse arrived that morning with bags of mail from Francis's lab addressed to Salk. That was just the beginning; over the next few days, cartons full of telegrams and letters were delivered. As Jonas and

Donna read the notes, the outpouring of gratitude astonished them. "You have given countless children a priceless gift," pronounced the Reverend Alvin D. Johnson of the First Baptist Church in Middletown, Connecticut.[35] "You have lifted a burden of fear from every loving father and mother in this country," wrote O. J. Fett of Roseburg, Oregon.[36]

In the end, the Salk family stayed in Ann Arbor for five days. Salk mistakenly thought he could finish the interviews and publicity shots before they left. When the Salks returned home, however, a welcoming committee of city and university officials met them at the airport. As Donna stepped out of the plane, the wife of the president of the Pittsburgh Chamber of Commerce presented her with three dozen red roses. Sipping a ginger ale, Peter remarked, "Boy, I sure have had enough excitement."[37] A chauffeur drove them home in the mayor's limousine with motorcycle police escorts. Donna asked the police to keep their sirens silent so as not to disturb the neighbors. It was too late. The Salks lived on a one-way street, and instead of going around the block, the police took them up the wrong way. Darrell loved the ride. "It was a great thrill, very exciting. Better than a roller coaster."[38]

"When we got home," Donna recalled, "the world had changed. And I must say, from our point of view, not for the better." Police patrolled the street, guarding their house. She overheard five-year-old Jonathan tell his friend Billy, "I'm back from my vacation and I'm famous and so is my dad."[39] The entire Salk family had lost its privacy. Strangers called day and night, forcing them to obtain an unlisted telephone number. Donna could now understand what the expression "living in a fish bowl" meant. "Mrs. Salk is busy tending again to their three-story twelve-room home," reported the *Pittsburgh Press Roto*.[40] Whenever Donna went shopping, clerks thanked her. "Aren't you so proud?" they asked. She received fan mail. "All the world is thinking of your husband as a saint," wrote a physician's wife, "but I know that you are the one who had to be a saint."[41]

When a reporter inquired how Salk felt now that the suspense was over, he replied, "There is little to say other than it would be nice to take a weekend off."[42] After that he wanted to get back to his lab; however, it had long since stopped being a sanctuary. When Lorraine returned, she could barely get into her office; bags of mail were stacked everywhere. Salk told her he felt a responsibility to the public; after all, they had supported his research through the March of Dimes. As in the past, he tried to reply to every letter, but when the number reached the thousands, that became impossible. The NFIP staff, responsible in large part for creating his hero image, seemed to have abandoned Salk, leaving him to deal with the public. Not O'Connor. Ten days after the Ann Arbor announcement, he sent a telegram inviting Jonas to Warm Springs: "Hop a plane Friday night and regain your girlish laughter."[43]

Freedom from fear—that is what Salk said he wanted to accomplish, and that was what he had done. What he had underestimated was how grateful the public would be and how long their appreciation would last. Communities rushed to immortalize him: a street in the Dominican Republic, an addition to the new Chicago Loop Synagogue, an activity room at the Parkside Community Center, a pharmacy in Paraguay, hospital wings, clinics, schools, babies all bore his name. Expressions of gratitude took many forms, including a 209-foot telegram signed by eight thousand residents of Winnipeg, Canada; a silver plow and an Oldsmobile from a Texas town; medallions, keys to cities, a new Cadillac, ballpoint pens, a chair, trees for Israel, a Miraculous Medal which had been blessed.[44] He kept nothing of monetary value; he sold the cars and sent the money back to the towns to buy vaccine. Still the tokens of thanks kept coming.

Notes of appreciation arrived from groups worldwide: the Phoenix Retail Merchants Association; the Metropolitan Water District of Southern California; the PTA of Pinellas County, Florida; the Southern Federal Savings and Loan Association of Pine Bluff, Arkansas; the Ladies Auxiliary to the Fraternal Order of Eagles, Elkhart, Indiana; the Interstate Shrine Club of Iron and Dickenson Counties, Michigan; the Upper Mohawk Council of the Boy Scouts of America; the Down-Town Jewish Orphan Home of Philadelphia; Loyal Order of the Moose, Johnstown, Pennsylvania; nuns of the Ursuline Academy; the Radio Club Argentino; the Operative Painters and Decorators Union of Australia; the Holy Blossom Temple Brotherhood in Toronto; and the East London and Border Society for the Care of Cripples, South Africa, to name a few.

Salk received letters from friends as well as those who knew him from the past. Murray Mintz's father owned the grocery store near the synagogue; Nate Jacobson remembered having their bar mitzvahs on the same day. Sidney Schwartz served with Jonas as a counselor at Camp Eutopia; Jane Heltzer Wagmen met him at his cousin Helen's sweet six-teen party. Dick Stein and S. J. Sindeba recalled their days together at Townsend Harris High. The head basketball coach of City College said if he were on his squad, he would put him in the starting lineup. And mail came from those who felt they had some small connection with him, such as "a fellow New Yorker," "a Mount Sinai alumnus," "a fellow Jew," "a parent."

He heard from relatives he hadn't seen in years, like Uncle Louis and Aunt Rachel, as well as relatives he didn't know he had. Ethel Salk of Chicago wrote that her father, Solomon, was a first cousin of his grand-father Harris, which made them second cousins once removed. Charles and Robert Salk said their late Uncle Sol and his father were cousins. Gertrude Salk, a cousin many times removed, sent a *New York Times* clipping, which quoted Temple Emanu-El's rabbi as saying, "The name of Salk will go down in our annals with men like Moses."[45]

Eddie Cantor, Helen Hayes, and Marlon Brando sent telegrams. Danny Kaye stopped by to meet the family. "The mail kept coming for a long, long time," Donna said—letters from bank tellers, waitresses, housewives, car mechanics. "And that was really more gratifying to Jonas and to me than all the celebrity feedback. This came from the heart."[46] She recalled sitting on the bed with Jonas opening notes on pink, blue, or polka-dotted stationary, some written with feeble hands, some with a flourish. Many started, "As a mother of two boys," "As a father of three." Mrs. Harry Specter of Los Angeles said she was one of the many moth-ers who dreaded every spring and summer. "I trembled at each slight fever and walked the floor in fear at each headache."[47] A Berkeley woman wrote, "Many, many times my heart has just shriveled with fear, looking at my son's bright little face."[48] Half of those who wrote said that Salk was in their prayers. One note simply had "Bless You" typed in the center of a single page.

Hundreds of children sent notes, as well, some in primitive block letters, others in careful cursive. Entire classrooms wrote to him: the sixth grade of New Columbian School in La Junta, Colorado; second-grade classes from North Miami Beach; schoolchildren from Rosaria, Argentina. They closed with "I like you very, very, very much" or "Your pal" or "I love you." Many said they prayed for him. "You, God, and Santa Claus are good," declared second-grader Becky Elliott of Pittsburg, Kansas.[49] Her classmate Cherre wrote she had a friend who had polio and couldn't wear dresses because of her leg brace. "So now with this vaccine," she reasoned, "I probably won't get polio and [can] always wear pretty dresses."[50]

The third graders of Hale Cook School in Kansas City, Missouri, sent Salk their photographs—girls in their Sunday best, boys on sleds, children holding a younger brother or sister or their dogs, a girl in her Brownie uniform, a Boy Scout saluting him. Donna and Jonas enjoyed the simple honesty of children. "Pinky Lee said to write you and thank you," wrote Glenda Casper of Sterling, Illinois.[51] "The reason I wrote this letter," revealed Linda Pietta of Huntington, West Virginia, "is because I was watching the Jerry Mahoney show. He is a dummy. He said that you are a great fellow."[52]

Some made them laugh. "My tongue is so twisted up with thanks I don't know what else to write," penned thirteen-year-old Lynn Vance of Kansas City.[53] "The polio injection medicine was pretty, but it didn't feel as good as it looks," observed a second-grader from Council Bluffs, Iowa.[54] "I would like to meet you but you ar to buzzzy," wrote another child.[55] Terry Doeblen of Milwaukee observed, "You are a small man with a big mind."[56] Paul Aaron of the Bronx sent a drawing of Salk, his mouth full of teeth, a lopsided grin, and one ear twice the size of the other.

Some letters touched them deeply. "I know how it feels not to be able to run, play games, or to scratch my nose," wrote fourth-grader Arthur Paul from Omaha, Nebraska. "I was in an iron lung for two months and seven days."[57] He thanked Salk for making the world safe. "My mother died of poli," wrote second-grader Randy Walker.[58] Richard Ray Manning sent a picture of himself in a striped T-shirt and jeans standing in front of his bicycle. An attached note read: "The disease cancer is just as bad. I wish there were a cure because my mother died of it on Saturday... at two o'clock in the morning. We were all very shocked."[59]

Along with the notes came a flurry of offers.[60] The Herman Fialkoff Agency proposed setting up a profit-sharing company to handle TV appearances, films, and the "highly lucrative field of lectures."[61] Lou Walters Enterprises Inc. offered to stage a benefit show at Madison

Square Garden; Salk could keep the proceeds. Editors at both Oxford University Press and Harper & Brothers suggested he compile a book; biographers asked to write his life story. Jack Warner of Warner Bros. said he would consider it an honor to make Salk's life into a motion picture. The next day, an agent contacted Tom Coleman about making *The Salk Story* in color and CinemaScope, with a budget of a million dollars. Producer Sam Engel of Twentieth Century-Fox also expressed interest; his choice to play Dr. Salk was Marlon Brando. Could he send a contract? Franklin D. Roosevelt, Jr., sent a note on behalf of his client Lester Cowan, who had produced W. C. Fields's most popular films. With three famous producers requesting the rights to his life story, Salk said, "I believe that such pictures are most appropriately made after the scientist is dead, and I'm willing to await my chances of such attention at that time."[62] With television appearances, movie offers, book proceeds, and gifts, Salk could have become a millionaire.[63] Yet he had never had that aspiration. The Salks would continue to live on his $25,000 annual salary.

The number of awards and invitations overwhelmed Salk: honorary degrees from the University of Pittsburgh, City College of New York, the Central University of Ecuador, the University of Michigan, and New York University; election to Phi Beta Kappa; an AMA resolution expressing its admiration for his monumental contribution; a citation from Mount Sinai Hospital, where he had done his internship. Artist Bernard Godwin painted his portrait to be hung in the New York Academy of Science. The Pennsylvania state legislature created a professorship in preventive medicine with Salk as its first recipient. Guatemala's president, Carlos Armas granted him the country's highest honor, the Order of the Quetzal. Pennsylvania's governor presented him with the Bronze Medal for Meritorious Service. He received Philadelphia's Poor Richard Award for distinguished service to humanity and the Mutual of Omaha Criss Award for his contribution to public health. The United Steel Workers of America gave him an honorary membership; the Borough of Moosic, Pennsylvania, made him honorary chief of police.[64]

His honors extended to the highest ranks of the US government. In a joint resolution, the Senate and House of Representatives awarded him the Congressional Gold Medal for his work.[65] He now shared a place in history with prior recipients George Washington, the Wright brothers,

Thomas Edison, and Charles Lindbergh. One side of the medal was engraved with Salk's portrait, the other with an allegorical figure protecting two children with a shield bearing a caduceus.

This intense period of veneration culminated in his trip to the White House to receive a presidential citation. On April 22, 1955, Jonas, Donna, and their sons attended a ceremony presided over by President Dwight Eisenhower in the Rose Garden. "No bands played and no flags waved," one reporter wrote. "But nothing could have been more impressive than this grandfather standing there and telling Dr. Salk in a voice trembling with emotion, 'I have no words to thank you.' "[66] Salk had been told that according to protocol he should say nothing except "Thank you, Mr. President." Yet he insisted on speaking. He attributed his success to the untiring devotion of his staff and many others. "I am sure you know how I feel," he continued, "when you single me out . . . to receive this Citation. You have been in similar situations, and I know that your thoughts were of the soldiers who crossed the Elbe and not of yourself." He concluded by saying, "On behalf of all the people in the laboratories, in the fields and those behind the lines, I gladly accept this recognition of what each of us has contributed."[67]

After the ceremony, Eisenhower took them into his office. "Mr. Eisenhower," Darrell asked, "what else do you do besides play golf?" When he replied, "I paint and fish," Darrell proceeded to describe a painting he had done in school.[68] The president gave the boys each a ballpoint pen and a pocketknife, advising Jonathan, "Don't use that knife until you're six."[69] (When they got home, Donna took away the knives.)[70]

Salk did not feel worthy of such attention. "There we stood, my wife, my three boys, and myself, in the Rose Garden of the White House," he told a reporter for the *New York Times Magazine*. "I thought to myself, 'What am I doing here?' "[71] As a reminder that he was as vulnerable as the next man, he found when he got home that someone had tried to siphon gas from their station wagon.[72]

Salk wanted to get back to work. Every morning when he awoke, he hoped the deluge would cease. Still it continued. Within the first month following the Ann Arbor announcement, he or the university on his behalf received more than ten thousand letters, telegrams, and phone calls. "I received an inordinate amount of attention and recognition," he reflected later in life, "out of proportion to what was contributed scientifically." Yet he understood. "It came about altogether because of the relief from fear. It was a human response on the part of the public."[73]

The one group from whom Salk received few notes was the scientific community. Although many practicing physicians wrote to congratulate him, few scientists bothered. Salk had made a vaccine that prevented polio; he should have been able to bask in the splendor of that incredible feat. Instead, a shadow had been cast over his achievement since the moment he walked off the Rackham Hall stage in Ann Arbor. During his presentation Salk had announced that in theory the 1955 vaccine and vaccination procedures could lead to 100 percent protection from paralysis. This statement annoyed Francis. "After Jonas was through talking," he later said, "I went over to him, sore. 'What the hell did you have to say that for?' I asked. 'You're in no position to claim 100 percent effectiveness. What's the matter with you?' "[74]

Salk's final conclusion also irritated Rivers, who thought it had eclipsed Francis's presentation. "Nothing should have detracted from the kudos that Tommy received that day," he said. "Salk should have kept his mouth shut. The dosage schedule didn't have to be changed on that day, dammit."[75] Salk thought it did. Nationwide vaccinations were to begin the next day. Rivers didn't stay mad for long, however. A few months later he wrote, "I have always supported you in the past because I thought you were right.... However, when I do feel I am supporting the right cause I can be pretty hard-headed.... My wife and I send you our love."[76]

If anyone had cause to be piqued, it was Salk. After he had developed the polio vaccine, Weaver and Rivers had appropriated the field trial and delegated its design and conduct to another investigator. To make matters worse, he had been compelled to continue his research, present his work to the scientific community, and answer public inquiries for an entire year with no idea how the trial was progressing. To top it off, the published results of the field trial did not even bear his name. The authorship listed Francis first, followed by eight others, mostly statisticians and epidemiologists. Rivers may have been angry that Salk "stole the day," but he had taken back what rightfully belonged to him.[77]

As for other poliomyelitis investigators, many grumbled that Salk had grabbed the limelight, neglecting to mention those who had laid the groundwork for his vaccine. Yet researchers did not usually review the accomplishments of others when presenting their own work. Francis hadn't, and no one criticized him in a similar vein. Many failed to notice that Salk had mentioned other polio scientists on numerous occasions. During *The Scientist Speaks for Himself*, as well as in his *JAMA* article on the vaccine, he had reviewed the history of polio research, giving them ample recognition. And on *See It Now*, Salk told Murrow that no one scientist could take credit for the vaccine. Even when he did mention other investigators in interviews, those statements often got cut. Newsmen, whether Edward R. Murrow, John Troan, or some rookie, knew the public didn't want to hear about David Bodian or Isabel Morgan, names unknown to them. Jonas Salk sold papers and pulled in the viewing audience.

The media were responsible in large part for creating the situation. Reporters had flaunted Salk's triumph, made him the centerpiece of the vaccine story. He didn't choose what questions they asked or what quotes they printed; he didn't edit their articles. To keep the public's interest, they exaggerated minor conflicts; portraying Salk as an outcast made good press.

Although Salk was the focal point for vilification, many attendees criticized the Ann Arbor meeting itself: "The information that had been gathered so painstakingly at the Evaluation Center," wrote John Paul, "did not deserve to be so cheapened by the outburst that ensued."[78] "Hoopla," "circus," "hailstorm," "chaos," "heyday for hucksters," and various other derogatory terms were used to describe the event. "The bedlam was revolting," complained one participant. "It was as if four supermarkets were having their premieres on the same day in the same parking lot."[79] Another called it an extravaganza set to the tune of "the rockets' red glare and flashbulbs bursting in air."[80] The *New York Times* said the symposium resembled a Hollywood premiere.[81] Writer Greer Williams likened it to "a TV spectacular," quoting a California physician who said, "It was a unique and distasteful experience . . . to wait shoulder to shoulder with a frenzied public for an announcement concerning a development in my own professional field." Williams reported a protest to the AMA that alleged that "undo fanfare" had violated traditional methods by which investigators critically review discoveries.[82]

A number blamed the NFIP, asserting it had incited the public's fears, raised their expectations, and then announced the consequences with a flourish. Granted, it had come close to becoming "the first agency to conquer a disease by popular subscription," Williams wrote. "Yet you cannot satisfy the needs of the showman and the scientist out of the same box."[83] The NFIP, however, had not had much of a hand in the arrangements; its public relations staff had been shunted aside. The University of Michigan had assumed control but hadn't controlled it effectively. Somehow, those in charge of the day, the university and Thomas Francis, remained untarnished. O'Connor felt he owed no one an apology. "To all the millions who contributed to the March of Dimes," he stated in the Annual NFIP Report, "the events of April 12, 1955, meant an accomplishment their dimes and dollars had paid for."[84]

Reproach for the NFIP "circus" spilled over onto Jonas Salk. "I was not unscathed by Ann Arbor," he reflected.[85] For whatever reason—insult, resentment, jealousy—disparagement of Salk's behavior surfaced. He was accused of showmanship, disregard, selfishness, greediness. An editorial in the *New England Journal of Medicine* warned that physicians should "resist the danger of being maneuvered into unscientific positions that put their prestige in jeopardy."[86] A palpable anti-Salk backlash had begun. "The worst tragedy that could have befallen me was my success," Salk later said. "I knew right away that I was through—cast out."[87] Disgusted by the affair and its instigators, from the press to the scientific community, O'Connor retorted, "He shows the world how to eliminate paralytic polio, and you'd think he had halitosis or had committed a felony."[88]

Despite the distortions and deprecation that followed in the wake of the Ann Arbor announcement, April 12, 1955, was a historic day. A disease that had stalked the nation's children for decades could be prevented. The moment that the public had hoped for, prayed for, given their dimes for, had finally come. Years later, people said they recalled the exact moment they heard the good news. "It was not unlike the ending of a war," many noted.[89] So for every child saved from an iron lung or an early grave, the controversy surrounding that day hardly mattered. Jonas Salk had set out to prevent polio, and he had succeeded. Nothing could diminish that.

The Cutter Affair

THOUSANDS OF CARTONS of polio vaccine were rushed across the country within hours of its approval. By week's end, millions of children were to be vaccinated, starting with those who had received placebo in the field trial, followed by the nation's first and second graders—those at highest risk for contracting polio. The NFIP had already ordered and paid for enough vaccine to inoculate nine million children before the school year finished. Parke, Davis and Company sent its first shipment to sixteen cities the day after the announcement; it planned to produce three hundred thousand shots weekly. Eli Lilly and Company had a hundred employees working fulltime on manufacturing vaccine, and on April 15 they dispatched 2.6 million doses to those sites designated by the NFIP. Cutter Laboratories shipped out one ton of vaccine within seventy-two hours of its being licensed; Sharp and Dohme sent its entire supply to the NFIP for distribution. Pittman-Moore announced it was interviewing personnel for a million-dollar expansion program.[1]

While American citizens awaited their shots, President Eisenhower, in a goodwill gesture, directed the State Department to send details of vaccine manufacturing to any nation requesting them, including those behind the Iron Curtain.[2] The Danish government announced its intent to vaccinate all children ages seven to twelve under the direction of scientists Herdis and Preben von Magnus, longtime friends of Salk. Pierre Lépine of Paris's Pasteur Institute planned to test his vaccine, made according to Salk's principles. Italy, Sweden, Germany, and South Africa announced the imminent initiation of vaccination programs. The United Kingdom's Ministry of Health did not rush ahead, concerned that Salk's vaccine might be ineffective against polio strains found in the Old World.[3] No thanks came from Russia either. A letter to the editor of a major international newspaper alleged that Russian scientist Josef Salkoff, influenced by the teachings of Comrade Josef Stalin, had made an antipolio vaccine in 1945. "There has been a false impression," it read, "created by false propaganda that the American Imperialist, Dr. Jonas Salk, discovered the vaccine."[4] Most of the world, however, expressed gratitude. "Dr. Salk's doings are commented upon in the Danish newspapers as if he was...the King of Sweden," Herdis von Magnus told Lorraine Friedman.[5]

American vaccination plans did not proceed as smoothly as hoped.[6] With the public clamoring for vaccine, the pharmaceutical companies could not fill the demand. A Michigan pediatrician reported receiving a call from parents every fifteen minutes; he had 650 children on his vaccination list but had received no supply. "Where's the Vaccine?" asked *Time* magazine.[7] The government had relied on the NFIP to do all the work up until April 12th. After that, O'Connor passed on oversight of production and distribution to HEW and Secretary Hobby who had underestimated the complexity and magnitude of the task. When later asked by a Congressional committee how she failed to anticipate the situation, Hobby answered, "I think no one could have foreseen the public demand."[8] This was not entirely accurate. Months earlier, when O'Connor had warned her that allocation of a limited stock could create a major problem, she had replied that the marketplace would dictate supply and demand. She felt no obligation beyond licensing the vaccine; after all, her department didn't control distribution of other licensed drugs.

The American system of free enterprise gave rise to chaos. Before the NFIP received the vaccine lots it had already purchased, half a million doses were shipped to private physicians. Price gouging became rampant. Although each shot cost about two dollars, physicians in High

Point, North Carolina, charged twelve dollars for the series of inocula-tions. Parents in other cities paid fees as high as twenty-one dollars. When it became apparent that families with means received shots first, those who had given freely to the March of Dimes expressed outrage.[9] To make matters worse, although Hobby had announced that the first lots of vaccine were reserved for first and second graders, employees of the pharmaceutical companies and physicians' friends and families were given priority. The president of Cutter Laboratories, informing stock-holders of the limited supply, wrote: "I want to be sure that you as a Cutter shareholder also have the opportunity to have your children or grandchildren under eighteen years of age immunized."[10]

Newsweek called the situation "The Polio Scramble."[11] In a brief period, the public's joy and relief had been replaced by frustration and anger. Under free market conditions, vaccine went to the highest bidders. Furthermore, vials of vaccine were reported missing or stolen. The *Detroit Free Press* ran a story about a New Orleans mother who took her child to the pediatrician for vaccination. When told he had no vaccine, she pulled two doses out of her pocket. "Never mind where I got 'em," she said. "Just use them."[12] The New York County Medical Center repri-manded six physicians for violating vaccine priorities.[13] The press ac-cused the government of graft and corruption. Parents called their congressmen, insisting upon federal control. President Eisenhower stepped in and charged Hobby with creating an equitable distribution plan. In a press release, Hobby reiterated that available vaccine had been committed to the NFIP for first and second graders. She expected that by September enough vaccine would be available for three-quarters of all children and teenagers. "It is a situation which will require very great patience on the part of everyone," she said.[14] But the polio season was under way. Near panic ensued.

Salk remained silent. He had hoped to move out of the spotlight. Nonetheless against his will, a political undertow pulled him into the middle of what would later be known as the "Cutter incident."[15]

◈

SALK RECEIVED A TELEGRAM from Surgeon General Leonard Scheele on April 27 requesting that he come to Washington immediately. Seven children had become paralyzed following polio vaccinations. Only then did Salk learn about the calamity that had emerged over the previous two days.

On April 25, less than two weeks after Americans rejoiced over the conquest of polio, Chicago's regional medical director notified William Workman, director of the Laboratory of Biologics Control, that a Chicago infant had been admitted to Michael Reese Hospital with paralysis of both legs. Eight days earlier, the baby had received a polio shot in the buttock. This would not be the first time a child had been infected with poliovirus prior to receiving vaccine, so Workman did nothing. On the following day, when an epidemiologist from the California Health Department reported paralysis in two seven-year-old San Diego boys who had recently received polio shots, he could not dismiss it as coincidental. A few hours later, the epidemiologist called back to report three more cases coming from Ventura, Napa, and Oakland.

At 5:30 p.m. on April 26, Workman alerted James Shannon, deputy director of the NIH. Within two hours, Shannon convened an emergency meeting of Public Health Service officials. Examining the details of each case, they found that all occurred within ten days of inoculation, that paralysis started in the arm or leg where the injection had been given, and that in each case the vaccine had been supplied by Cutter Laboratories of Berkeley, California. When the group looked at Cutter's manufacturing protocols, they found no obvious problems. They could not agree what should be done. At 2:30 a.m., Shannon notified Surgeon General Scheele.

Later that morning, Scheele held a telephone conference to seek advice from Thomas Francis, Jr.; Joseph Smadel; and William Hammon. Salk remained unaware of the situation. They considered three possibilities. Were the cases merely coincidental? They thought it unlikely, as no outbreak of polio had been reported from the communities in which the children lived. Had incipient polio been provoked by an injection after exposure to the virus? This hadn't happened in the field trial. Or had vaccine been contaminated with live virus? Without more information, the group was cautious about giving a firm recommendation. Scheele would have to make the decisions and accept responsibility for the consequences on his own.

Leonard Scheele already had experience with contentious health issues.[16] Appointed surgeon general at age forty by President Harry Truman, he had withstood a major public controversy when he introduced fluoridation of public drinking water in 1951. Antifluoride advocates had charged that fluoride caused mongolism (now called Down syndrome), cancer, even communism. In this case, however, the lives of millions of children were at risk. Scheele asked Cutter Laboratories to recall all its vaccine voluntarily, and he sent investigators to Berkeley. On the afternoon of April 27, he notified Jonas Salk and Basil O'Connor. By then, the two seven-year-old boys had been placed into iron lungs. "This is dreadful," Salk told his lab assistant, Don Wegemer. "I feel terrible. People are trusting me and all of a sudden this is happening to them."[17] Something had gone wrong; he suspected Cutter had not followed his specifications.

At a press conference later that day, Scheele reported that cases of poliomyelitis had occurred in a few children following inoculation with Salk vaccine from Cutter Laboratories. Trying to preempt widespread alarm, he said they had no proof the Cutter vaccine had caused paralysis; the children may have already been infected before the inoculations. Even so, Cutter had withdrawn its vaccine as a precaution. "I want first and foremost," Scheele said, "to assure the parents of children who have received an injection of poliomyelitis vaccine this spring that in the very best judgment of the Public Health Service they have no cause for alarm."[18] He urged parents to continue to get their children vaccinated.

The public was told to trust this tall, mild-mannered man, the country's surgeon general; even so, most did not recognize him. The man they did know—and trust—was Jonas Salk. They wanted his opinion. Informed of the situation just hours before, Salk made his first statement to the press at four o'clock that afternoon. Although shaken by the events, he appeared composed. "I have just learned of the decision by the Public Health Service," he said. "It is difficult to say whether or not the association between vaccination and the reported cases is one of cause and effect or one of coincidence.... What is being done is reasonable, namely that a thorough investigation of the reported cases is being made."[19] That evening Salk learned that five children from Pocatello, Idaho, had contracted polio following vaccination; a six-year-old girl had died.

On the morning of April 28, Salk rushed to Washington, where Scheele convened a group, composed of Enders, Sabin, Francis, Smadel, Paul, Hammon, Bodian, two state health officials, and himself to review the situation. The mood was tense. Sabin, Enders, Paul, and Hammon called for an immediate ban on all vaccine. Bodian and Salk disagreed. They thought their first task should be to determine what had happened at Cutter Laboratories. Vaccine from none of the other manufacturers had caused polio. After hearing all the arguments, the surgeon general agreed with the latter and appointed a technical advisory group to examine the problem in detail. At the same time, he directed the Communicable Disease Center (CDC) in Atlanta to set up a National Poliomyelitis Surveillance Unit that would collect and disseminate information regarding all cases of polio in vaccinated persons. Cutter had distributed its vaccine to only six states for the NFIP-supported school vaccination program; it had shipped truckloads to twenty-six states for commercial use. Between April 18 and 27, an estimated four hundred thousand, mostly children, had received the Cutter vaccine. If Cutter's product was contaminated with live virus, the number of poliomyelitis cases might mushroom.

Salk had just returned home when he received another telegram from Scheele. More cases had just been reported from Georgia, Louisiana, Illinois, Colorado, and Oregon, now totaling twenty-nine. Three had received vaccine prepared by companies other than Cutter. Health officials in California, Utah, and Massachusetts were halting all inoculations. Meanwhile, Enders, Sabin, and Paul were pressuring William Sebrell, Jr., director of the NIH, to immediately suspend all licenses and recall every lot. They advised the government to go public with details of the situation and accept responsibility for premature licensing of the vaccine. Those who had opposed a killed-virus vaccine used this opportunity to discredit Salk; Sabin called it the "Salk accident."[20] Salk knew there had to be some procedural problem with inactivating the poliovirus fully, likely a human error. But this did not lessen his grief. "Needless to say," Donna recalled, "it took an emotional toll."[21] Children were becoming paralyzed and dying from the vaccine he had developed to prevent this deadly disease.

On May 5, Salk returned to Washington to join Scheele's technical advisory group, composed of Bodian, Enders, Francis, Smadel, and

Howard Shaughnessy, an Illinois state health official. Salk reminded the group that millions of doses of vaccine had been given safely in the field trial. He pointed out that Canadian and Danish health officials had continued to vaccinate children with no mishaps. They should direct their attention to the problem with these particular lots, Salk stressed, not throw out the proverbial baby with the bathwater.

The investigators Scheele had sent to Cutter Laboratories reported to the group that vaccine was being manufactured according to the protocol; they could not determine what had gone awry. On further inspection of records, however, they learned the company had found live virus in nine of its first twenty-seven lots. Cutter scientists had not revealed this to the Laboratory of Biologics Control, as they were not required by law to do so. Instead, they had simply disposed of the lots. The investigators also noted that Cutter's protocol, although approved by the Laboratory of Biologics Control, differed somewhat from Salk's. Whereas Salk tested samples of the solution at five different time points to be certain inactivation of virus was proceeding at the proper rate, Cutter scientists had shortened their protocol to two. These findings troubled Salk; the company had taken shortcuts previously, and he had warned against such changes. Nonetheless, Scheele's investigators concluded that no impropriety had occurred.

As the technical advisory group reviewed data from the other licensed manufacturers, they made a disquieting observation: Each company had had trouble with viral inactivation at some point during vaccine production. They, like Cutter, had not notified the Laboratory of Biologics Control and just discarded tainted lots. Salk reiterated that if the companies had adhered to his principles and if the government had provided the same oversight he had, this would not have happened. At that, Enders leaned across the table and confronted him: "It is quack medicine to pretend that this is a killed vaccine when you know it has live virus in it." Salk remained silent. "This was the first and only time in my life," he later said, "that I felt suicidal."[22] The meeting ended at four o'clock in the morning. Scheele decided to suspend all further vaccinations until they had thoroughly checked each company and written more stringent regulations.

By May 7, fifty cases of vaccine-associated poliomyelitis had been confirmed, forty-four of them associated with Cutter vaccine. The following day, Scheele held another press conference. He announced he was post-poning all vaccinations even though he thought vaccine from the other manufacturers was safe. Going forward, the Laboratory of Biologics Control would be assessing all manufactured vaccine and clearing it for use on a lot-by-lot basis. "The undertaking of such a review," Scheele said, "does not arise from lack of confidence on the part of the Public Health Service in the fundamental safety of the Salk vaccine."[23] He reminded the public that five hundred thousand children had received vaccine the prior year without any problems and assured them that he considered the public's health his primary responsibility.

When O'Connor learned that some of Scheele's technical advisors had persuaded him to ban distribution of all vaccine, he began to pres-sure the surgeon general. He knew that suspension of the nationwide vaccination program could undermine the public's confidence in the Salk vaccine, perhaps setting them back years in their efforts to eradicate polio. O'Connor accused Scheele of concealing the facts and demanded open exposure. "He called me at all hours of the night," Scheele recalled. "He threatened to have me fired."[24]

The initial shock over the situation soon gave way to finger-pointing. Oveta Hobby received the initial brunt of the blame. When she stated that her responsibility was drug licensing, not distribution or oversight, she was accused of having licensed the vaccine prematurely, bowing to political and public pressure. Scheele received his share of scorn as well. The chief epidemiologist at the Communicable Disease Center called him "shilly-shally Scheele."[25] He was criticized for moving too slowly, too quickly, for wavering, for blundering. "People were frightened one day," a journalist for the *Democratic Digest* wrote. "They were reassured the next. They were cautioned the next day. They were reassured again. Then they were warned....At no time in the history of the land or its people has there been a muddle on such a grand scale."[26] The *Detroit Times* reported that the surgeon general "blew hot and cold on alternate breaths" and that he had "retreated behind silence or prepared interviews which didn't say anything."[27] During the entire Cutter affair, Scheele appeared unruffled, with one observer describing him as "a man of co-lossal restraint and shock-proof benignity."[28] For weeks, he shouldered a heavy burden, forced to make major decisions in the face of conflicting advice from the nation's leading scientists. "We had to operate in the public eye almost twenty-four hours a day," he later told a reporter for the *Saturday Evening Post*. "One morning I was greeted by a television camera as I stepped out of my office and by another as I entered the Capitol."[29]

The situation quickly turned political. Democratic congressmen blamed President Eisenhower for a lack of leadership. One *Time* reporter explained that vaccine used in the field trial had been triple-tested by Salk's lab, the Laboratory of Biologics Control, and the manufacturer's lab. He quoted the president as saying that this year tests were run only by the manufacturers, with the government making an occasional spot check in attempts to "short-cut a little bit."[30] Democrats initiated a congressional inquiry into the administration's handling of the vaccine. "The federal government inspects meat in the slaughterhouses," proclaimed Senator Wayne Morse, "more carefully than it has inspected the polio vaccine." Tennessee senator Estes Kefauver called it "one of the worst bungled programs I have ever seen."[31]

Some health officials criticized O'Connor for charging ahead with the field test before the vaccine's safety had been assured. "In retrospect," wrote a *Time* reporter, "a good deal of the blame for the vaccine snafu also went to the National Foundation which with years of publicity had built up the danger of polio out of all proportion to its actual incidence, and had rushed into vaccinations this year with patently insufficient preparation."[32] A humorist renamed the NFIP the "Infantile Foundation for National Paralysis."[33]

Cutter Laboratories became the main target. This was not the first contamination problem in its history.[34] Family-run, it had started as a veterinary business in the 1930s and then began producing vaccines, becoming the first company to combine diphtheria, pertussis, and tetanus vaccines into one inoculation. During World War II, Cutter Labs prospered, supplying blood products and penicillin to the armed services. In 1949, it pleaded nolo contendere to charges involving contamination of supposedly sterile intravenous solutions. Now Cutter Labs seemed to be the major source of contaminated vaccine. Reporters harassed the company's president, Robert Cutter. The press, he complained, "[tried] to make us look like people who didn't think a thing about killing a child if it meant a dollar to us."[35] His family was accosted, as well. One parent asked Cutter's niece, a schoolteacher, "How does it feel to be a killer of children?"[36]

Several manufacturers, including Cutter Labs, blamed Salk, saying that his straight-line theory of inactivation may have been accurate for small amounts of vaccine, but it didn't hold when manufacturing large quantities. His sterling reputation was becoming tarnished. The press took sides. Some science writers called the situation the "Salk Snafu."[37] Others came to his defense. "Dr. Jonas Salk is in the process of discovering that benefactors of humanity generally come in for as many kicks as they do commendations," read an editorial in a Vancouver newspaper. "Mankind has a nasty habit of beating up on the people who help it. It takes what they give, mauls it around, and finally accepts it, generally after the givers are dead."[38]

Salk knew his methods hadn't caused this crisis. "Somebody screwed up," Don Wegemer said, adding that Salk had realized that in the pharmacy world "they're out to make a buck."[39] Nonetheless Salk made no public statement; instead, he and Wegemer set out to determine what had gone wrong. The investigators Scheele had sent to Cutter Laboratories had said they could find no reason for the contaminated lots, but Salk knew that if inactivation of poliovirus had failed, something must have protected the virus from the formalin. In 1954, he had warned that if tissue fragments remained in the viral suspension, they could entrap viruses, harboring them from inactivation.[40] Such debris could be eliminated by proper filtration. He felt certain this was what had happened at Cutter Labs; he just needed some of their vaccine to prove it.

By May 11, inspection of Parke, Davis had been completed, and Scheele cleared its vaccine for use. Soon thereafter, he released lots from Eli Lilly. By then the public felt bewildered. If their children didn't get the vaccine, they might catch polio; if they got the vaccine, they might contract polio. Thirty percent of New York children whose parents had signed them up for inoculations didn't show up for their shots. Many turned to their family doctors for advice. Yet they, too, were perplexed. Practicing physicians had received no information on the problem to help them make recommendations for their patients. What they did know about the vaccine came via newspapers, magazines, radio, and television, not through the medical literature. So parents and physicians looked to Salk, who initially took the position that he had nothing to do with distribution and control of vaccine and thus could not comment. The public didn't accept that stance. "There are a lot of rumblings in the wind: name-callings, politicking, and anger over gross errors," a journalist and mother from Hackensack, New Jersey, wrote to Salk. "But sir, as a mother, and like other mothers, I'm not much interested in the politics and structure or control of the vaccine." In talking with others, she said, the questions foremost in their minds are: Would it help their child? Is it safe? "The people are waiting for YOUR WORDS!" she pleaded. "THEY WANT TO KNOW WHAT DR. SALK THINKS."[41] As he had many times previously, Salk wrote openly and honestly to a complete stranger. "I have searched my soul," he replied, "in seeking guidance for the course of action that I must follow."[42]

Although the surgeon general's technical advisors were under oath to keep their deliberations confidential, before long Salk tried to offer the public some explanation for what he thought had happened. Since his formula called for "cooking" the virus until it was killed, a reporter for *American Magazine* asked him, did that mean something was wrong with the formula? Salk replied: "Suppose you had a recipe for a cake, and every time you used it your cake turned out fine. Then you gave the recipe to your neighbor. You didn't stay in her kitchen to see what she did, but her cake was terrible. Now, would you blame the recipe?"[43] To date, this was the clearest account the public had heard.

Scheele scheduled the technical advisory group to meet again on May 23. Frustrated by this politically motivated, argumentative committee, Salk declined to attend. He sent Scheele a telegram saying he thought the problem could be solved expeditiously by a smaller group, one familiar with the problems the pharmaceutical manufacturers had experienced prior to the field trial. He would gladly assist with such a group, he added, confident that he, Smadel, Bodian, and Francis could solve the problem promptly. Scheele was in a quandary. The total number of paralyzed children had risen to seventy-eight, including the grandson of a New Orleans surgeon, Alton Ochsner, known for recognizing the relationship between smoking and cancer. Ochsner had obtained vaccine from Cutter Labs and inoculated his two-year-old grandson, who subsequently died.

To make matters worse, cases of polio were being reported in people who had never been inoculated. A twenty-eight-year-old woman from Knoxville, Tennessee, suddenly developed polio in the base of her brain and required an iron lung to breathe. Her children had received Cutter vaccine a month earlier. A mother from Atlanta and an eight-months-pregnant woman died of polio. In both cases, their children had recently been vaccinated. The CDC received reports almost daily of paralysis among unvaccinated parents, brothers, and sisters of children who had been inoculated with Cutter vaccine. It appeared that some vaccinees were excreting infectious virus even though they did not manifest signs of polio themselves. Then the disease spread into the wider community. An infant inoculated with Cutter vaccine, with no symptoms of infection, passed the virus on to her mother. Before the mother contracted polio, they had visited two other families. The father in one of these families and the mother and child in the other developed polio weeks after the infant got her shot. Children in those families had played with children in two other families; they also got polio. Health officials found a similar pattern of spread in a number of neighborhoods. They feared the Cutter vaccine had unleashed an epidemic. So Scheele yielded to Salk and appointed a small group to work with Shannon and get the job done.

Salk obtained vaccine samples from Cutter Laboratories and, after careful investigation of the contaminated lots, found what he had suspected.[44] At the bottom of several vials he discovered a fine granular sediment that could not be seen unless one was looking specifically for it. It was clear what had happened: From the beginning, he had specified that filtration of poliovirus solution before and after inactivation with formalin was a crucial step to remove any residual cellular debris from the kidney tissue culture, which might interfere with viral inactivation. For that he used a Seitz filter, made of layers of compressed asbestos. Cutter had used a glass filtration system which, although faster, had not been as effective. Some of the debris had slipped through the filter and formed a precipitate on the bottom of the flask. Live virus became entrapped in this precipitate, which provided a physical barrier against formalin inactivation. Cutter did not refilter the solution. At a later date, this protected virus, still alive, detached itself and contaminated the vaccine. Salk called the problem "filter failure."[45] Though the problem was serious, the resolution was simple—better filters and repeated filtrations before and after inactivation. Salk and the group worked swiftly to write stricter minimum requirements. On May 27, Scheele announced the vaccination program would commence again.

Salk was vindicated.[46] On June 8, however, when he read the white paper Scheele had written to summarize the entire Cutter episode, he found the surgeon general's interpretation troubling, if not deceiving. Scheele stated that although Salk's original concept of vaccine preparation assured a wide margin of safety, the manufacturers' experience revealed that the process of inactivation did not always follow the predicted course. Vaccine production had progressed from Salk's laboratory to large-scale manufacturing with unprecedented rapidity. This speed had created problems in biologics control. They had found no evidence to suggest that Cutter had been slipshod or cut corners deliberately; however, Scheele offered no explanation as to why the company had experienced such difficulty. In short, his report made the actual cause of the tainted lots appear mysterious. The report did hold the Laboratory of Biologics Control accountable for failing to supervise production. To Salk's dismay, the white paper implied that the main problem lay in applying his formulation to mass production, especially in the rush to release vaccine. "Events which in the traditional course of scientific development would have covered years," Scheele concluded, "were telescoped into months, and as a result, both success and failure have been magnified."[47]

Furious, O'Connor told the press the government's version of the Cutter incident concealed what really had happened. Salk was ambivalent. Although he may have been disappointed with Scheele's interpretation, he appreciated that the surgeon general had saved the vaccine from annihilation. Nationwide vaccinations had resumed. So publicly, Salk commended Scheele for his work. When asked how he felt about the Cutter affair and its resolution by *New York Times* reporter Jane Krieger, Salk replied: "You find yourself projected into a set of circumstances for which neither your training nor your talents have prepared you. It's very difficult in some respects, but it's a transitory thing and you wait till it blows over."[48] It wasn't a "transitory thing," however. Two weeks later his vaccine came under fire again.

On June 23, the House Committee on Interstate and Foreign Commerce held hearings on the vaccine. Its stated purpose was to decide whether the government should provide free vaccine for all those under the age of nineteen who could not afford it. At the hearing, which included a panel of experts, the discussion took a sharp turn from the economics of vaccine supply to a debate on the vaccine's safety. Once again Salk had to defend himself against Hammon, Sabin, Enders, and virologist Wendell Stanley. Stanley, Salk's old nemesis, cast doubt on the mathematical validity of his viral inactivation curve. "The chemist will tell you," he testified, "that in such a reaction it is theoretically impossible to wind up with a situation in which you have no active virus."[49] Stanley had disparaged Salk's work on many occasions, starting with his first research paper during medical school. Usually intimidated by this outspoken eminent scientist, Salk stood his ground this time. "I was a chemist once," he retorted, and as a chemist he had demonstrated over and over in the laboratory that a "point of no return" did exist after which no virus survived formalin inactivation. Then he spoke as a physician—something Stanley could not do—and reminded the congressional committee that he had produced a completely safe vaccine that had prevented poliomyelitis in the field trial. "I say these things," he concluded, "to counter some of the theoretical discussion, which is all very interesting and very nice, but let us not lose sight of the forest for the trees."[50]

Sabin testified that the Salk vaccine needed to be "completely overhauled."[51] He was testing a vaccine made with a weakened live-viral strain, he said, which would be safer and more effective. Enders and Hammon likewise joined his call for withdrawal of the Salk vaccine. Rivers chided Sabin, saying he had admitted Salk's vaccine was safe by voting to license it. "Right after that, he suggests that we stop making a safe vaccine and make a safer one." Sabin replied that as a young scientist, he had first studied viruses with Dr. Rivers. "Therefore I make my statement with trepidation.... But he has one ear in which he does not hear well, and I think this is the one." It was now clear, he continued, that "large lots of Salk vaccine can be prepared and given to millions of people with impunity. But the real issue is can the vaccine be prepared safely with regularity?"[52] Appealing to the congressmen, Rivers voiced his concern that if they stopped the vaccination program, it would be years before vaccine would be used again, and many children would die needlessly. When an unofficial vote was called, most agreed to proceed with the program. A green light from Congress only partially compensated Salk for having his work publicly denigrated by Enders, Stanley, and Sabin. John Paul wrote Salk afterwards, thanking him for his testimony: "I am not alone in appreciating what your help in this difficult assignment has meant."[53]

The congressional hearing and a subsequent AMA meeting gave Sabin a platform from which he tried to discredit the Salk vaccine. His behavior infuriated O'Connor, luring him into public debate. The NFIP director called Sabin's arguments "old stuff" that he had been voicing for years.[54] "Since the scientific method was established," O'Connor said, "every important advance in science has met with the twin obstacles, ignorance and envy."[55] He suggested Sabin had ulterior motives. Sabin replied he did not oppose vaccination for polio; he was opposed to the current Salk vaccine. Although the public debate ended there, Sabin and O'Connor carried on a heated private dispute. It culminated when Sabin wrote O'Connor, implying NFIP favoritism toward Salk. Furthermore, Sabin responded to O'Connor's accusations by quoting President Eisenhower: "If we allow ourselves to be persuaded that every individual...or party...that takes issue with our own convictions is necessarily wicked or treasonous...then indeed we are approaching the end of freedom's road."[56]

In a searing letter, O'Connor replied that Sabin had expended a great deal of energy trying to convince others that the path being followed by the NFIP and Salk was "wicked and treasonous." He questioned Sabin's morals as he repeatedly tried to persuade the public to refrain from receiving a safe and effective vaccine, and he maintained that Sabin was not acting as a scientist but as a propagandist. "No one has stood in your way, but you have made every effort to obstruct and stand in the way of others.... The victory that is in sight has occurred in spite of you and not because of you." He accused Sabin of public temper tantrums caused by envy. "If this be an unjust accusation, I can only say it is one that is shared by many."[57] Although the actual letter he sent conveyed the same sentiment, its tone had been modified.[58] In reply to O'Connor's attack on his morality, Sabin reminded him that as a result of the Salk vaccine, "there occurred the most tragic *manmade* epidemic of severe paralytic poliomyelitis which infected more than 100 individuals and caused many deaths."[59] In the midst of all this rancor, O'Connor's wife, Elvira, suddenly died of a coronary thrombosis.

⸭

WITH TIME, THE details of the Cutter incident became clearer. On April 12, 1955, as a result of the field trial, six pharmaceutical companies had been licensed to manufacture polio vaccine.[60] Commercial vaccine production, however, differed from that used in the field trial in several major ways. First, the triple testing for live virus performed by the company, the Biologics Control Laboratory, and Salk's lab had been reduced to one test—conducted by the company itself. The government laboratory had neither the funds nor staff to test all manufactured vaccine before its release. Thus, the extra safety nets had been removed. Second, although each manufacturer had followed the minimum requirements, those requirements did not specify the inactivation process in as much detail as they had for the field trial. And third, the Laboratory of Biologics Control no longer applied the "consistent performance" rule used in the field trial, whereby eleven consecutive lots had to be proved virus-free before the first could be released. Scheele's technical committee, spearheaded by Salk, found filter failure to be the problem and developed corrective measures. In the future, all lots had to be accounted for so companies could no longer conceal the number of faulty lots discarded.

In the end, between April 17 and June 30, 1955, 260 individuals contracted polio directly or indirectly from the Cutter vaccine. Ninety-four cases occurred among those vaccinated, 126 in family members, and forty among community contacts. Three-fourths suffered some form of debility ranging from a weak muscle to total paralysis from the neck down; eleven died. The Cutter incident would remain one of America's most tragic pharmaceutical catastrophes. And its victims numbered more than just those who had received contaminated vaccine; millions of children went unvaccinated in its wake.

Some states resumed their vaccination programs. More than a million children in New York received inoculations, and no cases of polio were attributed to the vaccine. During 1955, the incidence of polio remained low throughout the state. A different story unfolded in Massachusetts, where health officials had terminated the vaccination program based on advice from a panel of experts.[61] Harvard's John Enders and Thomas Weller said they could not recommend its use as long as it contained the Mahoney strain. At that point, only 138,000 children had received a single dose. In July of 1955, the state suffered an epidemic of Type 1 Mahoney virus. Four thousand contracted polio; 1,700 were paralyzed. Several other states closed their vaccination programs, as well. An epidemic hit Chicago at the end of June with 1,100 cases, eight hundred paralyzed, thirty-six dead. No one who had received all three doses of vaccine contracted the disease.

The public sought a scapegoat, and to a large extent they targeted Oveta Culp Hobby, nicknamed Oveta "Culpable" Hobby.[62] Those who chastised her for bowing to political pressure in licensing all six companies with such rapidity ignored one fact—a group of scientists had met with Workman, chief of the Laboratory of Biologics Control, immediately following the presentations and unanimously recommended licensing. Among them was Sabin. Hobby resigned, saying she wanted to spend time with her ailing husband. "Events seasoned with time are often mistaken and misunderstood," Salk wrote to her. "[You have] all my sympathy and understanding."[63]

Others in the Public Health Service connected with the Cutter tragedy resigned as well, including NIH director William Sebrell. James Shannon survived the upheaval to succeed him. Scheele closed the Laboratory of Biologics Control and retired its staff of thirty-five, including Workman. He replaced it with a new Division of Biologic Standards, a bureau with 150 employees, which had responsibility for controlling biologic products. Scheele resigned within the year. "I feel your departure from the Public Health Service as a personal loss," Salk wrote to him. "I am grateful, indeed, for us all that you were at the helm when the sea was stormy."[64]

At the year's end, most of the manufacturers did well financially. Eli Lilly made a thirty-million-dollar profit on Salk's vaccine. For Cutter, the blunder resulted in financial disaster. Its stock tumbled, and although it survived, the company never again manufactured polio vaccine.[65]

The true victims of the Cutter incident were those who were permanently disabled or died as a result of contaminated vaccine. Lawsuits followed.[66] Melvin Belli represented sixteen clients whose claims totaled five million dollars. Everyone awaited the verdicts in the first two, which did not go to trial until more than two years after the tragedy. They would set the tone for those who followed. At the Alameda County Superior Court in Oakland, California, a jury heard the cases of eight-year-old Anne Elizabeth Gottsdanker, daughter of a psychology professor at UC Santa Barbara, and four-year-old James Randal Phipps of Los Angeles, son of a missiles engineer. During the twenty-seven-day trial, doctors testified that Gottsdanker would have to wear a brace on her right leg and use crutches for the rest of her life. Phipps had irreparable damage to his stomach muscles. Cutter's medical director testified that they had produced vaccine according to the government's requirements. The defense counsel called virologist Wendell Stanley to the stand. He disparaged Salk's "straight-line theory" of inactivation and testified that the minimum requirements for polio vaccine production were "grossly inadequate."[67] The most damaging testimony for the plaintiffs came from Workman, who divulged that other companies had had difficulties with contamination and recalled several lots of vaccine.

The jury did not find Cutter Laboratories negligent. Although not explicitly stating it, the verdict implied that if negligence had occurred, it had resulted from Salk's method for inactivating the poliovirus used by all the manufacturers. The jury did find Cutter guilty of a "breach of warranty," concluding that the company had marketed a vaccine which had caused poliomyelitis in the plaintiffs.[68] They awarded Gottsdanker $131,500 and Phipps $15,800.[69] The Cutter Laboratories public relations group hailed the verdict as a complete exoneration. "A weight is off my shoulders," Cutter told a friend. "I'm going home and work on my camellias."[70] A disappointed Belli told reporters: "We will press the other 43 cases against Cutter. We will win those cases.... Next time we'll prove negligence, too."[71]

❖

"THE SALK VACCINE Appears to Be Proving Out," reported *Barron's* on September 12, 1955.[72] The summer over, data from six states showed a 75 percent reduction in poliomyelitis incidence in those vaccinated. Not a single case of paralytic polio occurred in New York State among children who received three shots. Outside the United States, Denmark reported inoculation of 430,000 children; none developed polio. Nine hundred thousand Canadian children got vaccinations, and polio occurred at one-fourth the rate of the prior year. In 1956, the secretary of HEW expanded the group eligible for vaccine to children up to age eighteen and pregnant women, reaching an additional thirty-five million persons. By 1957, only 5,894 cases of poliomyelitis were reported, one-tenth the number in 1952. By 1961, the total number of cases declined by 97 percent below the annual average in the prevaccine era. Six years following the introduction of the Salk vaccine, polio was almost eradicated in the United States.[73]

Jonas Salk remained the symbol for polio prevention. "In all the confusion surrounding the polio vaccination program," read an Atlanta editorial, "the one person who least deserves to be a victim of the maelstrom of bickering is Dr. Jonas Salk, the man responsible for the vaccine. The country sympathizes with this scientist whose great discovery failed to get the kind of reception it merited because of the disorder in Washington."[74] Over the span of a few weeks, Salk had plummeted from the heights of glory to the brink of scientific disgrace. He had tried to remain above the fray, or at least he projected a reserved persona. To some he appeared too passive. When an associate encouraged him to contest an article in *Business Week* criticizing his work, Salk wrote back: "We may be aroused at times by unreasonableness and irrationality but we must choose the arena in which we do battle."[75]

Yet he must have felt some antipathy toward those who had made his life miserable. When Van Riper told him that they were going to have "some fun in the coming months after the beating we have taken for the last year and a half,"[76] Salk responded, "I think that the fun will come just by sitting by quietly and watching those who have gotten themselves out on a limb struggling to get back."[77] Van Riper accused him of reading one of those psychology books that makes one love his enemies.[78] Salk was more open with Herdis von Magnus. After a long-awaited vacation, he wrote, "My sense of humor is somewhat more stable these days, largely because those who are inclined to disturb it also must be on vacation."[79] When she insisted Salk attend the upcoming World Health Organization conference on poliomyelitis in Stockholm, he replied, "The invitation may be for a lynching, and I would like to avoid such unpleasantness."[80]

Salk's tribulations did not go unappreciated in Washington. "The year-end review leads me to a simple conclusion," Shannon, now director of the NIH, wrote to him. "It was rough—but without your unselfish help, it would have been impossible, at least to me."[81] Of all Salk's correspondence during this turbulent period, among the most apropos came from a Pittsburgh colleague who sent him a copy of Kipling's poem "If—." Parts of it spoke directly to Salk.

> If you can keep your head when all about you
>   Are losing theirs and blaming it on you,
> If you can trust yourself when all men doubt you,
>   But make allowance for their doubting too;
> If you can wait and not be tired by waiting,
>   Or being lied about, don't deal in lies,
> Or being hated, don't give way to hating,
>   And yet don't look too good, nor talk too wise:
> . . . .
> If you can bear to hear the truth you've spoken
>   Twisted by knaves to make a trap for fools,
> Or watch the things you gave your life to, broken,
>   And stoop and build 'em up with worn-out tools:
> . . . .
> If you can fill the unforgiving minute
>   With sixty seconds' worth of distance run,
> Yours is the Earth and everything that's in it,
>   And—which is more—you'll be a Man, my son![82]

"I would like to be able to measure up to Kipling's standards," Salk replied. "I shall try."[83]

Fame and Its Consequences

ON THE EVENING of April 12th, 1955, Edward R. Murrow had warned Salk, "Young man, a great tragedy has just befallen you....You have just lost your anonymity."[1] He soon learned not only how right Murrow had been but also how enduring the wisdom was. Baffled by his new standing, Salk told one reporter he was "treading water till the waves recede."[2] But the waves didn't recede. Jonas Salk was a public figure, and no matter how hard he tried he could not shed this new identity. Newsmen, following the adage "Names make the news," had used Salk to personify the events surrounding the polio story and in doing so had turned him into a national hero. Pictures of him appeared regularly in daily papers, women's magazines, and children's weeklies; articles about him sold papers. By revealing as much about his daily life as they could find (or make up), the media created a false sense of intimacy between him and the public. Salk couldn't enter a restaurant or hotel without causing a stir like a movie star.

Throughout 1956 and 1957, he continued to receive stacks of mail.[3] Correspondence included enough poetry to fill an anthology. "Jonas Salk conquered polio while I was reading a book," began a poem from an eight-year-old. Nine-year-old Charles Baumann sent a poem entitled

"Thoughts on Being Shot."[4] Some conveyed their thanks in music. Teofilo Gleytas, a Paraguayan music teacher and grandfather of three, sent a march he had composed in Salk's honor. Cuban composer Hector Garcia wrote the "Dr. Jonas Salk Waltz."[5] Salk was warm and thoughtful in his replies, especially to children. "It was kind of you to select me for your 'brotherhood buddy,'" he wrote ten-year-old Robert Ritter of Allentown, Pennsylvania.[6] With some he showed his humor, as with the Harvard student who sent "The Ballad of Jonas Salk," admitting that he had taken some poetic license.[7] A representative stanza ran:

> He was just a Flatbush kid, a precocious little Yid
> And his Ma and Pa came over on the boat.
> So when Senator Pat McCarran starts in a-swearin,
> About foreigners, he really gets my goat.

"After reading this ballad," Salk quipped, "I shall now take with a grain of salt some of the things I have learned about Davy Crockett."[8]

Much of his mail included requests for pictures, autographs, and advice. Natalie Hatch of Los Angeles sought guidance on how to become a laboratory technologist. Joan Anderson was writing an essay for English class and requested information on his vaccine before the Christmas holidays, since her essay was due in January. A Brooklyn high school student wanted Salk's "first-hand" notes on his experiments for a biology project.[9] An equal number of people suffering from polio and other illnesses asked for help. Despite his growing weariness, Salk remained sensitive and sympathetic. When M. Alpert of the Bronx wrote that a few months after the polio vaccine announcement, her husband contracted polio, Salk replied, "Please take heart."[10] Physiotherapy could help patients regain function. To Mrs. L. Valchuela of the Bronx he wrote, "I am quite certain there is no correlation between heart disease and the wearing of tight sox."[11] And to an Australian woman he responded, "It was very kind of you to write me of your observations [on your health] over the past twenty years."[12] Salk's heartfelt thanks to individuals around the world—old or young, in big cities and the smallest towns, his willingness to answer questions from simple to complex was remarkable. What he didn't realize was how much reaching out to the public fanned the flames of celebrity.

Salk continued to receive a staggering number of honors: the Murray-Green Award from the AFL-CIO; the Salvation Army Citation for Humanitarian Service; the Great Cross of Our National Order of Carlos J. Finley from Havana; awards from the Milk and Welfare Fund of Chicago for the Tuberculosis Poor, from the Grand Lodge of the Knights of Pythias in Swampscott, Massachusetts, to name a few. And each day brought a new request for Salk to be a guest speaker from a variety of organizations: the American Women's Medical Association, the New York Academy of Medicine, the Pakistan Medical Association, the Arizona House of Representatives, the Mount Lebanon Council of the Knights of Columbus, the International Supreme Council Order of DeMolay in Kansas City, and on and on. Most events entailed a banquet and tour, the news media and autograph seekers following in his wake.

Although touched by every expression of gratitude, Salk was suffo-cating. Eventually he created a printed thank-you note, after going through many drafts to get the sentiment right. And he decided to de-cline all invitations to award ceremonies except those from universities and colleges with which he had some association. Finally, he planned to attend only those conferences related to his work. In declining invita-tions, Salk tried to be courteous and forthright, yet his letters reflected the toll celebrity was taking on him. "The tax upon my conscience of being arbitrary when invitations are received from all who are equally sincere, is a difficult one for me to bear," he wrote the president of Hebrew Union College. "The things that are appropriate to be and to do at twenty, forty, and sixty are not all the same....Too much has happened too quickly."[13] He wrote many such letters, baring his soul to strangers. Salk thought people would understand his predicament. And most did. Nevertheless, some felt slighted. "When he refused invitations," Friedman said, "he was often misunderstood; many thought he felt he was too good, too important to grace them."[14] When the National Father's Day Committee attempted for a third time to name him Father of the Year, they wrote: "You twice rejected the nomination as Father of the Year for reasons of your own."[15]

The requests kept coming. Some had no relationship to his work, as if his scientific success imparted wisdom in other fields. Could he attend the Senate hearings in support of a bill to create a National Medical

Library? Would he participate in a discussion on voting for the American Heritage Foundation, sign a statement proposing solutions to the Middle East crisis? Salk stuck to his policy no matter who made the request. When Benjamin Spock asked him to serve on the Committee to Protect our Children's Teeth, he replied he didn't question the value of the project; however, for him to survive this period he had to decline all requests.[16] When John Enders pressured him to accept an award from Filene's, the well-known Boston department store, he wrote back, "Although the causes for which they seek help and for which I have become a highly prized commodity are good in principle…these are not pleasurable occasions.…The situation in which I find myself is not one of my own seeking nor one that I would wish to espouse."[17]

Occasionally Salk found the public's perception of him amusing. He told a journalist about the time he had sat through a tedious, contentious scientific conference, after which he decided to go down to the beach for a swim. "Sure that's Dr. Salk," he heard a boy telling his friends. "I saw him on television."

"The hell it is," another boy argued. "What would Dr. Salk be doing in a bathing suit?"[18]

Stardom did give Salk access to other famous people. He could have mixed with movie stars, heads of states, sports legends. If he wanted, high school classmates who had excluded him from their select club, undergraduates who had snubbed him, and scientists who had belittled his work all could see him dining with Helen Hayes, laughing with Eleanor Roosevelt, throwing out a ball on opening day in Yankee Stadium. Although the temptation must have been great, Salk rarely succumbed. He declined a special seat at the Academy Awards, a dinner with the Jewish Theatrical Guild honoring Jimmy Durante, the Ambassador's Ball in honor of Israeli diplomat Abba Eban, a dinner given by Secretary of State John Foster Dulles for the prime minister of Burma, Harry Truman's seventy-fourth birthday party.

Among the most persistent in their requests were Jewish organizations. Could he attend the First Annual Donor Dinner Dance at Menorah Masonic Temple in Brooklyn or speak at the cornerstone exercises for the new B'nai B'rith building in Washington? Would he dedicate a clinic for the Jewish Social Service Agency, sponsor an art show for American

Friends of Hebrew University? Salk had become a symbol of humanitarian success for Jews. "And what Jew is there who cannot note with an inner glow the fact that Dr. Salk is of the faith?" asked an article in the *Jewish Criterion*.[19] Urging him to accept an honorary degree from Hebrew Union College, a friend wrote: "Don't minimize the feeling of pride you have given our people all over the world.... Even Einstein...made a great many concessions in this direction because he felt deeply his relationship to the Jewish people (despite the fact that he was about as 'religious' as you are.)"[20]

Most wearing on Salk was the media. *Perfect Home* asked for recollections from childhood; *Esquire* asked him to contribute to a feature article, "The Summer Job I Had as a Boy"; *Family Weekly* wanted to know his New Year's resolution. *Current Events* asked him to tell young readers the important events that had occurred during his youth, and *Better Homes and Gardens* wanted to know the most memorable book he had read as a child. When Salk did not answer their questions, writers speculated what he would have answered. At times the media so exasperated Salk he let his annoyance show. "You do not have my permission to publish the article you sent me," he wrote an editor from *American Weekly*. "I cannot accept the position in which you have placed me. I was willing to give you the facts and opinions so that you could be accurate, but I cannot give you myself."[21]

Several authors rushed to write his biography, but Salk refused to cooperate. "I know that someday I will be the victim of a biography," he told Robert Coughlan of *Life*. "[But] to have a biography written about myself at 'our age' would seem to me in poor taste."[22] The popular television program *Masquerade Party* sought his participation; ABC's *Treasure Hunt* was devoting a quiz section to his life. Salk could have made substantial sums of money from television appearances, movie rights, and speaking engagements. Though he did not consider capitalizing on his celebrity, that didn't keep others from exploiting him.

Lorraine Friedman began receiving calls to confirm Salk's support of an air sanitation system from the Glycolator Manufacturing Company. When she wrote to the president of Glycolator to complain, he said he would "brief" the salesman who had made this claim.[23] A registered assayer inquired about Joe Bassick, who professed to be an electronics scientist with a large research lab and ties to Salk as evidenced from a picture of them together in a newspaper. One of her clients was planning to invest $100,000 in Bassick's venture, based on Salk's endorsement.[24] Bassick turned out to be a fraud who had stood next to Salk when a journalist started to photograph him. The Albany Chamber of Commerce sent a telegram that read: "Inquiries received here indicate your appearance being used by fundraisers to sell program advertising and tickets to Jewish War Veterans dinner dance, March 21. Advise your plans."[25] Aside from Friedman, Salk had no one to protect him.

Fame attracts a number of strange people, and Salk was not immune. Dr. John E. Fratzke of Chicago wrote that since he had supplied Salk with modifications for processing the polio vaccine, which had resulted in longer immunity and less danger, he knew Salk would be willing to do him a favor. He had been approached by an organization interested in financing production of his leukemia formula. They requested a letter from Salk confirming Fratzke's role in the polio vaccine processing. When Salk wrote back that there must be some confusion, Fratzke replied that when he had divulged his polio formulation to Salk over the phone, he had another party listening as well as the operator, who knew his voice from his TV appearances. "I know that you are too BIG a man to try and contradict our verbal agreement," he went on to say. "My word is my bond when I make a verbal agreement, and I do hope that yours is the same."[26] He insisted they meet. No one had warned Salk that when the media creates a luminary, people can delude themselves into feeling they are on collegial terms with the celebrity. By replying to his letters, Salk had reinforced Fratzke's delusions; when he ignored Fratzke, the harassment stopped.

Salk was experiencing the dark side of fame. The emotional toll from Fratzke and other con artists, obsessives, and stalkers must have been enormous. "The pinnacle of any career is fame," a psychologist wrote. "Or is it?" He quoted Picasso as saying that "of all the unpleasant things he had known in life—poverty, disapproval, unhappiness—fame was not only the worst, but worse than all the other things put together."[27]

Fame burdened Salk's family, as well. Their lives had revolved around him and his work; now they had to accommodate to his stardom. His three young sons had to don their suits and attend formal events where they heard their father praised again and again. And Donna was called upon to stand at his side, coerced by the media to play the role of his First Lady. She detested the expected public display of charm and congeniality. Perhaps more difficult than having a legendary husband or father was becoming a celebrity by association. As introverts, Donna and Peter shunned the spotlight. Still, the public had an insatiable curiosity about Salk's family, and, somewhat oblivious, Salk did not protect them as much as he should have. "I wasn't anonymous anymore," Peter later recalled. "People looked at me and interacted with me differently, even when I played little league. I was a marked person." Success in a parent begets expectations for the children; accordingly some teachers and relatives anticipated the Salk sons would emulate their father. "It was really uncomfortable for me within my class," Peter said. "I certainly wasn't a star, but there was no way to melt into the background. I came with a tag."[28]

When Salk's middle son, Darrell, was asked in retrospect how it felt to have a famous father, he replied, "Hey—he made me practice the piano when I didn't want to." In a more reflective tone, he continued, "There may very well be a perception among the public that this wonderful thing happened to this family overnight, and everything was rosy, meeting the president and all of these wonderful things. [But] it was an ordinary life with these things thrown in on top, which is stressful."[29]

No matter how much Salk resisted the temptations of fame, they had to have affected him. He wasn't the same father and husband as he had been before April 12. "My memories of my father are divided into prevaccine and postvaccine," Jonathan recalled. "Prevaccine, I have images of a warm guy. I remember sitting on his lap, playing with the hair on his chest. When we all bought moccasins, mine were just like my dad's." Jonathan considered the Ann Arbor announcement a turning point. "After that," he said, "I have the sense that he wasn't around much anymore, mostly mentally. He just wasn't present in that same way."[30]

The family trip to Europe in the summer of 1957 epitomized how their lives had been altered. The boys looked forward to summer vacations at their cottage on Deep Creek Lake in Maryland, where they swam and played games with friends. That summer, instead, thirteen-year-old Peter, ten-year-old Darrell, and seven-year-old Jonathan traveled aboard an ocean liner to tour Europe, leaving as soon as the school year ended and returning after Labor Day. What may have been described to Donna and the boys as a family trip seemed weighted with social functions. They stopped in New York en route for an affair celebrating the dedication of the Dr. Jonas E. Salk Ward at the Shaare Zedek Hospital in Jerusalem. Again the family listened to Jonas being praised. "By your presence," Reverend Asher Hirsch said, "you have given us the opportunity to say the following blessing: 'Blessed be he who hath given from his wisdom to the mortal.'"[31]

Aboard the ocean liner, they could not relax either. They traveled with Basil O'Connor and his charming new bride, Hazel Royall, director of functional therapy at the Georgia Warm Springs Foundation. The couple planned to interrupt their honeymoon just long enough to attend the Fourth International Poliomyelitis Conference in Geneva. To the dismay of the Salk boys, every dinner required formal attire; their father wore a tuxedo with a boutonnière just like O'Connor. Photographers followed them everywhere. "Of all the people I could have been born to in life," Peter lamented, "I was born the son of this famous man."[32]

Once in Europe, the itinerary didn't ease up.[33] Rather than staying in charming inns or bed and breakfasts, the Salk family was booked into the Grand Hotel Zermatterhof in Zermatt, the Excelsior Hotel Italie in Florence, the Hôtel de Savoie in Grenoble, the Hôtel de Crillon in Paris. In Zermatt, their father participated in a scientific symposium; in Rome, he visited the Instituto Superiore di Sanità. From July 8 to 12, while he attended the Fourth International Poliomyelitis Conference in Geneva, Donna and the boys may have envisioned visiting the Clock and Watch Museum or Nestlé's chocolate factory or the Chillon Castle with its dungeons. Instead they had to attend a number of social events: On July 8, the Swiss Federal Council held a reception at the Art and History Museum. The next day, O'Connor hosted a buffet at Hotel des Bergues. On July 10, Madame Bodmer-Naville invited Donna to a tea, followed by an evening cruise on Lake Geneva. And the next evening, they attended a banquet at the Palais des Expositions. Hazel Royall O'Connor may have thrived on such gala events, but Donna would have preferred to be lying in a hammock at Deep Creek Lake, reading.

To add to the family's exasperation, the press chronicled their trip. The *New York Times Magazine* printed pictures of them riding in a paddleboat in Nice. "Salk back from Europe, antique buyer Bobo too" read headlines from the *New York World-Telegram and Sun*, referring to socialite Bobo Rockefeller, a former model and showgirl who had inherited five million dollars when she divorced oil tycoon Winthrop Rockefeller.[34] The *New York Herald Tribune* reported that the Salks had boarded the SS *United States* in Southampton along with 1,730 other passengers, including railroad executive Harold Vanderbilt, president of the American Stock Exchange, and a member of the America's Cup team.[35]

Photos of the crossing show the boys in suits playing bingo, wearing funny hats at a dinner party. Peter and Darrell appear bored; only Jonathan seems to be enjoying himself, his broad smile displaying a missing front tooth. The photographers caught Jonas laughing with Bobo, a glamorous blond, dressed in an open-necked white dress. Another picture shows him dancing with an attractive young woman in a strapless evening gown. Donna never became accustomed to her celebrity status and refused to oblige the paparazzi. In every picture she wears a plain dress buttoned up at the neck with minimal makeup, her dark hair parted in middle and pulled back in a bun. Shots of Donna alone with Jonas show her gaze averted, his brow furrowed, depicting a marriage strained by celebrity.

⁜

SALK WAS SUFFERING under fame's heavy load. "His life did change immediately with the April announcement," Darrell later said, "but it just took him time to realize it."[36] The interruptions and obligations were overt, the altered relationships subtle. People looked at and treated Salk differently. He never knew whether they were interested in Jonas Salk the person or Jonas Salk the icon. Old classmates and friends didn't hesitate to call upon him for favors. Every letter, no matter how pleasant, seemed to have some underlying agenda. To make matters worse, one question always hovered: What great feat would he accomplish next? If Salk submitted any new data, it made headlines, embarrassing him. At a meeting of the New York Academy of Sciences, when he mentioned the idea of a vaccine against a number of viruses that attack the nervous system, the press announced: "All Virus Vaccine Eyed by Dr. Salk."[37] When a reporter said, "I hear you're trying to find an anti-cold vaccine,"

Salk replied, "All I'm trying to do is keep my balance."[38] "Balance" meant returning to his laboratory work uninterrupted.

There he faced an immediate problem; few of his staff remained. Initially the Pittsburgh team had felt "elated," lab assistant Donald Wegemer recalled.[39] Julius Youngner told a reporter he considered his role in preventing polio the highlight of his career. "This was like a rocket going off," he said, "a space shot."[40] In Ann Arbor, however, a wave of discord had started to build. Members of Salk's research team attended the meeting as honored guests, their trip paid for by the NFIP. They waited for recognition as Salk went through his long list of acknowledgments. "This opportunity would have no meaning," he finally said, "if it were not for the devotion with which each of the … group that comprises our laboratory contributed and shared in that which needed to be done."[41] He did not name them individually. That night on *See It Now* he paid tribute to his laboratory coworkers again, but after years of dedication, some considered this recognition insufficient. In his glorification, they felt Salk had risen above them, and some started referring to him as "Jonas E. Christ."[42]

The team left Ann Arbor without fanfare. No reporters flocked around them; no special celebration had been planned. Julius Youngner got drunk on the plane to California. Byron Bennett and James Lewis took a train back to Pittsburgh with Bennett in tears. Youngner, the most vocal, told a journalist that while Salk raised research funds, fought with his scientific opponents, and dealt with the public and the press, he stayed in the lab and conducted the experiments.[43] In a later interview with historian David Oshinsky, Youngner offered a litany of complaints that had been festering for years, painting a portrait of Salk as an insensitive autocrat who not only failed to give him proper recognition but also stole his work.[44]

Not everyone felt this way. Don Wegemer disagreed with Youngner's claims: "[Salk] recognized people's abilities and gave them credit. Some people figured they should have got more credit, which is a problem for them."[45] Lewis, too, painted a different picture of his boss. "It seems I will always be a part of the place," he wrote Salk after taking a position elsewhere. "This feeling comes to all of us who were associated with you, chiefly because you have left us feeling this way."[46] It is hard to discern where the truth lies years after the fact. "Sharing research is an evolving process," noted Campbell Moses, one of Salk's Pitt colleagues, "and for every discovery of note someone probably feels a little left out."[47] Others thought Youngner more than a bit self-promoting. Although Salk instilled a sense of purpose in his group, he did not shower them with praise. No one recalls lab parties or dinners at the Salks' home. But every person in his laboratory could have left at any time. Yet they had stayed— at least until April 12.

Salk tried to make amends. He broke protocol when he insisted on recognizing "the untiring devotion of my staff" while receiving his presidential citation.[48] In an interview for the *Pittsburgh Press*, he talked about the team effort, commending his dedicated group of fifty, naming Percival Bazeley, Byron Bennett, Ulrich Krech, James Lewis, Elsie Ward, and Julius Youngner, in alphabetical order.[49] But these attempts did not appease those who felt bruised. Youngner left Salk's lab to work in the microbiology department. Lewis took a job with the National Drug Company. Bazeley and Krech, in the United States on visas, had to return to their respective countries. By the spring of 1957, only Elsie Ward, Donald Wegemer, a few technicians, and Lorraine Friedman remained of Salk's original team. When a prominent British pathologist requested to visit the lab, Salk expressed a bit of embarrassment. "I will tell you quite candidly that we are in a state of transition."[50] With Bazeley, he spoke more candidly about the upheaval. "I have learned," he wrote, "what happens to one's energies and how they can be drained extravagantly, and unprofitably, by unwise selections that have been allowed to continue too long."[51]

When Salk did return to academic life, he found a chasm had developed between himself and the scientific community. He shouldn't have been surprised. In the year following the announcement, amid all the mail and calls he received, few came from researchers with whom he had previously collaborated. Although he did not overtly crave awards, he must have noted how few of the elite scientific societies honored him. "Jonas received a lot of recognition from the public," Darrell observed, "which was very gratifying. He did not receive similar kinds of recognition from his peers, which is for anybody a hurtful kind of experience."[52]

Some scientists considered his behavior—posing with movie stars, giving television interviews—unbefitting a prominent researcher. "He had become too public for some people," Friedman said. Several resented Salk's favored position with O'Connor. Others thought the sensationalism surrounding the polio vaccine had debased medical science, and they blamed Salk. "He was the public's darling," Friedman said, "but he was a pariah of sorts in the scientific community."[53] He did win the Albert Lasker Award, which recognizes the nation's most accomplished scientists. When a friend sent his regards, Salk replied, "It is still nice to be recognized by one's colleagues even if one may have caused discomfort or disturbance, unintentionally and unwittingly."[54]

Several researchers thought Salk deserved the Nobel Prize. Much of the public thought he already had been awarded this prestigious scientific award. In his 1895 will, wealthy industrialist Alfred Nobel stipulated that a substantial portion of his capital should be used to set up a fund at the Royal Swedish Academy of Sciences to award yearly prizes in five areas "to those who during the preceding year have done the greatest benefit to mankind."[55] He further indicated the award in physiology or medicine should be given for the most important discovery. Although nominated several times, Salk never received this most coveted prize. Many have speculated that Salk was denied the Nobel Prize because his was not a "discovery" in the true scientific sense. Others contend that politics played a major role. The details of his nominations were revealed after his death by the permanent secretary of the Royal Swedish Academy of Sciences, who obtained permission to access the previously closed archives according to the fifty-year secrecy rule.

Each year a five-member committee sought nominations from select individuals, reviewed their accomplishments, and proposed a candidate to the fifty members of the Nobel Assembly for the final decision. Sven Gard, professor of virology at Stockholm's Karolina Institute and one of the five members of the Nobel Committee, had a major influence over the selection process during the 1950s and 1960s. He called John Enders's discovery "the most important in the whole history of virology."[56] In his 1955 evaluation of Salk's nomination, Gard wrote that although the field trial results had been compiled, a complete report was not yet available; he proposed Salk's work be subjected to "exhaustive analysis" first.[57] In his review a year later, he wrote that Salk's most important contribution was the demonstration that inactivated poliovirus vaccine conferred immunity, which he considered "nothing new." Furthermore, Salk had "exploited discoveries made by others." In his most damning statement, Gard said he had not been able to reproduce Salk's inactivation data himself, and rigid adherence to his hypothesis had likely been responsible for the accidents associated with the mass immunizations (i.e., the Cutter incident). He concluded Salk's work on the polio vaccine was not "prize-worthy."[58]

Salk likely did anticipate an invitation to join the National Academy of Sciences, the elite society of investigators established by President Lincoln in 1863. The academy elects members "in recognition of their distinguished and continuing achievements in original research," although there are no specific guidelines as to what constitutes "original."[59] Membership represents one of the highest honors bestowed upon a scientist. Almost every researcher who received the Lasker Award has been inducted into the academy. But no invitation was forthcoming for Salk. It remains unclear why this was the case, as election proceedings are never made public, and strict secrecy is maintained throughout the academic community. Members submit nominations for new inductees, after which five membership committees prepare a rank list of nominees to be considered. "A vigorous partisan or opponent on the class membership committee," a science writer learned from one of the academy's presidents, "can mean the difference between an individual's eventual election or defeat."[60] It may have been at this stage that Salk's nomination was checked. After a mail ballot is sent to all members, a formal vote is taken at the annual meeting to elect new members. Only members of the academy can be present. Names of newly elected members are flashed up on a screen, and the president asks if anyone has reason to oppose a candidate.

Salk's election could have been blocked for a number of reasons. Some said his work did not merit induction into the academy because it represented a technical piece of work, lacking scientific creativity. "Salk was a kitchen chemist," academy member Albert Sabin had sniped. "He never had an original idea in his life.... You could go into the kitchen and do what he did."[61] And most academy virologists believed only a live vaccine could impart lifelong immunity. In addition, several blamed Salk for the Cutter incident. Others felt differently. "The real reasons for refusal," historian Aaron Klein wrote, "were the press conferences, radio and TV appearances, the *Life* magazine spreads, the mad scenes at Ann Arbor...the outpouring of public adoration and all the other violations of the scientists' unofficial code of behavior."[62] "I think people were jealous of his success," academy member Paul Stumpf concluded.[63] Whatever the reason—failure to contribute original science, behavior unbecoming an academician, or jealousy, Salk was blackballed.

Salk must have anticipated election every February, only to be disappointed. "He was hurt," Pitt colleague Campbell Moses recalled, "but he wasn't shocked."[64] He knew his relationship with the scientific community—uneasy to begin with—had changed in ways he had never expected. Nonetheless, Salk stood behind his belief that scientists should reach out to the public about issues that affected their health. He had dared to step out from behind the walls of academia and communicate with the common man. He tried to dismiss the ostracism that followed. "It is not the awards made by men that give us the greatest reason for doing," he told Mary Lasker.[65] Later in life he was less generous. Speaking of Ann Arbor, he reflected: "I was neither a politician nor a performer. Those remarks were simply made by colleagues who at that time were reacting as is perfectly natural in professional circles, particularly in the field of science where the coin of the realm is recognition. I was being recognized; they were not."[66]

Although Salk tried many times to share the credit, the public and the media had made him the icon for polio prevention. With the introduction of the vaccine came a wave of celebrity accorded few scientists in the history of medicine. Though Salk was undeniably ambitious, his desire had been to accomplish something great, not necessarily to be someone great. And while other scientists may have blamed him, the attention was not primarily of Salk's own choosing. "He was embarrassed by his fame," Professor Moses maintained.[67]

Nevertheless, historians debate the level of Salk's humility and naiveté. "Salk was very private, very shy," argued John Troan. "He dealt with us because he had to, not because he wanted to. He'd much rather have been left alone."[68] Historian David Oshinsky disagreed. "Salk, in truth, was more than an innocent bystander," he contended. "One of his great gifts was a knack for putting himself forward in a manner that made him seem genuinely indifferent to his fame, a reluctant celebrity, embarrassed by the accolades, oblivious to the rewards."[69] Perhaps most reliable are the observations of his longtime secretary, Lorraine Friedman, who had watched the drama unfold close-up. "He wasn't looking for fame," she maintained in an interview months before she died. "It cost him an awful lot personally. Many in the scientific community just didn't believe he was the innocent he claimed to be." At one point, Salk had confided in Friedman, "I wish this had never happened to me."[70]

Act II

JONAS SALK, NOW forty-three years old, stood at a crossroads. "You must decide whether to spend the rest of your days enjoying your fame or working," Alan Gregg, vice president of the Rockefeller Foundation, told him after the Ann Arbor symposium. "You will be unable to do both. You can spend your life traveling, reading papers, accepting awards, and being comfortable. Or you can have the courage to turn aside publicity, the courage to resume your work, the courage to face the possibility that you may never again be able to do a piece of work as important as the [polio vaccine]."[1] Salk rejected—or tried to reject—the celebrity route and declined an administrative role as well, turning down a number of offers to chair departments or direct national organizations. Considering what to do next, he recalled Gregg's final words of advice: "Jonas, do only that which makes your heart leap."

Salk knew what made his heart leap—solving problems that afflicted mankind. Besides that, he wasn't sure. Consumed by the press, his fans, and the politics of polio prevention, he hadn't had time to think about science. When television commentator Dave Garroway asked what he planned to do next, Salk replied, "Satisfy my curiosity."[2] When Garroway asked what he was curious about, he didn't have an answer.

Other issues were demanding his attention. While traveling in Europe in July of 1957, Salk received a letter from Assistant Attorney General Robert Bicks, informing him that the Antitrust Division was conducting a grand jury investigation into the distribution and pricing of the Salk poliomyelitis vaccine by the six manufacturers.[3] Back in 1953, a Detroit newspaper had reported that Parke, Davis and Company had contracted with Salk to make a polio vaccine for which he had received payment.[4] It was bad enough that the company had embarrassed him at the moment of his scientific triumph by implying he had given it exclusive information; now that false claim had come back to haunt him. Salk assured Bicks that he had no consulting arrangements with any company; payment for the work that led to the polio vaccine came from the people through the March of Dimes.[5] His main association had consisted of technical advice. Despite assurances from Salk, the NFIP, and the companies, the Department of Justice charged five drug manufacturers with conspiracy and price-fixing. "It is incredible that as a postscript to one of our greatest achievements," the president of Eli Lilly and Company wrote Salk, "we should now have to face this fantastic suit."[6] (Two years later, after Salk spent an inordinate amount of time testifying, the federal judge dismissed the case.)

Finally, Salk returned to his Pittsburgh laboratory, where he needed to wrap up some polio research, which included determining how long antibody levels persisted, finding a substitute for the virulent Type 1 Mahoney virus, and improving his tissue cultivation and viral inactivation techniques. While he and Elsie Ward were searching for a more efficient way to grow poliovirus, an unexpected finding intrigued him.

To date, poliovirus was being cultivated in monkey kidney tissue. This was not ideal; besides the expense, restricted access to monkeys intermittently curbed vaccine production. Seeking a substitute, Salk tried a recently reported technique whereby monkey heart cells were grown in culture, after which they underwent transformation, developing the ability to multiply indefinitely. If he could cultivate poliovirus on this self-perpetuating line of cells, it would obviate the need for additional live monkeys and facilitate vaccine production. He and others had a major concern: since the cell lines had unrestrained growth, the signal characteristic of cancer cells, vaccines prepared from virus grown in these cell lines theoretically could cause cancer in the recipient. To study this, Salk and Ward inoculated two hundred monkeys with transformed heart cells. Although they found no evidence of cancer, several monkeys did develop large benign tumors at the injection site, which spontaneously disappeared a few weeks later. Instead of abandoning this approach as not feasible for human use, Salk investigated. What he found astounded him. When the rapidly dividing heart cells formed a tumor at the site of inoculation, the monkeys developed antibodies to the heart cells, causing the tumors to regress.

When they reinoculated these animals with heart cells, no new tumors appeared. It seemed the animals had become immune as a result of the first inoculation. "The outcome of experiments to date," Salk wrote to Peter Bazeley, "particularly the immunologic phase of it, is so exciting as to overshadow almost all else."[7] While trying to enhance vaccine production, Salk had slipped into the nascent field of tumor immunology. Although scientists going back to the 1900s had tried to treat cancer with vaccines, their rudimentary techniques had failed. A vaccine against cancer remained elusive.

So far, Salk had observed that he could immunize monkeys with small amounts of transformed heart cells and measure anti-heart-cell antibodies. If he reinoculated the monkeys with large amounts of these cells, tumors didn't grow. He postulated that antiserum from these animals, which contained antitumor antibodies, might be able to kill other tumors, maybe even malignant ones. To test this, he and Ward grew three different types of cancer cells in culture and treated them with the antiserum. It killed every one.

In December of 1957, a premier research journal, *Science*, published their findings in an article entitled "Some Characteristics of a Continuously Propagating Cell Derived from Monkey Heart Tissue."[8] Just over a page in length, the paper described their techniques and results but drew no conclusions. Such a preliminary report normally would have gone unnoticed by the media, except that in this case its author was Jonas Salk. The public was waiting for the next great discovery from this scientist whose prowess had reached mythical heights. The press realized the implications of his observations—a cancer vaccine. "May Have Stumbled on Way to Cancer Victory," read the headline in one newspaper.[9] "Salk's New

Anticancer Claim," read another.[10] News of Salk's purported break-through circulated worldwide.

Eight months later, trying to avoid the media, Salk inoculated sixteen patients suffering from leukemia, lymphoma, and melanoma with a suspension of transformed monkey heart cells and tested for antibody. If he thought he could conduct this study unnoticed, he was mistaken. The Pittsburgh's *Post and Times-Star* printed a picture of a mother and her cancer-stricken child. "Mrs. Dolores Paul of Pittsburgh braids the hair of her daughter, Mary Ann," the caption read, "who is one of four children receiving test injections from Dr. Jonas Salk in a cancer research project. Mary Ann, however, is more interested in what will happen Saturday. She will be six years old."[11]

With his brief report in *Science*, Salk leapt from polio researcher to cancer researcher to cancer expert in the eyes of the public. As news of his clinical study leaked out, this perception intensified. A Pennsylvania congressman asked Salk to recommend therapy for the state police chief's sister, who had eye cancer.[12] A Pittsburgh physician asked him to treat his English setter's melanoma.[13] Letters from desperate patients and families arrived from Malaya, Brazil, Germany, Colombia, Italy. H. Bzuro of Tel Aviv wrote that his thirty-seven-year-old wife had widespread breast cancer. Polish Jews, they were the only members of their family to survive the Nazis. "Honorable Doctor," he wrote, "I know that you are working on new techniques and new preparants....This is my last hope."[14] G. Waters from Poplar Grove, Arkansas, said he was suffering from metastatic colon cancer but could still walk and drive; he would go anywhere and submit to any treatment. "I am pleading for you for help."[15] R. Maxia, wife of a young pediatrician from Sardinia, wrote that her husband was dying from pancreatic cancer. "I beg you to do whatever is possible for this colleague of yours, a father to five children."[16]

Salk regretted the answer he had to give. "It is unfortunate that newspapers, in recent weeks, have carried stories suggesting that we may be on the verge of a cure for cancer," he wrote H. Crum of Banner, Kentucky. "This is not true." He and his team were doing basic research on the nature of cancer cells. "This is a far cry from a cure for cancer."[17] He wrote hundreds of such letters, saddened and frustrated. Lashing out at the media in a press release, he contended that cancer evoked such strong emotional responses that it placed significant responsibility upon scientists and journalists alike. "Why are news reporters permitted to quote out of context," he demanded, "and essentially re-write the meaning intended by a carefully worded report to colleagues in science?" Such license was disturbing to scientists and "grossly unfair" to cancer victims. "Is the right of the free press so much greater than the rights of scientists to work freely and unhampered by the consequences of exaggerated reports for which they are not responsible?"[18]

In the end, the sixteen cancer patients in Salk's study did not respond to the injections as the monkeys had. No report of a cancer vaccine was forthcoming, and the hoopla died down.

◈

WHILE SALK WAS attending banquets, signing autographs, and writing thank-you notes, another chapter in the history of polio was unfolding.[19] Salk had expected his vaccine to eradicate polio, but in 1957, six thousand children and adults in the United States became infected. Just a fraction of the public had been inoculated since the vaccine's release in 1955. Advocates for the live-virus vaccine used these figures to disparage the killed vaccine, saying the public deserved a more effective preparation. Their arguments included biological as well as socioeconomic concerns.

Poliovirus was known to enter the body through the mouth and multiply in the intestinal tract, from which it spread into the bloodstream, subsequently invading the brain and spinal cord. The killed vaccine stimulated formation of antibodies that intercepted the virus in the bloodstream, thus preventing paralysis. The live-virus vaccine, given orally, introduced a weakened, live virus into the intestines, where it multiplied, simulating a low-grade infection. This activated antibody production not only in the bloodstream but also in the intestinal lymph tissue, generating two sites of attack on the virus. Advocates for this approach argued that the immunity generated by a live virus developed more quickly and lasted a lifetime. Initially dispensed in milk, then in a teaspoon of cherry syrup, then in a sugar cube, the oral vaccine eliminated the cost of needles and syringes and required fewer trained personnel. In addition, the requisite three shots made the Salk vaccine impractical in rural areas and developing countries. Several scientists were rushing to be the first to make a safe live-virus vaccine.

Initially, Hilary Koprowski of Lederle Laboratories had taken the lead, reporting in 1951 that he had administered a rodent-adapted strain of poliovirus to twenty volunteers. Most excreted virus in the stool, and all developed antipoliovirus antibodies with no ill effects. He neglected to say the "volunteers" were disabled children from a state institution. The public would have been repulsed had they known he fed the children infected rat brain and spinal cord tissue mixed in chocolate milk.

Albert Sabin, at the University of Cincinnati, was also working on a live-virus vaccine. He had selected three poliovirus strains and grown successive generations in tissue culture, until the virus became weak enough to stimulate antibody formation without generating polio. He had approached Tom Rivers about using his NFIP grant to test his oral vaccine in children, but Rivers tabled the request, saying too many safety issues remained unresolved. Subjects excreted live virus in their stools, which could infect others. Worse yet, weakened virus could regain its former strength, termed "reversion to virulence." Despite these concerns, Sabin gave inmates at the federal reformatory in Chillicothe, Ohio, live poliovirus mixed in milk.[20]

He then proceeded to immunize his two young daughters, neither of whom had received the Salk vaccine. "He considered us clean slates," his daughter Debbe said. When she and her sister, Amy, read a historical account of how their father had agonized over the decision with his wife before proceeding, they looked at each other and said, "You know that never took place." They didn't remember a civil conversation between their parents; Debbe recollected that her father just called her and her sister into the kitchen and instructed them, "Take this." They would never have considered disobeying their father; his temper was legend. They detested the throat swabs, blood draws, and stool cultures that followed. "Here I am going to elementary school," Debbe said, "and I had to take a stool cup to save samples for virus shedding."[21] Her father held clinics in their kitchen, where he vaccinated cousins and neighborhood children well before his vaccine was licensed.

By the end of 1956, Sabin had immunized 133 subjects with his vaccine. Neither he nor Koprowski could conduct a large field trial in the

United States, however, because of the widespread use of the Salk vaccine. They needed collaborators in other countries. Koprowski teamed up with George Dick, a microbiology professor at Queen's University Belfast, who fed Koprowski's live, attenuated virus to 190 children, reporting increased antibodies and no ill effects. Before long, Dick discovered that reversion to virulence had ensued. The presumably weakened, harmless virus regained strength and infectivity; virus recovered from the children's stool paralyzed monkeys. That meant those vaccinated with Koprowski's vaccine could start a polio epidemic. Dick terminated the British trials. By then, Lederle Laboratories had spent $13 million on live polio vaccine research; the company and Koprowski abruptly parted ways. Koprowski assumed directorship of the Wistar Institute in Philadelphia and promptly initiated a trial in the Congo, using a new Type 1 strain.

Herald Cox, director of research at Lederle, continued work on an oral vaccine. Although warned of its potential danger, he immunized a half million young adults in Dade County, Florida, and began a trial in Berlin as well. Meanwhile, Sabin fed vaccine to the entire child population of Toluca, Mexico, a city of one hundred thousand. He also sent vaccine to Czechoslovakia and Singapore, where outbreaks had occurred. His most impressive trials, however, took place in Russia.

Sabin's opportunity to introduce his vaccine in the Soviet Union came about in part due to a tactical error by Salk.[22] Mikhail Chumakov of Moscow's Poliomyelitis Research Institute had visited Salk's lab in the fall of 1956, after which they communicated regularly. The following year, Chumakov invited Salk and his wife to visit the USSR to discuss a vaccination program. Donna refused to go, and Salk said the home situation made it impossible for him to come. He later regretted the decision, as that trip might have entrenched the killed vaccine in Russia. Instead, Sabin, with his Russian roots and fluency in the language, collaborated with Chumakov and Anatoli Smorodintsev, director of virology at the USSR Academy of Medical Sciences in Leningrad, to initiate what would become the landmark trial for oral vaccine. Both Russians later received the Lenin Prize for their work.

With the initiation of the Russian trial, Sabin soon pulled ahead of his competitors. A political upheaval interrupted Koprowski's Congo study before its completion, and when Cox's live vaccine caused seven cases of paralytic polio in Dade County and twenty-three in West Berlin, Lederle dropped his vaccine. Millions of Russian children swallowed Sabin's live vaccine without mishap. In September of 1959, at the Sixth European Symposium on Poliomyelitis in Munich, Sabin announced that 4.5 million people in the Soviet Union, Czechoslovakia, Mexico, Poland, and Malaya had received his vaccine. Smorodintsev and Chumakov presented data showing elevated antibody titers, no toxicity, and no reversion to virulence.

Some virologists questioned the veracity of the Russian data.[23] Rumors began to spread that Russian physicians had been told not to report polio cases in patients who had received the vaccine. Sabin blamed anti-Soviet sentiment. At a National Institutes of Health workshop, he was aghast when, after the Soviets presented their data, Charles Armstrong, an old-time polio researcher, said he was not prepared to accept their safety data since he did not think the Soviets "had a very great regard for life." Before Sabin could defend his Russian colleagues, Viktor Ahdanov, the deputy minister of health, replied: "Dr. Armstrong, I would like for you to know that the regard we have, the feeling for the well-being of our children in the Soviet Union is no less than the feeling which you have for your own children."[24] To settle the concern, the World Health Organization (WHO) dispatched Yale epidemiologist Dorothy Horstman to Russia to review the data. After three months, she sent the WHO a "guarded but favorable" report.[25] Preparations to vaccinate the seventy million Soviets under age twenty ensued.

Salk now realized that if he wanted use of the killed vaccine to continue, he would have to go on the offensive. If economics, not scientific logic, drove vaccine choice, he needed an innovative way to make his vaccine more appealing. By adding mineral oil adjuvant, he could achieve the same antibody levels with one shot that previously had required three. And since adjuvant allowed him to use a reduced amount of antigen, he could add diphtheria, tetanus, and smallpox to the single shot to prevent the major childhood diseases. Nevertheless, Salk knew mineral oil adjuvant would be a stumbling block for US trials, as the Biologics Control Laboratory had declined to approve it for his influenza vaccine. So, looking beyond American borders, he suggested the Israeli Ministry of Health add adjuvant to their country's vaccine.

By this point it was too late. On April 24, 1960, Sabin initiated "Sabin Sundays," when thousands of Cincinnati residents lined up outside churches and schools to take what they understood to be a life-saving vaccine. Debbe Sabin recounted how the slogan "Sabin Oral Sunday" was posted across Cincinnati. "People wore SOS badges, and SOS signs were put up on buses and billboards as newspapers promoted vaccination days."[26] The "sugar cube vaccine" was given to 180,000 children, and the surgeon general pronounced the live, oral preparation effective and harmless. Henceforth, it was referred to as the Sabin vaccine.

Sabin began campaigning vigorously for a switch to his vaccine. The health commissioner of Hamilton County, Ohio, complained to Surgeon General Luther Terry that Sabin was pressuring him to participate in the distribution of his oral vaccine to the point of harassment.[27] That summer, when three adults developed paralysis and died after taking the oral vaccine, some physicians worried that Sabin had unleashed live virus in the community. He contended that they did not have polio. "We were there to do the autopsies," he stated.[28] Use of the vaccine continued.

Salk was circumspect in his pronouncements, at least at that point in time. When interviewed on *Meet the Press*, he said, "What I try to do is simply to present the facts and then it is up to those who practice medicine to make the decision."[29] Yet the major medical advisors and decision-makers were moving toward the Sabin vaccine. So Salk paid a visit to the AMA, where he emphasized to the executive vice president that the principal problem with the killed vaccine was "failure to *use* vaccine rather than vaccine failure." Recent outbreaks had been confined largely to poorly vaccinated neighborhoods. "It is clear from the foregoing that we are confronted with a social problem not a technical or scientific one," he said.[30] He urged the AMA to consider mandatory vaccination with the killed vaccine.

On June 28, 1961, the AMA House of Delegates formally endorsed the Sabin vaccine, recommending mass, community-wide vaccination. Salk sent a lengthy critique of their action, expressing surprise at the AMA's departure from its long-established policy of not recommending one biological over another.[31] When he asked if he could present additional information to the AMA Council on Drugs, he was told, "Your appearance before the full Council would not be practical at this time."[32] Instead he could send comments to the council secretary. Some physicians thought this egregious. "To cause such action to be taken," one wrote the AMA president, "without even having Dr. Salk present is the most shameful treatment of this humble, devoted scientist who only a few years ago was honored by your association, the nation, and the world for his epoch-making contribution to mankind."[33] The president responded that the "majority of virologists" felt the Salk vaccine could never eliminate polio.[34]

David Bodian did not agree with the "majority of virologists." In a widely circulated journal, the Johns Hopkins virologist wrote that the AMA document recommending a change to the Sabin vaccine contained statements that were unproven in some cases, erroneous in others.[35] Three crises had arisen already regarding its use, Bodian pointed out. First, the vaccine had been implicated in cases of paralysis. Second, investigators had reported finding a new virus, SV40, contaminating the monkey kidney tissue in which poliovirus had been grown. Not much was known about the effects of this virus on humans, but it did cause cancer in hamsters. Third, the Type 3 strain appeared unstable and could revert to its original virulence. He called the AMA recommendation "rash" and "irresponsible."[36] When asked about Bodian's objections, Sabin said, "David Bodian [is] the voice of Basil O'Connor," suggesting he parroted the NFIP director's opinions.[37]

In July of 1961, Pfizer Ltd. of England offered the first commercial Sabin vaccine. A year later, the UK minister of health announced the decision to make oral vaccine routine; Canada followed, then others. In addition to the hundred million people immunized in the Soviet Union and its allied countries, another thirty million around the world received Sabin's vaccine that year. Perceiving an imminent change in US policy, Salk sent Surgeon General Terry a note in early August saying that if Terry planned to license the oral vaccine, he would like to speak with him first and make his case against such a move.[38] The surgeon general met with Salk on August 13. Four days later, he licensed Type 1 Sabin vaccine; two months after that he licensed Type 2.

Meanwhile, the AMA president told Salk that he could expect to see a revision of its statement in the near future. "I hope that I will not again learn of the Council's revised report via the newspapers," Salk wrote, requesting a copy prior to publication.[39] The reply to his request did not come from the president but from John Youmans, director of scientific activities, who appeared to be the president's hatchet man: "With regard to your hope that you will not again learn of a Council on Drug report 'via the newspapers,' you seemed to imply that you were entitled to special consideration in the matter." They were not obligated to furnish him with prepublished reports. Youmans went on to admonish Salk for stretching the truth. "You did not," he wrote, "as you imply, learn of the Council's report of last June via the newspapers"; a telegram to the AMA suggested that Salk knew of the report before it had even reached the AMA House of Delegates. Furthermore, he did not know how Salk had obtained what was a private communication. "Your actions concerning the report, were not, in my opinion, in keeping with either good taste or good ethics."[40] Salk was shocked by this vitriolic scolding— obviously reflective of the medical community's attitude toward him. He sent back a note acknowledging receipt of Youman's "astonishing" letter and included the newspaper clipping from which he had learned about the AMA's decision.[41]

In January of 1962, Salk attended the WHO meeting in Geneva, where he met with Viktor Zhdanov, director of Moscow's Institute of Virology. "I gathered from him," Salk wrote to David Bodian, "the failure of the incidence of polio in the USSR to show the expected decline and the large number of individuals who...developed paralytic polio was somewhat disappointing."[42] Zhdanov expressed an increased interest in using the Salk vaccine in the USSR. "The story from Russia is fascinating," Salk told O'Connor. "The last word has not yet been uttered on live virus vaccine—but when it is, the word may be—DEAD."[43]

Acceptance of Sabin's vaccine, however, was accelerating. On March 27, 1962, the surgeon general licensed Type 3, leaving the choice of vaccine—Salk or Sabin—up to the individual physician. The AMA agreed, modifying its prior stance, which had favored Sabin's vaccine. Three days later, Pfizer announced the availability of oral vaccine in the United States. Sabin recommended that all children and adults get vaccinated, even those who had received the Salk vaccine, since there was no proof that it provided lifetime immunity. And if an entire city received vaccine on the same day, it was more likely to "break the chain of transmission."[44] Omaha, Nebraska, followed Cincinnati in initiating Sabin Oral Sundays. Ninety percent of Cleveland's population turned out to take the oral vaccine, and it was credited with halting polio outbreaks in Syracuse and San Antonio. Sabin was emerging as the new face in the fight against polio. The media portrayed him as the son of poor Russian immigrants, "a man who has fought hard for everything he has accomplished and, in a sense, is still fighting."[45]

Among those few who sided with Salk in opposition to the oral vaccine was the director of the Communicable Disease Center, Alex Langmuir. The number of polio cases had fallen to 2 percent of that prior to the field trial. He saw no reason to revaccinate those who had received the Salk vaccine. O'Connor agreed and held a press conference at which he vehemently opposed revaccination and leveled his guns at the surgeon general. Saying Terry was "flying in the face of facts and for reasons that might not best be questioned," O'Connor accused him of "withholding from the public the true picture of the need…to promote the preferential sale of the second vaccine to do what's already been done by one.…Half-truths and nonscientific innuendos and implications" had no place where the health of the public was concerned.[46] He sent a letter to the editor of *Washington Star*, decrying the advice to revaccinate those already protected with the killed vaccine. "There is no sane or scientific basis."[47] Yet widespread oral vaccination continued.

On June 14, 1962, a fifty-six-year-old man stopped at a mobile polio vaccine station in Brooklyn, where he and his wife were given a sugar cube laced with a red liquid, the Type 3 Sabin vaccine.[48] On July 3, he suddenly began dragging his left foot. By the time he got home from work, his entire leg was weak. He had a fever and went to bed. When he awoke, he couldn't move either leg; he was paralyzed from the hips down. His case puzzled doctors, who performed a number of tests, including multiple lumbar punctures. A month later, his spinal fluid tested positive for poliovirus.

In December, a physician wrote Eli Lilly about an unusual situation in a colleague.[49] This previously unvaccinated forty-five-year-old ophthalmologist had taken the Sabin vaccine. Fourteen days later, he developed a severe headache and paralysis of one arm. Over the next three days, he deteriorated, experiencing paralysis in the other arm, double vision, confusion, and difficulty breathing. A tracheotomy was performed, and he was now on a respirator. His spinal fluid was teeming with the Type 3 poliovirus. The physician asked if Eli Lilly had encountered this in other vaccinees.

More cases followed. Sabin denied a link to his vaccine; a certain number of people, especially in epidemic areas, could have contracted the disease prior to taking the vaccine. The mere fact that a paralyzed person excreted live virus in their stool did not mean the vaccine had caused the paralysis, since those vaccinated were expected to excrete virus. Besides, several other neurologic diseases had the same clinical findings as polio. Nonetheless, Canada withdrew the vaccine containing Type 3 poliovirus from its market.

When the number of reported cases of paralysis reached sixteen, Surgeon General Terry appointed a review committee, which included Sabin but not Salk. The group found that most vaccine-associated cases had occurred in adults who had received Type 3 poliovirus. They recommended that mass vaccination programs using Type 1 and 2 vaccine in all age groups should continue but that Type 3 be limited to children and adults at high risk, which included those traveling to hyperendemic areas or living in epidemic areas. Terry followed their advice.

In response, O'Connor wrote to Anthony Celebrezze, President John F. Kennedy's secretary of Health, Education, and Welfare, with a copy to the president. Government figures had shown that by the end of 1961, polio had been reduced by 97 percent with the killed vaccine. "In these circumstances," he stated, "I am at a total loss to understand why the Surgeon General has so ardently supported the idea for some time that all the people of this country should be treated with live polio vaccine *even though they have received a full course of the killed vaccine* and even though during this period the Surgeon General admitted there was a *'very small risk'* in using the live virus." After enumerating a number of other problems with the oral vaccine, he concluded: "The fact that he would encourage the use of *any* vaccine that had any risk connected with it, except in what may be described as a 'disaster situation,' is quite frightening to one who is just a layman."[50] Nonetheless, after 1962, the Sabin vaccine became the polio vaccine of choice in the United States.

◈

WHILE TRYING TO treat cancer with antiserum and devise a oneshot polio vaccine, Salk undertook yet another endeavor, the creation of a research institute.[51] He believed his life's purpose was to help aid suffering humanity. A challenging list of problems—infectious diseases, cancer, heart disease, disorders of the nervous system—presented itself. He had nearly eradicated polio because he had been granted the academic freedom and funds to pursue his ideas. Given the same circumstances, with the obstacles removed, innovative scientists could start to rid the world of these other ills.

Salk set forth to change the academic research paradigm. He envisioned an institute of experimental medicine, a scientific haven within the University of Pittsburgh where the results of basic biological research would be applied to human disease. Investigators working side by side would have a far greater effect than the sum of their separate contributions. Although he defended the autonomy of the investigator, Salk believed that an understanding of societal ills should underlie their work. "Since it is not for the glorification of the individual," he had written in a note to himself in May of 1957, "but for the service of humanity that these activities are or should be oriented, the goal should be to solve a problem and not merely to work on a problem."[52]

The concept was not new. Prominent research institutes included the Pasteur Institute in Paris, Philadelphia's Wistar Institute, the Carnegie Institution in Washington, DC, and the Rockefeller Institute for Medical Research in New York. Salk had visited many of these, but he considered his model unique. Investigators would not be restricted to one area of study, such as at Philadelphia's Henry Phipps Institute, which concentrated on tuberculosis, or the Carnegie Institution, which focused on the origin of life. Nor would research be prescribed, such as at the Mellon Institute, which hired scientists to solve specific industrial problems. Academic freedom would prevail. Most scientists spent valuable time writing research grants; at his institute research costs would be covered, providing "unencumbered time for work and contemplation," Salk proposed. "The only limitation that should exist would be in the imagination."[53]

Salk had anticipated full endorsement from Dean McEllroy and Chancellor Fitzgerald, but the players were changing. When Fitzgerald retired from the University of Pittsburgh in 1956, forty-two-year-old Edward Litchfield succeeded him. An ambitious administrator, Litchfield vowed to transform Pitt from a mediocre school into a premier university. He hadn't been in office long before Salk approached him. When he began to unfold his proposal for a research institute, Litchfield saw that this world-famous scientist was offering to help him realize his aspirations, and they came to a cordial understanding.

The trouble began when they started to work out the details. Salk proposed a staff comprising four senior researchers, plus a number of junior faculty, all with appointments in the medical school, guaranteed salaries, and complete scientific freedom. When he recommended a self-governing institute with its own funding, Litchfield began to hear grumbling from the faculty. "Jonas was a very independent operator, and he wanted to run his own show without anyone telling him what to do," the chair of the Department of Medicine Jack Myers said. "We had a team, and it was important that we held together to build the school without feathering our own nests. Jonas was more interested in his own nest."[54] Engrossed in his work, Salk had never taken time to develop close relationships with other faculty. That single-mindedness, which contributed to his success, led some faculty to consider him arrogant and secretive. "They considered Jonas a threat," recalled Bernard Fisher, a Pitt cancer surgeon.[55] Sensing potential trouble, the chancellor put together a committee, composed of nationally known researchers and industrialists, to advise him. This move troubled Salk. Litchfield had delegated his institute's future to an advisory committee in which he had no say.

This latest setback weighed heavily on Salk, and his spirits reached a low point. He had been drawn back into the politics of polio vaccination; his cancer work was proving less fruitful than anticipated; and now his dream for an institute had been delegated to a committee. He struggled with depression and in November of 1957 wrote O'Connor, "I recognize that the disease that has enveloped me is moving deeper and deeper into the relationships that have sustained me." He feared it might even alter his relationship with O'Connor. "I know the futility that I have felt, time and again, in dwelling on how to resolve what seems to be something insoluble." He didn't specify if he was talking about his work or his marriage, or both. "I shall bear in mind," he continued, "the primary purpose of my life—to be of service to society." He knew he had injured others in living such a focused life. On the other hand, if deterred, he would no longer be of value to the public. He called this a "grim prospect" and thanked O'Connor for his affection during this "crisis." In closing, he assured his great friend, "I've not lost hope."[56]

After two months, Litchfield's advisory committee sent their report, but the proposal for a research institute remained in what Salk called "a state of suspension."[57] Litchfield's true colors began to show as he centralized authority at Pitt; faculty started calling him "King Edward."[58] Salk no longer considered him a crusader leading his faculty to great heights, but a dictator who would not cede control. "His view," Salk complained, "was that one could administer a science institute as one did a prison, a university, a church."[59] Eighteen months had passed since he had first presented his vision to the chancellor. During that time, Salk had wavered between feeling euphoric and pessimistic, hopeful and ultimately discouraged. In April of 1959, he told Vice Chancellor Edmund McCluskey, "I've had it."[60] He was leaving for Europe and would not be back until early June. He hoped to gain perspective while away.

Salk traveled alone to Amsterdam, London, Rome, Stockholm, and Copenhagen, where he attended ceremonial dinners and award banquets and met numerous dignitaries, much of which he disliked. His reasons for the trip were unclear. Perhaps the frustrations with the chancellor and his strained marriage made him seek an escape. Maybe he planned an anti-live-virus-vaccine campaign, or his conscience urged him to fulfill his obligations to the many who had been gracious in recognizing him but whose invitations he had declined. Most likely he was searching for an answer to his private dilemma—what to do with the rest of his life. Whatever motivated him, when he was abroad he found himself beloved, appreciated, his ideas accepted.

Salk returned home with a fresh outlook and renewed spirit. His dream for a research institute had not died. "What was great about this place," he said of the University of Pittsburgh, "was that one could pioneer. It was one of the last frontiers of medicine east of the Mississippi River."[61] Still, Salk recognized that the time had come for him to leave.

Two Cultures Under One Roof

"I HAVE NEVER been so comfortably ensconced and so ready to work at this hour of the morning as at this moment," Salk wrote in a note to himself in the summer of 1959.[1] He may have been submerged by the politics in Pittsburgh, but he had resurfaced. Refreshed by his travels abroad, he once again thought about founding an institute. Except now Salk's concept had a new dimension.

While he was in Europe, the English physicist and novelist Sir Charles Percy Snow had aroused the academic community when he delivered a public lecture at Cambridge entitled "The Two Cultures." "We are living in the middle of two cultures," Snow had proclaimed, "which have scarcely any contact at all—the traditional non-scientific culture and an up-and-coming scientific one. They are startlingly different, not only in their intellectual approach, but even more so in their climate of thought and their moral attitudes."[2] These two groups, literary intellectuals and scientists, rarely communicated, and when they did, they were unreceptive, often antagonistic. Lawmakers, for example, seldom took into account the implications of science when determining public policy, and scientists didn't always consider the best interests of mankind when conducting research. Snow's writings on the topic generated widespread debate throughout Europe and America.

Snow's ideas did more than resonate with Salk; published as a book, *The Two Cultures and the Scientific Revolution* became his bible. "It is not only that the gap exists, but that the posture of scientists and artists seems to be back-to-back, rather than face-to-face," he wrote a colleague. "As each of them moves forward in his own way, the gap increases."[3] This was strikingly visible at many of the finest universities, where each discipline was anchored in a separate department; scientific institutes and intellectual think tanks stood as isolated silos. "There ought to be a place," Salk thought, "for biological studies but which also contained the conscience of man."[4]

That summer, the family was vacationing at Deep Creek Lake, where Donna likely hoped to recapture her husband's attention. Yet there were no walks in the woods, family games of Monopoly, or evening chats around a campfire. C. P. Snow's ideas preoccupied Salk. "This is being dictated in the quiet of the early morning while sitting in front of our lake cottage," Salk wrote a British friend that summer. "My eyes rest on a view that induces the kind of serenity one likes to feel even if only from time to time. The quiet of the lake…and the beauty of the hills in the distance make this as close to heaven as I will ever get."[5] He wanted a setting like this for his institute—a place whose natural splendor engendered an atmosphere conducive to harmony and creativity. As he gazed at the lake, his spirits rose. The quest to fulfill his dream began to take the form of a crusade.

What seemed easy while lying in a hammock at Deep Creek Lake would present enormous challenges. An institute required substantial resources, and when he left Pittsburgh, Salk would relinquish financial support from wealthy community benefactors. Still, he had an ally in Basil O'Connor. "There are many more great gifts still within you," Salk wrote to his old friend, "of which mankind, and even you yourself, are still unaware."[6] With polio almost vanquished, the NFIP had to reposition itself. It dropped "Infantile Paralysis" from its name, becoming the National Foundation (NF), and was trying to engage its volunteers in taking on birth defects and arthritis when O'Connor suddenly announced his intent to introduce a sense of social accountability into science. He told his puzzled staff that gifted scientists needed a place where they could work in "an atmosphere of intellectual imagination," free from academic restrictions. Such a vital endeavor should not be left to the government or universities to fund, however. "Time is appropriate for the creation [of such an institute] by the public," O'Connor said, meaning the National Foundation.[7]

Although the NF board may have wondered where this unexpected pronouncement had come from, O'Connor and Salk had been talking about the possibility privately for at least two years. In May of 1957, while relaxing together at Warm Springs, Salk had proposed a partnership between the NF and an institute devoted to the evolving problems of humanity. A year later, he had sent O'Connor a thirteen-page letter making his case. He was not proposing that the NF build and operate its own institute, although he could see how a properly configured institution could further the goals of the Foundation by tackling birth defects, arthritis, and other diseases in which it had an interest. "The future of the NF," he contended, "would be less at the mercy of unoriented, undirected, and inadequately motivated scientists than is presently the case." He visualized an independent, autonomous administration, "with the understanding and control exercised through the transfer of funds for the support of research." NF-supported investigators would have censured Salk had they known he was proposing to siphon off Foundation research dollars. And as Salk knew, no self-respecting scientist would agree to join an institute in which O'Connor held the controlling stock. So Salk never revealed the bargain struck between the two when he began to recruit scientists and trustees. That would become apparent— and a problem—with time. For the moment, however, it seemed to be the means to reach his end. After three years of feeling adrift, Salk told O'Connor, "This is the answer to the question as to what it is I would like to do."[8]

With O'Connor's encouragement, Salk began to seek the ideal location for his institute. When word of his intent became public, a number of cities welcomed him. Initially he found Palo Alto, California, adjacent to Stanford University particularly appealing; the medical school had recently relocated to the main campus and already boasted a number of Nobel laureates. Although the faculty's reception seemed lukewarm, the liberal atmosphere and temperate climate attracted Salk. O'Connor confirmed the National Foundation's support to Stanford's president, and

Salk told Donna and the boys to prepare to move to Palo Alto. That was when Leo Szilard, a nuclear physicist who had played a major role in developing the atom bomb, suggested he consider La Jolla. Szilard, then at the University of Chicago, had been talking with Salk about institutes for some time. Now he informed Salk that the University of California planned to construct a new campus in San Diego County, and he had reason to believe the school would welcome him and his institute.[9]

Salk found it hard not to like San Diego—a sparkling white city situated on a natural harbor dotted with sailboats, average temperatures ranging from fifty-five to seventy degrees year-round, and cloudless skies.[10] Its economy had been based on its canneries, and with the location of a large naval base and Consolidated Aircraft Corporation there, San Diego had grown from a small town before the war to a city of a half million by the 1950s. Located at the southern tip of California, it had a similar kind of frontier feel to Pittsburgh, which initially had attracted Salk. On his first visit to San Diego, he noted the strong sense of community, although he found the intellectual climate somewhat unformed. The city had made national news when one of its citizens, Theodor Geisel, better known as Dr. Seuss, published *The Cat in the Hat*; Jack in the Box opened its first drive-through restaurant; and *Some Like It Hot*, starring Jack Lemmon and Marilyn Monroe, was filmed at Hotel del Coronado.

La Jolla lay to the north of San Diego. Its seven-mile stretch of coastline, with some of the most beautiful beaches in the world, made La Jolla worthy of its name, initially spelled La Joya, which means "the jewel" in Spanish. The Scripps Institution of Oceanography is located there, and in 1956 the University of California (UC) regents and President Clark Kerr authorized the establishment of a new campus, similar to Berkeley, in La Jolla. Roger Revelle, director of Scripps, assumed leadership for UC San Diego. Construction was set to begin in 1960.

When they first met in August of 1959, Revelle told Salk about the proposed campus and about his vision: the university community, Scripps, a growing number of electronic groups, and Salk's institute would form a "City of the Mind."[11] Revelle told Kerr that their plans had impressed Salk. "On our side, we liked him a great deal," he said, "both as a man and as a scientist."[12] He described Salk as modest, serious, idealistic, and experienced. And he had money in hand for an institute. If one of the world's most famed scientists moved to San Diego, bringing a cadre of elite researchers, it would lend distinction to the nascent university at a critical stage.

For his part, Salk found Revelle welcoming. He wrote Edward R. Murrow that he was taken with the beauty of the coast, the climate, and the opportunity "for pioneering...without being surrounded too tightly by the past and by academic prejudices in an already established university community."[13] And when he visited Torrey Pines Mesa, a spectacular tract of land overlooking the Pacific Ocean, he was mesmerized. Located adjacent to a state nature reserve, it was populated with indigenous, picturesque Torrey pine trees. Although he had settled on Palo Alto, the possibilities he saw in La Jolla were so powerful that he told Murrow, "I found myself quite tortured for some weeks thereafter."[14]

In the midst of this indecision, Salk's father underwent elective back surgery, after which he developed an acute arrhythmia. "My father had a coronary," he wrote Hazel O'Connor on November 25. "Complications from this developed, and he's rallied twice. However, the situation is very grave."[15] Daniel Salk died the next day at the age of sixty-nine.

Salk continued to pursue La Jolla as a possible site for his institute. On a subsequent visit in early January of 1960, San Diego mayor Charles Dail, a polio survivor, showed him several potential areas he would be happy to offer him.[16] At the end of the day, Dail took him to see lot 1324 on the Torrey Pines Mesa. They arrived just before sunset as the azure sky took on shades of yellow and orange. Standing on a cliff, looking out to sea, Salk saw waves breaking in lines on the sandy beach with streaks of gold flashing through the water. "Looking back upon the land behind me," he reflected years later, "I saw a breathtaking site."[17] The craggy terrain with its deep ravines was dotted with Torrey pine trees, grown crooked from the ocean breeze. With almost no other structure in sight, its tranquility moved him deeply. "I instantly recognized it to be what I had been seeking." Here at the juncture of land, sea, and sky, spirits could soar; imagination could thrive. Here he would build his institute.

❦

TO START, SALK sought an architect who could design a structure that reflected his vision. When he viewed the works of those recommended to him, he found them pedestrian. Then a colleague called to say he had just heard Louis Kahn lecture about a research building he had designed for the University of Pennsylvania. Salk had to meet him.

In 1901 Kahn was born Leiser-Itze Schmuilowsky in what is now Estonia.[18] He became scarred for life at the age of three when he reached into the stove and picked up some embers, which flared up, scorching his face and hands. His family emigrated when he was five, settling in Philadelphia, where his father changed the family name to Kahn and his son's name to Louis. In grammar school, Louis's teacher noted his talent for drawing, and he was selected to attend Philadelphia's Public Industrial Art School. Enthralled by design in high school, he studied architecture at the University of Pennsylvania. Kahn's first job was as a draftsman for a city architect. Feeling constrained by what he considered the old guard, he helped found the Architectural Research Group, composed of young architects who embraced the social consciousness of European modernists. Kahn spent the next decade designing public housing. Although charismatic, he was quixotic and at times uncompromising; his temperament curtailed nearly every partnership.

Initially, nothing distinguished Kahn's work. That changed in the early 1950s after he spent three months as an architect in residence at the American Academy in Rome. Visiting ruins in Italy, Greece, and Egypt, Kahn studied how ancient architects considered light and form in their colossal structures. Upon his return, he developed a unique style in which he created structures monumental in appearance yet practical and comfortable for those who would inhabit them. At the age of fifty, he entered the most productive period of his career. The Yale University Art Gallery, designed in 1951, is considered his first great work. It was the awe-inspiring Alfred Newton Richards Medical Research Laboratories at the University of Pennsylvania, however, that brought him renown. Discarding the traditional laboratory design, he constructed interconnected towers of precast concrete in a pinwheel formation. Its open, studio-style laboratories, which facilitated the conduct of research while fostering connectedness between investigators, changed the way architects thought about science buildings. A 1961 solo exhibit at the Museum of Modern Art would place him in the vanguard of American architecture.

Though embraced by mainstream organizations such as the American Institute of Architects, Kahn remained a maverick, conducting his private life with the same abandon as his art. Although not physically attractive—short and heavyset, his face disfigured by his childhood burns, his prematurely white hair unkempt, and his clothes always rumpled—three women devoted themselves to him and bore him children. In 1930, he married Esther Israeli, with whom he had one daughter, Sue Ann Kahn. In 1945, he began an affair with Anne Tyng, his architectural partner, who bore him another daughter, Alexandra. Later, he added a third family with landscape architect Harriet Pattison and their son Nathaniel. "Clearly he chose perfection in his work at the expense of his personal life," Nathaniel indicated in his award-winning documentary on his father's life.[19]

At their first meeting in December of 1959, Salk comprehended why Kahn had gained a reputation as a philosopher among architects. "Lou had a way of capturing people and their imaginations," his young associate, Jack MacAllister, recalled. When they toured the Richards Medical Research Laboratories, Salk felt Kahn was the architect who could actualize his vision. "There was never any question from that day on who his architect would be," MacAllister said.[20] Two months later, as Salk, O'Connor, and Kahn stood on the Torrey Pines Mesa, looking out to the Pacific Ocean, Kahn said that he envisioned a monument to science and humanity infused by light with the blue sky and sea as a backdrop. Captivated by Kahn, Salk wanted his institute built straightaway. Assuming imminent full endorsement by the University of California and the city of San Diego, he moved ahead.

On March 15, 1960, the National Foundation granted Salk's institute an endowment of one million dollars a year for ten years and another one million annually to support operations.[21] Mayor Dail offered Salk seventy choice acres on the Torrey Pines Mesa in lot 1324. Two days later, Salk announced his resignation from the University of Pittsburgh. His plans had been set in motion. That's when the trouble began.

Revelle thought that the land Salk coveted had been promised to UC San Diego. In addition, he was starting to fret about having an institute that touted freedom from university constraints built in his backyard. Initially unaware of these concerns, Salk first learned of the brewing conflict from headlines in a local newspaper. "I've just returned to Pittsburgh," he wrote Revelle, "from where I wanted to see, with the additional perspective of distance and time, the events of the past week. It seemed until then that pleasant dreams were about to be fulfilled. The events of the days that have just gone by for me have been like a nightmare." Revelle's seeming about-face baffled him. "That which attracted me...upon my first visit," Salk continued, "was your friendship and interest....I was taken with your idea of contributing in a missionary sense to a larger cause." On his second visit, Salk had detected some coolness to the concept of a separate institute. Before he left, however, they had had a long talk, and he thought they understood each other. "If I had had any idea whatsoever that our interest in the Torrey Pines Mesa location would have led to the situation that developed last week, I can assure you all this would have been prevented." He had been led to believe no confusion existed over the title of the land. "Perhaps I assumed too much and have taken at face value a great deal that I should have seen through and beyond. I neither want to come to La Jolla, at all cost, nor do I want to look at something that would be less than optimal."[22] If they could not resolve their differences, he had a crucial decision to make. He continued like this for eight pages. There is no indication that he ever sent the letter. Perhaps it served as a means of venting. It was clear that he never intended to give up the La Jolla site.

Once again the press chronicled the drama swirling around Salk. While the La Jolla city council, the San Diego city manager, and UC regents were arguing, Salk received letters from Amarillo; Colorado Springs; Lake Placid; Miami; Chatfield, Minnesota; and other places offering large parcels of land for his institute. But he had fallen in love with La Jolla and specifically with the Torrey Pines Mesa.

Over the next three weeks, a series of negotiations took place between Mayor Dail, President Kerr, and Salk. On April 8, 1960, they reached an agreement. Salk would receive property in an area adjacent to the original lot.[23] He may have thought the furor would die down now, but the new lot included public parkland, and a group of citizens tried to block the land transfer in court.[24] Given that a gift of public land required voter agreement, Salk was advised to hire a public relations firm to help secure approval on the upcoming ballot. The firm recommended circulating a

brochure that described the proposed institute, publishing twenty-five fea-
ture and news stories, talks by Salk to the Chamber of Commerce, Pacific
Beach Town Council, and Lions Club, and a televised panel discussion.[25]
Salk took their advice. A flurry of favorable reports resulted.

Less than two weeks before the June ballot, the press announced
that a new compromise agreement had ended the feud between the La
Jolla City Council, the University of California, and Salk. He had withdrawn his request for the parklands. The new proposition would authorize granting city-owned land on Torrey Pines Mesa to be shared by
the institute and UC with twenty-seven acres each. It passed on June 7.[26]
In the end, Salk received the piece of the land at the ocean's edge with
which he originally had been enamored.

⁂

WHILE KAHN WAS designing the institute, Salk began recruiting the
scholars to populate it. Resident fellows, a cadre of humanists and scientists, would work there, fully funded for life; nonresident fellows would
remain at their home universities and come to La Jolla at intervals as a
retreat from their workaday world. Salk's wish list read like a who's who
of the most eminent minds. Once they had learned of his plans, some
scientists smirked behind closed doors; others openly derided him. Salk
was not a member of the National Academy of Sciences nor a serious
Nobel Prize candidate. How did he expect to attract academic lumi-
naries, getting them to leave their posts at top universities or research
institutes and relocate to a relatively small West Coast town with no
university or scientific community? And why would they consider moving
to a hypothetical institute, which was still just a tract of bare land, to join
this pied piper who had the crazy idea of uniting the "two cultures" under
one roof? Perhaps because Salk offered independence from university
regulations and guaranteed funds that required no grant-writing, no paperwork, and no strings. In other words, he offered total academic
freedom.

Among the first Salk pursued was humanist and mathematician
Jacob Bronowski, whose book *Science and Human Values* had caught
Salk's attention.[27] A philosopher of science, Bronowski contended that
science and art were impoverished if segregated. Born in Lodz, Poland,

in 1908 to a haberdasher, Bronowski and his family fled to England as
the Nazis rose to power. While studying mathematics at Cambridge, he
coedited a literary periodical. "All his life, he treated art and science as
the same expression of the human imagination," according to his wife,
Rita Coblentz, a sculptor for whom he had once posed.[28] During World
War II, Bronowski worked in operations research, forecasting the economic impact of bombing, and afterward was sent to Japan to investigate
the consequences of the Hiroshima and Nagasaki attacks. Seeing the
havoc created by the atom bomb firsthand, he became passionate about
the role scientists must play in decisions such as the one that destroyed a
large segment of the Japanese population. Two books, *The Common Sense
of Science* and *Science and Human Values,* followed.

Bruno, as his friends called him, stood less than five feet tall, with
thick glasses and bushy hair. When he talked, he held his hands in front
of him, "the finger-tips touching," the Welsh writer Gwyn Thomas
wrote, "as if guarding a shrine of golden perceptions."[29] He was eloquent
and witty. "I have met a number of brilliant men," MIT professor Bruce
Mazlish said. "Bruno was about the only one who…made you feel after
talking to him, that you, too, had been part of a brilliant exchange."[30]

Bronowski was working as the director of the British National Coal
Board when Salk contacted him. At their first meeting in July of 1960,
Bronowski told Salk, "You have changed the course of my life."[31] He accepted the offer to join Salk's institute, predicting a lasting friendship
between them. Salk had an almost mystical interpretation of Bronowski's
quick response. "Events had caught us in the stream of time," he wrote,
"and brought us together for a purpose."[32] He thought he had found a
soul mate.

Salk's initial list of scholars also included Francis Crick, who with
James Watson had codiscovered the structure of DNA.[33] Crick was born
in Northamptonshire, England, where his father ran a boot factory. As a
child, science fascinated him, and, after an inauspicious start, he secured a
position at Cambridge's Cavendish Laboratory, where he investigated
protein structure using X-ray diffraction. His garrulousness and grating
laugh irritated the director, who said he looked forward to the day Crick
finished his work, got his PhD, and left. But Crick was in no hurry to
leave, and in 1951 Watson joined the laboratory. Fast friends, they set out

to decipher DNA's configuration. Two years later, they determined its double-helix structure and predicted that the precise sequence of the bases was the code that carries genetic information. At thirty-five and still a graduate student, Crick had helped initiate the field of molecular biology.

"I have never seen Francis Crick in a modest mood," Watson wrote.[34] A fair-haired, slender, ebullient man, Crick was described by colleagues as brash and lacking humility. Yet he was kind to Salk. Knowing Crick wanted to continue his work at the Cavendish Laboratory, Salk invited him to become the first nonresident fellow, and Crick accepted. Within the year, he received the Nobel Prize. Those who had laughed at Salk's ambitions stopped laughing.

Next he approached Leo Szilard, the sixty-four-year-old Hungarian-born physicist who had suggested he consider La Jolla for his institute.[35] Szilard and his colleague Enrico Fermi had generated the first controlled, self-sustaining nuclear chain reaction, after which Szilard helped initiate the Manhattan Project, making the case to President Roosevelt that the United States must develop an atom bomb before Germany. He never intended for the bomb to be used against Japan, however, and was so horrified by its decimation that he spent the rest of his life campaigning to control nuclear weapons. Szilard exemplified the melding of the "two cultures." He was a scientist—a physics professor and member of the National Academy of Sciences—and a humanist, the author of *The Voice of the Dolphins and Other Stories*, in which he addresses the nuclear arms race and promotes disarmament. His efforts toward averting war lead to an Atoms for Peace Award. Brilliant and eccentric, he said he conceived his best thoughts in the bath. When Szilard agreed to become a nonresident fellow, he added another luminary to Salk's group.

Jacques Monod, the third scientist Salk invited to become a nonresident fellow, was a French biologist, accomplished cellist, and philosopher of science.[36] For his role in the French Resistance he had been named a knight of the Legion of Honor. His discovery of the regulation of DNA transcription into proteins would lead to a Nobel Prize. Certain to become director of the Pasteur Institute, Monod brought yet more prestige to Salk's institute.

"I am making good progress on the dream we've been dreaming," Salk wrote O'Connor, "and preliminary indications are that there will be no refusals."[37] Attracting nonresident fellows seemed almost effortless. After all, they could continue working in their home laboratories, taking no risk. It was far more difficult to recruit resident fellows, who had to relinquish their academic positions, close their laboratories, and move to La Jolla. These senior scientists had a lot more to lose if Salk's endeavor failed.

High on his wish list of potential resident fellows was Theodore Puck, a University of Colorado geneticist who had determined the number of chromosomes in humans. Salk's courtship dragged on for several years, until Puck eventually declined the proposal. In the meantime, Salk contacted Renato Dulbecco, a world leader in viral carcinogenesis.[38] Born in Catanzaro, Italy, the same year as Salk, Dulbecco now conducted research at the California Institute of Technology (Caltech). In the late fifties, his trainee Howard Temin had stimulated his interest in tumor viruses. They would later share the Nobel Prize with David Baltimore for determining how viral genes are incorporated into a normal cell's genetic material, leading to malignant transformation. Dulbecco would add enormous scientific depth and luster to the institute.

After their first encounter in late 1960, Dulbecco told Salk he found the concept of the institute compelling, but he felt conflicted about accepting the position. Salk tried to entice him with a spacious laboratory overlooking the ocean. At the same time, he appealed to Dulbecco's social conscience, saying he seemed to want to make a contribution and sensed the opportunity in La Jolla. Dulbecco told Salk he could not reach a decision, and since he could not "tolerate this state of uncertainty any longer," he asked to be withdrawn from consideration.[39] Salk replied that he was glad Renato would have "a period of relief from torment"; he had faith in the "healing and clarifying power of time."[40] He had not given up on Dulbecco.

As yet Salk had secured only one resident fellow, Jacob Bronowski. He proceeded to discuss appointments with three other esteemed scientists: Seymour Benzer, Edwin Lennox, and Melvin Cohn. Thirty-nine-year-old Benzer, the son of Polish Jewish immigrants, would one day be known as "the man who took us from genes to behavior."[41] A professor at Purdue University, he was designing one of the first genetic maps. Benzer's enthusiasm for moving to La Jolla was, in large part, linked to that of two other scientists on Salk's list, Edwin Lennox and Melvin Cohn. Salk had already begun conversations with Lennox.[42]

Born in 1920 in Savannah, Georgia, Lennox came from a family of Jewish scholars, including a number of rabbis. Having read Paul de Kriuf's *Microbe Hunters* in his youth, he aspired to be a scientist, not a rabbi, and was now a microbiology professor at New York University. His studies on mechanisms of antibody formation intrigued Salk. A tall, thin man, Lennox was mild-mannered and articulate. Salk was delighted with his enthusiasm. "I think all of us loved the idea of starting something new," Lennox recalled, "with a structure that would be different from the usual structure of universities, and that we would do research and not have other duties." He also embraced the concept of blending the two cultures. During the war, Lennox had worked at Los Alamos on the atom bomb. "All of us who were there had in some sense bad consciences," he said; they wished to make some positive contribution to society.[43]

The third member of the threesome, Melvin Cohn, had received a PhD in biochemistry from New York University.[44] He spent five years working with Monod at the Pasteur Institute, where he was considered Monod's inspiration and the leader of the lab.[45] He then took a professorship at Washington University in Saint Louis to work on antibody production and genetic mechanisms of protein synthesis. Colleagues described him as smart, imaginative, and gregarious. He had just moved to Stanford University when Lennox encouraged Salk to talk with him.

Though Lennox had just started a sabbatical at the Pasteur Institute along with Cohn, Salk continued to court both of them, his efforts bolstered by meetings with Monod, Crick, and Bronowski. Nobel-laureate Paul Berg, another scientist on Salk's list, recounted a visit to Paris during which he spent time with Lennox, Cohn, and Benzer: "We all sat in the cafes, and I listened to these guys with their dreamy visions. Nobody would have any administrative work; they would do their great science, think great thoughts, and somebody else would pay the bills." Berg was skeptical.[46] "In some sense," Lennox said, recalling those days, "we were very innocent to think we would put together an institute like that."[47]

Candidates got caught up in Salk's vision initially, but when reality set in, they wanted to see the organizational structure, including the duties of the board, director, and residents, spelled out in the bylaws before they would agree to join him. The request underscored one of Salk's weaknesses—moving from lofty ideals to practical details and committing them to writing. He sent a draft of the bylaws to Dulbecco and Cohn in the fall of 1960. Dulbecco thought the trustees' charge and its relationship to the scientists was sound, however, he took issue with the director's position. He thought the director should be a resident scientist who represented the fellows' opinions to the trustees. Furthermore, he insisted new members be selected by the entire scientific group. On this, Salk had been vague. "Let us be clear and outspoken," Dulbecco wrote. "This is the crucial point which will decide my future part in the Institute."[48]

Mel Cohn had similar problems. Although he wrote of his respect and affection for Salk, he thought the bylaws did not reflect the goals or spirit of the institute as he understood them. The director seemed to have ultimate power. Cohn preferred more democratic decision-making. "It's entirely unfair," he wrote, "that you, who will certainly be our first director, should be burdened with all of the responsibilities and decisions implied in benevolent despotism while we should be 'kept scientists.'"[49] Salk told Dulbecco he felt the group had "ganged up" on him.[50] The rosy path to his utopia had become overgrown with thorns. He wrote Cohen that his son Darrell, fourteen at the time, had sensed his discouragement and left him a touching note: "Dad, about the institute, you should remember that success is a journey, not a destination."[51]

Meanwhile, with advice from O'Connor, Salk had been assembling the board of trustees. He first asked C. P. Snow who agreed, instructing Salk to drop the "heraldic titles" and stop calling him "Sir Charles."[52] Just as he was planning to come to La Jolla, however, Snow suffered a cardiac arrest during eye surgery. Although his poor health precluded his participation, Snow and Salk remained lifelong friends.

For chairman of the board, Salk wanted the country's best-known scientific administrator, Warren Weaver.[53] A mathematician and civil engineer, Weaver held top administrative posts at the Rockefeller and Alfred P. Sloan Foundations, where he helped advance the careers of young scientists and strove to improve the public's understanding of science. For his work, he won numerous awards, including membership in the National Academy of Sciences, the US Medal of Merit, and being

named an officer in the French Legion of Honor. An ardent book collector, Weaver became fascinated with Lewis Carroll's *Alice in Wonderland*.
He acquired 160 editions in forty-two languages and published a book
on its history.

This would be a difficult recruitment. Weaver had publicly criticized
Salk's model for luring top scientists, who should be training the next
generation of researchers, from their academic teaching duties. On the
contrary, Salk told Weaver, the melding of scientists and humanists should
contribute far more to higher education. At their first meeting, Weaver
questioned Salk sharply. He had seen a number of attempts to set up institutes end in a stalemate. Yet he found himself more enthusiastic than he
had anticipated. The flexibility and freedom in Salk's self-governing community of scholars sounded appealing, as did the conduct of basic biologic
research in a humanitarian environment. He called it the "perfect culmination of what [he] had been struggling to do in the Rockefeller Foundation
since 1932." And he was deeply impressed by Salk. "I thought this is a
perfectly wonderful young man," he recollected, "a very gentle person
[with] a beautiful artistic mind....He spoke almost in parables, almost
using similes and metaphors that a poet might use."[54]

After Salk left, Weaver worried he had been too blunt. "I wonder if
I'll ever see him again," he thought.[55] The next day Salk called to say how
much he enjoyed their conversation and that he appreciated the issues
Weaver had raised. Moreover, he invited Weaver and his wife to La Jolla,
where he used the beauty of the area as a drawing card. Weaver accepted
Salk's offer, which placed one of the country's top scientific administrators at the helm. In addition, Salk made Weaver a nonresident fellow.
The remainder of the board was quite impressive as well: besides Weaver
and O'Connor, it included Gerard Piel, publisher of *Scientific American*;
Edward R. Murrow; and a dean, a judge, and other notables from the
public sector.

Salk now needed to incorporate the institute in order to transfer the
deed from the city and to set up a corporate account so that he could pay
Kahn. Though still facing resistance from his fellows, Salk told Dulbecco
and Cohn that the bylaws could be changed after incorporation. On
December 1, 1960, the institute was established as a nonprofit corporation
in California, and the board of trustees appointed Salk as its director.

To date, all Salk had offered the prospective resident fellows was a promise that the institute would be built, that research funds would be provided for life, and that he would lead the institute in the direction they advised. Nothing was set in writing. Salk knew he needed to provide the fellows a definitive proposal, backed by the National Foundation, with a specific operating date. When he discussed such a proposition with the scientists, he told O'Connor, "Their enthusiasm and morale reached such new heights as to have created a spirit that has not existed heretofore." If they received such assurances, they were willing to make a commitment by July 1, 1961. "If this cannot be done, I will not be able to presume upon this group any longer." Besides the personal stress and the effect on their work, they had to contend with "the additional factor of their colleagues in the academic world who question the wisdom of continuing to have faith and turn down other opportunities."[56]

Money had become a major problem. Although the National Foundation had agreed to donate one million dollars annually toward an endowment and another million annually for operations, Salk still needed to raise funds for construction and equipment. He hired a New York public relations firm run by Victor Weingarten, who assured him the task would be easy, given Salk's popularity. A few months later, Salk received a distressing letter from Weingarten. "In thirteen years' work with an impressive variety of clients, I have never before even remotely experienced such a total bust." Their failure to solicit funds baffled him. Weingarten had started with foundations. "Not one has had the courage of Basil O'Connor." As an alternative, he suggested Salk apply for federal dollars or seek donations from individuals in small amounts. "Saying that I share your disappointment," Weingarten wrote in closing, "doesn't ameliorate the fact that we haven't raised any money."[57]

In his Director's Annual Report a decade later, Salk explained what happened next: "At the end of April, I went to Mr. O'Connor to say that I was forced to abandon the pursuit for the Institute idea because I had tried and had failed to raise even $1 for construction." To his surprise, O'Connor offered to help obtain funds for the buildings if he would agree to one condition—the Institute had to bear his name. Until then it had been called the Institute for Biological Studies. "I was most reluctant to comply with the name change," Salk said.[58] Tom Rivers had warned him that it would appear self-serving and damage his reputation. O'Connor insisted he could not raise money without Salk's name. Although he finally capitulated, Salk decided to put off informing the resident and nonresident fellows as well as those to whom he had offered positions until a more propitious time.

The staff of the National Foundation were shocked by O'Connor's pledge, especially at a time when the Foundation was itself on the brink of bankruptcy. In trying to understand his move, senior staff member Charles Massey surmised it stemmed from a practical agreement: "Jonas saw in O'Connor a way to achieve the financial support that he needed, and O'Connor saw in Jonas a way to maintain the popularity and support of the March of Dimes."[59] Others believed more than that was involved. "I think that O'Connor felt himself as kind of an adventurer and maverick in terms of public health and the application of science to public health problems," March of Dimes archivist David Rose postulated. "Consequently, I think that the idea and enterprise of the Salk Institute for Biological Studies was a great adventure in science for the two men."[60] And, as Massey added, "O'Connor was philosophically susceptible to Jonas's dream of what he called an 'institute of man.'"[61] O'Connor wanted to see it created, and since the National Foundation was an autocracy, that was what would happen.

Confident O'Connor would secure building funds, Salk sent Cohn, Benzer, and Lennox formal offer letters with a generous salary and full research support for life. Cohn hesitated. Salk was asking him to relinquish his position at Stanford University and trust him completely. This he could not do. His decision hinged on a change in the bylaws: the director must share administrative responsibilities with the resident fellows. "[I will] give you the chance now to tell me whether or not we pull together," he wrote Salk, signing the letter, "Affectionately, Mel."[62]

In the fall of 1961, the prospective fellows met with Salk in Paris to try to reach consensus regarding the bylaws. A major sticking point was their relationship with the trustees: they wanted to avoid power struggles; they did not want to accept unilateral decisions made by the board. A document, drawn up on October 23, set forth the basic principles they felt must be incorporated into the bylaws: (1) Current fellows would nominate all potential fellows and the director with the board's approval. (2) Although the board would elect new trustees, the fellows would hold veto power. Salk agreed.

Then on December 8, Salk sent a letter to the group intimating that the proposed changes to the bylaws had to be set aside for the time being. Exasperated, Cohn, Benzer, and Lennox sent a letter signed by all three, reminding Salk that after two years of discussions they had come to an agreement in Paris, yet no modifications to the bylaws had been forthcoming. So they were setting a new deadline: by the end of February 1962, the trustees needed to ratify the changes. "If this understanding cannot be the basis for our association," they wrote, "then a quick response will spare us all further indecision, for in that case, we would definitely withdraw."[63]

Salk's plans were starting to unravel. Jacques Monod, who had already accepted a position as a nonresident fellow, sent Salk a letter saying the cornerstone principle upon which they had agreed in Paris and on which everything else hinged was that the permanent fellows, together with the trustees, constituted the corporation. As Salk had rightly emphasized, he continued, "what is wanted is not only just one more center for research, [but] a community of 'scientist-citizens.' "[64] There was no hope of achieving such a goal if the creative members of this community were excluded from the body that owned and legally represented the institute. His acceptance remained contingent upon the adoption of these principles.

The changes to the bylaws that had been suggested in October reduced the director's role, in a sense, to that of spokesperson for the fellows. Current fellows would nominate all prospective fellows, including the director. Consensus, democracy, equality were the bywords. Up to this point, Salk had been reluctant to share power. On the one hand, he may have been trying to spare these scientists the drudgery of administrative work, and assuming the role of a benevolent dictator would diminish the burden imposed by a democratic process. On the other hand, Salk may have wanted total control over his institute. Likely painful memories of working on the polio vaccine still plagued him; the Committee on Immunization had impeded his every step. He was justifiably leery of rule by majority. Yet he had this group of esteemed scientists within his grasp, and in the end he relinquished control. Now he faced the drudgery of rewriting the bylaws. "I look forward to bringing poliovirus an antiserum," he wrote Cohn, "with far more pleasure than I do amendments to Bylaws."[65] Fortunately, he had strong allies in Francis Crick and Jacques Monod. Although busy with their own work, these two wrote the majority of the revisions. Both wanted the institute and the ideals on which it was founded to come to fruition.

The bylaws amended, Salk returned to Paris and achieved consensus among the prospective fellows. Then in rapid succession, O'Connor swept aside Salk's two biggest impediments. On February 26, 1962, the National Foundation signed a formal agreement with the Salk Institute for Biological Studies, making available $15 million for construction and equipment in addition to the $2 million annually for operating costs and endowment.[66] Salk agreed to initiate another fundraising effort to raise $7 million to help cover building costs. A week later, the board of trustees ratified the new bylaws.[67] With that, Dulbecco accepted Salk's offer. "The log-jam has been broken," Salk wrote Bronowski.[68] "Institute born 7 March," read his telegram to Cohn, Benzer, and Lennox. "Infant vigorous. Parents and family exhausted but happy."[69]

On May 19, 1962, Salk arranged a meeting in New York with all the resident and nonresident fellows to whom he had made offers. This was a bold move; the meeting could have served as a forum for individuals to express their misgivings, spreading concern to others. Nonetheless, Salk's sense of purpose and idealism infused the group, and Warren Weaver as chairman of the board kept them on course. At the end of two days, Salk secured his institute. "I think all of us recognize that this success is the just outcome of your unflagging zeal," Bronowski wrote to him. "It was a fine day to see you bring the ship into harbor all flags flying."[70]

On June 1, 1962, the popular journal *Science* announced the creation of the Institute for Biological Studies in La Jolla, California. Resident fellows included Seymour Benzer, Jacob Bronowski, Melvin Cohn, Renato Dulbecco, Edwin Lennox, and Jonas Salk. Francis Crick, Jacques Monod, Leo Szilard, and Warren Weaver comprised the nonresident fellows. Jonas Salk would serve as director, Gerald Piel as president, and Warren Weaver as chairman of the board of trustees. "I've seen a list of several of the people that Dr. Salk hopes to get," a colleague had told

Weaver a couple of years earlier. "If Dr. Salk could get half of them, this would instantaneously be the best place in the world! But I don't think he can."[71] Salk had done better than that. The man whom the American scientific community had shunned was able, in over just two years, to attract nine of the world's most creative scholars, the first step in fulfilling his dream of uniting the two cultures under one roof.

18

The Price of a Masterpiece

WHENEVER LOUIS KAHN and Jonas Salk met, their vivacity filled the room. In Kahn, Salk felt that he had found the perfect architect to give his vision structure. When he articulated his desire that the institute be a work of art in which great minds could flourish, Kahn understood. Collaborators from the start, they shared each other's "metaphors and allusions," architectural scholar Daniel Friedman wrote, including "monastic seclusion and spirituality, peripatetic learning, the scientific and mystical body."[1] Kahn assured Salk that he would design a functional building. Yet any architect could do that. This building needed to be infused with humanism and spirituality.[2] Salk agreed. Perched on the cliff overlooking the sea, it should stimulate the fellows to see themselves from different points of view. Such discussions inspired Kahn. "There are few clients who can understand philosophically the institutes they are creating," he told architectural historian Esther McCoy.[3] "Dr. Salk is an exception." And on his relationship with Kahn, Salk reflected thirty years later: "Lou was a poet, a mystic but a realist as well, someone who combines the intuitive with the rational.... We could express ideas freely and, whether his or mine, they soon took form.... Our encounter transformed us both."[4]

Kahn's design team included Spanish architect Carlos Enrique Vallhonrat, his chief assistant; Fred Langford, an expert in architectural concrete; and Jack MacAllister. Only twenty-two at the time, MacAllister met with Salk weekly to decipher his wishes. Concerned that Salk might not want to work with someone so young, MacAllister grew a beard, trying to look older. He need not have worried; he found Salk to be a gentle, considerate man.

With its undulating terrain and division by a ravine, the twenty-seven-acre mesa on which Salk's institute would be built proved to be challenging.[5] On March 15, 1960, Kahn presented his initial concept—an arrangement of three elements: the working spaces which comprised the laboratories and studies; a meeting house which contained a communal dining room, auditorium, seminar rooms, library, and recreation center; and residencies for fifty visiting scholars. He considered the laboratories to be the site for "independent discovery" and the meeting house as the setting for "collective reflection."[6] These three elements were positioned around a central canyon, with the labs overlooking its southern end, the residencies along its western edge, and the meeting house at the north end on a cliff above the ocean. As they talked, Salk recalled the peaceful cloisters he had seen at the Convent of Saint Francis in Assisi, Italy. That was what he wanted—a cloistered garden and a colonnade. He suggested that the studies be placed alongside the laboratories, "like a necklace strung along a building," providing the basis for the colonnade.[7] And he insisted each lab have a view of the ocean, every study a view of the garden court. "I would like to invite Picasso to the laboratory," Salk said.[8] Kahn promised to deliver.

Salk, Kahn, and MacAllister traveled to New York to present the plans to O'Connor. When O'Connor saw what amounted to an enormous compound, of much larger scale and greater expense than he had been led to believe, he quipped, "Even your name can't raise that kind of money, Jonas."[9] Kahn assured O'Connor that the plans would be scaled back—"more realistic as I develop the architectural interpretation of space requirements," he said.[10]

Kahn and Salk's relationship, which had radiated with conviviality and collegiality, began to fray a bit as their differing temperaments surfaced. Determination defined Salk. Once set on a goal, he wanted it realized expeditiously and rarely deviated from his course. Kahn seldom adhered to a timetable, a trait Salk had failed to discover from those who had previously engaged the architect. If he had talked to those involved in construction of the Richards Medical Research Laboratories, Salk would have learned that the project finished late, way over budget, and with substantial tension between Kahn and the faculty who would work in the labs.[11] And Salk may have heard Kahn described as spontaneous, disorganized, whimsical. Perhaps Kahn's rumpled suit and unkempt hair should have forewarned him. "Architecture's not about chewing pencils and spitting out ideas," Kahn used to say.[12] Ideas had to incubate.

Salk insisted on involving himself in all aspects of the design. "My father was obsessed with details," his son Peter said, recalling the time his mother asked him to clean the stove.[13] She came in later to find the stove pulled away from the wall and his father cleaning the screws on its back side. Salk's intrusion in matters, from the significant to the picayune, began to annoy Kahn's staff. "Show me how you arrived at that decision," he repeatedly asked.[14] Kahn seemed to thrive on questions and challenges. His staff did not.

Years later, Salk described the Institute as "a work of art to serve the work of science."[15] He never talked about its painful genesis. January 18, 1961, had been the deadline set for the submission of the architectural plans prior to the transfer of the deed. Six months later, Salk still had no blueprints and had to request an extension from the city manager. Occupancy had been scheduled for the summer of 1963. Deadline after deadline passed, and the beginning of 1962 saw Salk empty-handed. In attempts to reduce the mounting friction and obtain resolution, the board of trustees hired a general manager, Charles Wilson. As one of his first directives, he insisted that Kahn cancel a trip to Israel and complete the work. Summarizing his first meeting with Kahn's staff, he wrote: "There is no doubt but that it was wise to call off Mr. Kahn's trip to Israel, but in confidence, the telephone conversation was so upsetting that Mr. Kahn was unable to work effectively for three days." Wilson secured a new timetable for the drawings. "It is felt that a visit by Dr. Salk to Philadelphia at this time," he wrote, "will be cause for... aesthetic ramblings which will delay the work which needs to be done."[16]

For eight months, Kahn had been struggling with the second version of his design, and by April of 1962 he had determined the spatial and functional requirements for the laboratories and meeting house. Assuming that blueprints would soon follow, Salk signed a contract with the George A. Fuller Company of New York. The June 1962 ground-breaking ceremony should have been a joyous event. Yet as the shovel dug into the soil, Salk still had no architectural plans—two years after they had been promised.

One reason for the delay was Kahn's obsession with the meeting house. The central focus of the Institute, it was to be the space in which humanists and scientists commingled, a bridge between the two cultures. Draft after draft ended up on the floor. He finally conceived of a five-sided base with a great central hall, surrounded by the other components, reminiscent of a Roman villa. Exterior concrete walls, perforated with large geometric openings, surrounded glass-walled rooms, leaving a space open to the outside. Kahn said he was wrapping the building in ruins. As a final touch, he added cloistered gardens, bisected by a water-course with fountains at each end. Here everyone would dine together, attend concerts, exercise, reflect. To complement the meeting house, he designed the residencies to look like a Pompeian village with its forty-eight apartments connected by a labyrinth of paths and gardens.

Salk, too, shared responsibility for slowing progress. Kahn and his team had finished the draft of the laboratories, depicting four buildings, set in pairs, with two garden courtyards. After signing the contract with Fuller Construction Company, Salk revisited the Torrey Pines Mesa at twilight. "I sensed that something was not quite right," he later reflected, "but could not identify what it was that troubled [me]. My mind stirred restlessly in the night."[17] The next day, Salk told Kahn that they couldn't have two courtyards; it would lead to A people and B people. And standing on the mesa the night before, he had sensed the need for better balance between buildings and space. Kahn's team, now numbering twenty, had been working eighteen-hour days for months. "There was almost mutiny in the office," MacAllister recalled. Kahn calmed them. "It's an opportunity for us to do even better," he said.[18] So they started over.

Salk's intrusions extended beyond the architectural design. When Kahn contemplated using stone for the exterior, Salk said he preferred concrete, "so as not to destroy the monolithic character."[19] He wanted a warm color that blended with the surrounding landscape and suggested

Kahn look at the Kips Bay Towers on Second Avenue in Manhattan.[20] Salk stood by as twenty-five concrete test slabs were poured on the site.[21] A scientist visiting that day recounted how "Jonas was hopping around like a gazelle," asking him, "Should I pick this one or this one? This one is too grey; this one too mottled, this has a bit of yellow."[22]

In an attempt to expedite the project, the National Foundation sent Dale Harvey, a top staff member, to serve as their representative during construction. He and Charles Wilson met regularly with the architectural team, represented by MacAllister. Hoping to avoid further unnecessary delays, they excluded Salk and Kahn. But that didn't stop Salk from involving himself in every decision, from the ventilation system to the overhead rolling grille to the wiring. Even though they had hired an experienced laboratory design consultant, Salk sent equipment specifications directly to Kahn. When Harvey found out, he gently reprimanded him: "It will be Mr. Wall's responsibility to see that the scientists' requirements are properly set forth."[23] Two weeks later, Salk was advising Kahn about the design of the studies. He imagined a humanist's studio such as that depicted in Vermeer's painting *The Astronomer*.[24] A week after that, he requested calculations of the heat gain from five autoclaves operating simultaneously in each lab. In frustration, Harvey sent the team a memo, stating, "Dr. Salk should divorce himself from any construction matters other than design, services, and general appearance now that the concept is set."[25] More frustrating was Salk's attitude toward the financial consequences, which tended toward laissez-faire. Kahn was constantly over budget. "If it had been left up to the accountants," Salk said, "the Institute would never have been built."[26]

As the end of the year approached, they still had no architectural plans. Costs were mounting, and the fellows were tired of waiting. If construction were delayed further, the Institute would incur tax penalties. Salk usually avoided confrontation, but on November 16, 1962, prompted by the board, he wrote Kahn: "I have been called to account by the Board of Trustees and by others regarding responsibility for the present demoralized state of the Institute building program." Not acknowledging his own part in the delays, Salk presented a list of demands: All working drawings and specifications must be completed by December 31. A time schedule must be submitted along with weekly progress reports and establishment of an architect's unit on site. "Unless this schedule is adhered to and the 31 December 1962 date is met, continuation of our present association will no longer be under my control."[27] Salk sent copies of the letter to O'Connor, Fuller, and Harvey. The conviviality and collegiality between Salk and Kahn seemed to have ended. MacAllister wasn't surprised. "That's the way architecture works. It's inevitable. When you are in the conceptual state of design, it's easy to have a honeymoon, because nothing is grounded in reality. So two dreamers can get together and dream, and everything's possible. The further you go down the line, when contractors and building codes come in, things become less and less possible, and that can become contentious. That's when relationships break down."[28]

That December Salk and his family spent their first Christmas in La Jolla. Although Salk told Warren Weaver, "My move here has had the most liberating effect, as you so wisely knew," the day after New Year's, he had to send an uncomfortable telegram to Kahn.[29] "Plans and specifications not yet received. Does this indicate noncompliance with earlier agreements? Unexplained delays demoralizing."[30] A day later, Harvey received the long-awaited blueprints. The package contained only eleven sheets, with no structural, mechanical, or electrical drawings.

The fellows were getting increasingly restless. Their appointments had been announced, their resignations from their current positions pending. Weaver tried to explain the delay, saying that they had an extremely talented architect, "but something of a dreamer who is bored by time schedules, who loves to keep thinking of new and better ideas, and who is therefore very hard to pin down to a calendar." Thus, he explained, "We are paying a price, namely a disappointingly slow start for architectural beauty and for the functional convenience which over the long haul will certainly justify the price."[31] He estimated that the laboratories would be ready to occupy by July 1, 1964, a year later than planned.

Salk thought it would help to have Kahn explain his concepts to the fellows and arranged a meeting. They weren't as captivated as he had been. "There are two things about architects," Lennox observed. "One is what they say, and one is what they do."[32] He watched Crick roll his eyes as Kahn talked. They preferred dealing with MacAllister; he listened to them.

Harvey tightened the reins on Kahn, sending him a new set of deadlines. Again nothing transpired, and, fed up with the dysfunctional situation, he quit. "It is my personal feeling," Harvey wrote O'Connor, "that Mr. Kahn and his architectural organization will never complete an acceptable set of working drawings and specifications on this project."[33] Shortly after his departure, George Fuller, president of the construction company, sent Salk a list of grievances. When he had tried to pin down Kahn regarding specifications for the concrete walls, Kahn had replied, "We must make concrete in this building say 'I am expressive of the hands and forms that held me in place until I could grasp my inner steel and gain the strength and power that I now possess.'"[34] Fuller had never worked with such an exasperating architect. They had been on the job almost a year with nothing to show but a few footings. He had put other projects on hold, and his company was losing money. He, too, was on the verge of quitting.

At that point, O'Connor stepped in. He called Kahn. "We're going to fire you," he warned him. "The project's late; you're over budget."[35] Only if Kahn put MacAllister in complete charge of the project, moving him and his staff to La Jolla, would they consider continuing. Furthermore, O'Connor told Salk to give Kahn a financial incentive, offering a larger fee if the plans arrived by a specific date. It worked. Architect Louis Kahn, *Life* magazine reported, "is putting off commissions on three continents to transform Salk's dream into three-dimensional reality."[36]

With the building almost two years behind schedule, Salk needed to maintain a virtual institute lest the enthusiasm and camaraderie he worked so hard to attain with the fellows start to fade. When recruiting them, Salk had sent congenial, thoughtful letters; they had a number of festive meetings at the Carlyle Hotel in New York where they ate smoked salmon and other delicacies. Now the fellows seemed to be left out of crucial discussions and decisions. "The only person who talked to the source of money, which was Basil O'Connor," Lennox complained, "was Jonas."[37] More upsetting, they had not been consulted about a change in the Institute's name. Early on, the fellows had gone through several exercises to choose the name that would best reflect its character. Then one day the press announced that it had been changed to the Salk Institute for Biological Studies. The fellows received no explanation.

Benzer informed Salk that he had second thoughts about coming. Salk had spent too much time on the ventilation system and color of concrete and not enough on creating a community among the fellows. At Weaver's insistence, he hired William Glazier, a professional economist, to facilitate communication and encourage camaraderie.

While trying to appease the fellows, Salk made a near-fatal blunder. He allowed a *Life* magazine reporter to publish a piece entitled "The Great New Dream of Dr. Salk" in its February 8, 1963, issue.[38] The article called the Institute "an experiment on a grand scale, an intellectual adventure almost without parallel in the history of science." Around the subheadline "Get-together of Fine Fellows" were pictures of Salk's "all-star team" with a description of each fellow's work. Salk was quoted as saying he expected them to be concerned with the "philosophical implications of their work," an area of study he called "biophilosophy." He hoped they would be asking questions such as "What will be the effects of biological advance on the arts and education? What about the cosmic meaning of biological striving?" The article reported that each fellow would have a spacious lab as well as a study and gardens "in which to stroll or meditate." It went on to say that Salk thought of the Institute as a living organism, and he considered each fellow to be "an enzyme which will catalyze the activities of the others." Although ostensibly about the Institute, the article featured Salk and his family, displaying pictures of them at Deep Creek Lake—Jonas sailing, Jonas swimming, Jonas cutting a steak at a barbecue. Under the subheadline "A Jaunty Sailor and a Cautious Skier," a bare-chested, tan, Salk in sunglasses looked quite the celebrity.

Salk was used to the press with their hype and poetic license. The fellows were not. Most had never been subjected to the popular press; angry letters followed. "The article in *Life* has profoundly disturbed me," Dulbecco wrote to Salk, "[and] has left me wondering about the true aims of our undertaking." Looking at the photographs, which is what most of *Life*'s readership did, Dulbecco said he felt like "a rare specimen in a zoo or a circus."[39] He was also disturbed to realize that the public identified the Institute almost solely with Salk. When Salk tried to explain that contact with the public helped raise funds, Dulbecco pointed out, "The complete failure of the previous fundraising campaign that was based on such an assumption shows its fallacy."[40] Equally outraged, Mel Cohn thought the article could damage their reputations. In a letter to the fellows, he quoted from a journalist friend: "If I might offer some free public relations counsel to the Salk Institute...let's have less of Salk in the sunset and more of him in the lab with that not-so-fresh white coat."[41]

All Salk could do was apologize. The fellows insisted that henceforth Bronowski would monitor public relations for the group; however, he soon found the press was not so easily controlled. A subsequent article in the *Los Angeles Herald-Examiner* called the Institute "a fortress where war is waged on disease" by "Commander Salk and his eight generals."[42] The resident fellows concluded that time had come to begin functioning as an institute, namely so they could have a greater say. Having realized how precarious things had become, Salk agreed. He obtained temporary space from the University of California and urged the fellows to join him there while their labs were being constructed. Dulbecco and Lennox announced their move to La Jolla in the summer of 1963; Mel Cohn wrote: "D-Day November 30 we arrive!"[43]

So far, Salk had been carrying most of the administrative burden. During the Institute's early development, he and Lorraine Friedman had been, in effect, the entire staff. He had recruited the fellows and trustees; conferred with city officials, attorneys, and contractors; tried to raise funds; bought equipment; represented the Institute to the media. He had not heeded Edward R. Murrow's admonition: "Your duty and your destiny is to inspire and encourage those who seek to extend the human horizon. Don't become an administrator. You would probably be a bad one."[44]

The fellows began complaining that Salk ran the Institute single-handedly. "Dr. Salk must be relieved of the necessity of his giving personal attention to housekeeping business and general managerial details," Weaver wrote in response to their concerns. "Hour by hour decisions in these areas are neither his forte nor his desire."[45] The board of trustees appointed Bronowski as deputy director, which pleased the fellows. Although Bronowski did relieve Salk of some duties, such as choosing the Institute's stationery and letterhead, Salk could not—or would not—curtail his involvement in most decisions. In his September Director's Report, he advised that administration be centralized by filling the posts of director and president with the same person.[46] Within three months, Salk had assumed both positions.

Salk's most pressing problem continued to be money. He had signed an agreement with O'Connor to initiate a fundraising effort to help defray the costs of construction, with its goal set at $7 million. Promotion attempts included talks to the Baltimore Advertising Club, the Tulsa Chamber of Commerce, and an American Legion convention in Las Vegas; a New York press conference with science writers; and an address at the Seattle World's Fair, where O'Connor would unveil a model of the Institute. In a two-month period, Salk attended dinners with prospective donors in Chicago, Detroit, Los Angeles, San Francisco, and Albuquerque. Society pages showed him, tuxedo-clad, posing with members of the Women's Association for the Salk Institute, or in a turtleneck, chatting with the popular folk singing group the Brothers Four at a fundraising concert. Salk complied with every request. He had to; he was beholden to the National Foundation, which held the purse strings. After almost $5 million of the original NF grant had been expended, Salk put plans for the meeting house and residencies on hold. Kahn's meeting house, over which he had labored for so long and which was considered by many architectural historians to be one of his masterworks, would never be built.

By August of 1965, construction of the labs was nearing completion. Two mirror-image buildings were separated by a large courtyard. Both contained three floors of spacious laboratories. Between the floors, Kahn designed what he called "servant spaces."[47] High enough to walk through, these mechanical spaces housed the wires, pipes, and ducts. This provided flexibility, allowing each scientist to configure his own space. Ten towers, containing thirty-six studies, edged the laboratories. To isolate these office-studios, which Kahn conceived of as monastic cells, he connected them to the labs with bridges. His sawtooth arrangement of the towers assured unobstructed views of the ocean. These towers "stood like giant hollow columns," architectural historians David Brownlee and David De Long wrote, "lining and defining the space of the central court with basilican authority."[48] The concrete exterior gave the building the monolithic character Salk and Kahn had envisioned. "Kahn raised concrete to a new level," architecture professor Robert McCarter wrote, "virtually reinventing the material."[49] He took advantage of the joints between the concrete levels and symmetrical plugs from the steel bolts to add texture to the surface; teak shutters contrasted with the concrete. His design created an artistic display of light and shadows across the walls.

The courtyard remained unfinished. Although he and Salk had envisioned a tree-lined garden, this design troubled Kahn for some time. Impressed with the work of Mexican landscape architect Luis Barragán, Kahn invited him to La Jolla. As Kahn recounted the story: "When he entered the space, he went to the concrete walls and touched them and expressed his love for them, and then he said as he looked across the space and towards the sea, 'I would not put a tree or blade of grass in this space. This should be a plaza of stone, not a garden....If you make this a plaza, you will gain a façade—a façade to the sky.' "[50] Kahn and Salk both knew Barragán was right.

One entered the plaza through a grove of trees into an expanse of Italian travertine edged by the towers. A channel of running water bisected the space. It originated in a fountain on the entrance side, spilled into a pool at the other, then cascaded into a sculptured basin on a lower terrace. The play of light upon the travertine, water, and concrete towers, particularly at sunset, was breathtaking. Architectural scholar Kent Larson called the plaza "perhaps the most sublime space of the twentieth century."[51]

The fellows had mixed reactions "Frankly," Lennox remarked, "I did not wish an architectural treasure. I wanted a lab to work in."[52] Although his study was exquisite, as a scientist he spent most of his time in the lab. Some resented the amount of money spent on the building, arguing that it could have been better spent on research. And Kahn had overlooked some practical things like proper downspouts. When it rained heavily, water gushed over the edges of the building to the floor below. One scientist complained he had no bathroom on his floor. "There were man-traps all around the building," another said, "all kinds of places to fall into and tumble over."[53] Paul Berg, who spent his sabbatical at the Institute, felt differently. He was amazed that a building could be so elegant yet functional. When he arrived, a crew reconfigured his lab overnight by moving partitions and interior floors. At the same time, its beauty enthralled him. "I could sit at my desk," he reminisced, "and look out on the courtyard. As the sun moved, the shadows that it created on the ver-tical surfaces became like a cubist sculpture. It was a work of art."[54]

No one was happier than Salk. He thought Kahn's masterpiece approached perfection.[55] "He was in love with that building," his son Peter recollected. "He would touch it with tenderness."[56] Many consider it Kahn's finest work, evoking images of Greek temples and Roman vil-las, blending the ancient and the modern. The constant flow of visiting architects, likened to pilgrims, attests to its place in architectural history. "No matter who is talking about it," Friedman wrote, "all seem to say the same thing: 'Salk stirs the soul.'"[57]

Seeking Shangri-La

DESPITE THE SHAKY beginning, the Institute fellows thrived, igniting each other's imaginations in the ways Salk had hoped. A National Institutes of Health director, after visiting La Jolla, told Salk he found the fellows "engagingly open and absorptive, willing to go along a path even though the point of departure and destination were not entirely clear." They represented, he said, "the finest models of truth seekers I've ever encountered."[1] At the same time, they enjoyed each other socially. Ed Lennox found Francis Crick entertaining, Jacques Monod a charmer, and Leo Szilard wildly imaginative. An esprit de corps was developing among the fellows, their ebullient mood dampened only by Szilard's sudden death on May 30, 1964, from a heart attack at the age of sixty-six.

The Institute's constellation of resident fellows grew brighter when Leslie Orgel accepted Salk's offer that September.[2] The British chemist was investigating the synthetic reactions that had generated life on Earth. Crick called Orgel "one of the keenest intellects in molecular biology."[3] Over the next two years, three more academic stars joined the nonresident fellows: Harvard neurophysiologist Stephen Kuffler, who had determined how nerve cells carry out their functions, initiating the field of neurobiology; Jerome Wiesner, dean of the School of Science at the Massachusetts Institute of Technology (MIT), who had served as President Kennedy's special assistant for science and technology; and MIT microbiologist Salvador Luria, who would be awarded a Nobel Prize for determining the genetic structure of viruses. "Has Dr. Salk's Dream Come True?" asked *Medical World News*.[4] Among the eleven resident and nonresident fellows, five had received or would receive a Nobel Prize, and all who were US citizens were members of the National Academy of Sciences—except Salk.

Although the fellows fired each other's imagination in ways Salk had hoped, he began to feel excluded from their coterie. The fellows thought him modest, friendly, and warm-hearted, yet no one called him "wildly imaginative" or "one of the keenest intellects" or "engagingly open." Somewhat reticent, Salk didn't connect with them scientifically, socially, or personally. According to Lennox, "Jonas never quite became part of the group."[5] He suffered from the isolation and consulted his friend Joel Elkes, a psychiatrist, who recalled "a sense of urgency in the conversations, a sense of anxiety."[6] Salk had successfully recruited academic giants and built them a splendid refuge with almost unparalleled freedom—a scientific Shangri-La. Now he felt alienated, and he didn't understand why.

One reason may have been that while spirits flourished, finances continued to flounder. Salk barely could keep the Institute afloat, and fellows began to worry about their financial health. Other than their own research grants, O'Connor provided most of the Institute's funding. "Jonas kept much of the details of what he was doing with O'Connor from us," Lennox complained. "That was his private arrangement, and we were not part of it. It was galling." Added to that, Salk's leadership style annoyed the fellows. "He gave the pretense of participatory democracy," Lennox said, "but it wasn't."[7] Salk talked to fellows individually about issues, rather than seeking consensus. And he often acted alone, which generated considerable uneasiness.

Weaver realized that Salk had taken on responsibilities for which he was ill-suited. He lacked the skills to be an effective manager; he avoided confrontation and had difficulty making decisions. "When he did make decisions," Weaver said in his oral history, "they tended to be very gentle and kind…influenced more by his heart than by his mind."[8] Weaver cared deeply for Salk and concluded he must persuade him to relinquish his position as president. Although Salk could not perceive his managerial limitations, he realized he had not succeeded in creating a utopia, free of concerns that impair creativity. He told Weaver he embraced the idea of hiring a president and chief executive officer with administrative experience. "I think that Jonas has come to see he must not waste his time playing his weakest cards," Weaver told a trustee.[9]

The board of trustees appointed Dr. Augustus Kinzel, vice president of research for Union Carbide, to be the new president and CEO. Having faced crisis after crisis, Salk suddenly seemed at peace. "For reasons too numerous and too obvious to enumerate," he wrote Weaver, "there has occurred a great settling—even though major problems still face us."[10] He told Elkes, "I always knew that I needed a respite but did not know how badly this was needed until now when I am beginning to feel qualified to rejoin the human race."[11] Although he stated publicly that he had stepped down so he could devote himself to his scientific work, the press portrayed Salk as having "fallen from grace."[12]

On August 1, 1965, Kinzel took office. The sixty-five-year-old mathematician and engineer had outstanding credentials: seven honorary degrees, a member of the National Academy of Sciences, first president of the National Academy of Engineering, six years as president of Union Carbide Research Laboratories.[13] He would assume all responsibilities related to administration, financial affairs, and fundraising for the Salk Institute. As director, Salk would continue to oversee academic programs. When Kinzel arrived, however, the fellows informed him that their group constituted the Institute's academic body, and as such they would make all programmatic decisions and pass recommendations to him for action. Salk's single-handed control had ended.

One function Salk looked forward to relinquishing was fiscal affairs. The buildings had cost far more than anticipated, $16 million thus far, and the south wing still stood unfinished. He had had no choice but to dip into the endowment. "I was appalled at the amount of money that was going to go initially into capital expenditure," Weaver related. "I knew there was no use to talk about this, because there were emotional and other factors involved."[14] Resentment festered among the fellows; that money was supposed to have been reserved for future research and operations. "There was a big endowment," Lennox said, "that got gobbled up by what we thought was an excessively expensive building."[15] Resident fellows had been granted lifetime contracts that couldn't be broken until they died—"Not until retirement," scientist Paul Berg emphasized, "but until death." The appointment letters guaranteed a substantial amount of money each year, referred to as the fellows' estates. "They carried around this letter," Berg recalled, "which endowed them with certain inalienable rights and privileges, like it was the Bible."[16] Now the Institute didn't have enough money to honor that commitment fully.

During this time, Salk's relationship with O'Connor became strained. The NF had expended millions on the Institute and as yet had seen no scientific discoveries that had direct application to the public's health. Salk didn't quite comprehend the basis for his friend's apparent detachment. Upset, he proposed they spend some quiet time together. O'Connor agreed. "Since my return from our visit," he wrote "Doc" in June of 1966, "I have felt like a new person....Thank you for the wonderful days together. Just being with you makes things clear, brings perspective, and fills me with the energy and courage to go on."[17] Their discussions had reminded him of the Institute's original aim. He had been remiss in keeping O'Connor apprised of its academic growth, and he would press forward to appoint a fundraising chairman.

Despite Kinzel's experience and Salk's intent, the Institute continued to face significant fiscal problems. At the annual fellows' meeting in February of 1967, Kinzel reported that they needed to raise $6 million to maintain the present level of operation or $22 million to develop more fully the academic program and finish planned construction. As the Institute continued to depend on the NF for solvency, Salk had to perform a task he loathed but which he knew O'Connor expected of him—courting donors. That he complied with so many requests showed the extent to which he would go to appease O'Connor and save the Institute.

Using many of the March of Dimes fundraising techniques, they capitalized on the relationship between the Foundation and the entertainment industry. Burt Lancaster hosted a gathering of friends at which Salk talked about his work.[18] Andy Williams gave a benefit performance along with Henry Mancini, Dean Martin, and Bob Newhart at the San Diego Civic Theater.[19] Williams held a charity golf tournament and donated proceeds from his album *Born Free* to the Institute.[20] Although some of these events appeared demeaning, such as thanking two hundred teenage graduates of Wendy Ward Charm School who held fashion shows across the country to raise funds,[21] or greeting the fifty-one candidates of the Mrs. America contest, Salk acquiesced.[22] Even with these efforts, the 1967 donations totaled $666,000, the next year only $577,000.

Although Salk thought he and O'Connor had renewed their friendship at his visit in June of 1966, O'Connor remained aloof. Having received frequent effusive letters and telegrams from his dear friend over the years, Salk began to note their absence. "It is almost two months since I've talked with you on the telephone," Salk wrote in February of 1967.[23] Again he suggested they go away for a few days. "We need to be together long enough to reinstate the basic communication between us and to clear away the subjects that have accumulated as residue and refuse that remain after a building has been completed. I know that you are very unhappy. You know I am too."[24] Three months passed with no response, so he wrote again: "In spite of whatever you are feeling, underneath it all you must know the deep feeling of respect and love I have for you."[25] He sent telegrams: "When greatness as well as strength is called for, you are the one to call upon. And when a generous spirit is needed and the cause is in the public good, you are always there. As always and ever."[26] O'Connor remained silent.

Meanwhile, Salk was trying to help Kinzel steer the Institute through some rocky rapids, starting with an art exhibit on May 1, 1967. The show was to feature the works of Sandra Woodward-Baltimore, wife of David Baltimore, a young scientist in Dulbecco's lab. Woodward-Baltimore had chosen two other local artists to join her in displaying forty-seven pieces. The evening prior to the opening, Kinzel was looking over the exhibit. He was shocked with what he saw. One statue, *American Death Scene*, contained part of the American flag. The painting *Self Portrait and Thought* portrayed a woman draped in a robe of stars and stripes with a man clinging to her knees, a knife in his back. A sketch depicted a nude male holding an elongated penis. Horrified, Kinzel had the pieces removed. The artists threatened to cancel the show. Calling the works of art "an abuse of our hospitality," Kinzel told them he was not censoring art, just protecting the Institute.[27]

As the story unfolded, it turned out that a week earlier, there had been rumors that some pieces might give offense "on grounds of propriety."[28] Orgel and Bronowski, representing the fellows, had reviewed the artwork and asked Mrs. Woodward-Baltimore to omit one painting. Instead, she modified it. When they learned what Kinzel had done, an immediate outcry ensued. Orgel called Kinzel's act "a breach of conduct" of the academic community.[29] "Hassle Ends Art Show at Institute," read a headline in the *San Diego Union*.[30] "Artists, Salk Official Row over Paintings," announced the *Los Angeles Times*.[31] Baltimore said he would resign in protest if the three pieces were not put back in the show. "It seems oddly inconsistent for an organization such as the Salk Institute to dedicate itself to the quest for scientific truth," the UCSD Chairman of Philosophy wrote Kinzel, "and yet...to impose constraints on those who seek such goals."[32]

Kinzel replied that he was not trying to repress the artists but to safeguard the Institute. Both he and Orgel sought legal advice; both received the same answer: *American Death Scene* breached the Military and Veterans Code of the State of California; the nude male, who appeared to be masturbating, violated the California antiobscenity statute. "Each of said violations," Orgel's lawyer wrote, "could result in criminal prosecution against the entity and its responsible officers exhibiting said works."[33] Baltimore's lawyer told him "ornamental pictures" were exempt.[34]

The situation quickly acquired political overtones. "Whether or not the Military and Veterans' Code outlaws any works in this show is irrelevant," Woodward-Baltimore and sculptor Hubert Duckworth wrote the fellows. If intellectual and artistic freedom were to be defended, censoring works of art should not be tolerated. If the Institute did not take a stand, they insisted, it would fail to be the intellectual leader that it sought to be in the community. The two artists offered some alterations: They would obscure the portion of the flag in *American Death Scene*; they would set *Self Portrait and Thought* and the drawing of three nudes in a separate room labeled "For Adults Only"; and they would post a disclaimer saying that the Institute didn't necessarily endorse the views expressed in the works.[35] Kinzel agreed. But that was not the end of his problems.

Although the fellows understood the legal issues, they thought Kinzel's actions represented an attempt to usurp their authority. Orgel composed a letter from the fellows to the board of trustees, charging that President Kinzel had overruled them in matters of academic policy, their province. They considered the situation "inimical to free intellectual expression."[36] Mel Cohn refused to sign the letter.

Built to bridge the gap between the sciences and humanities, the Salk Institute had become a battleground. "That was just one of those sixties things," scientist Walter Eckhart recalled.[37] "It was a test of how open the Institute was to fringe ideas," added Berg. "In that sense, it failed."[38] It may have been "just one of those sixties things," but for Kinzel, it was a humiliating, trying affair. And for Salk, it was devastating. He watched his utopia split into factions. He would have turned to O'Connor for advice, but their relationship had cooled. When asked, as a member of the fellows' group, to sign the letter of protest to the board of trustees, he procrastinated. In the end, he could not do it and wrote a lengthy letter explaining his position.

"It was from Adlai Stevenson I first heard 'I am too old to cry, and it hurts too much to laugh,'" he began. "I know how he felt." He proceeded to review the entire history of the Institute: "We suffered all the pains of childbirth, and there were a number of times when I was sure that neither mother nor child would survive. They did—and I daresay all bear the scars of the early struggle." He called the current situation "unfortunate." "But, need it be one that can very well destroy us even before we get off the ground?" Then he poured out the sentiments he had kept private for so long: "One of my many regrets has been that my unavoidable preoccupation with the many urgencies with which I have had to deal limited my opportunities for contact with many of you." He did not sense the collegial spirit he had envisioned. "We have divisions: we have those who are 'in' and those who are 'out'; we have the academic vs. the administrative." As scientists, they knew that not all cells are the same. "Unless the liver cell respects the spleen cell…the heart cell respects the lung—they are in trouble. And so we are. You know it. I know it." The fellows felt strongly that an individual has the right to express himself freely. "I share these feelings," Salk continued. "But this freedom applies to all—equally to the one who expresses himself via criticism and the one who expresses himself through the creative act. There has to be room for both." This was the belief on which he had founded the Institute.

He would not sign the fellows' letter because in doing so, he disavowed this principle. In closing, he said, "I will not destroy this institute—I would hope you do not."[39] His impassioned letter might have astonished the fellows; its honesty could have forged a new relationship with them; yet there is no indication he ever sent it. Likely he was too exhausted and sad to bare his soul.

Just as the brouhaha over the art exhibit was subsiding, a visiting fellow sued the Institute for breach of contract. Seventy-year-old Leonell C. Strong, well-known in the scientific world for his mice colony, had spent decades developing forty-one strains of inbred mice for research.[40] Scientists working on the immune system and cancer depended on these strains. For that reason, when the opportunity arose, Salk invited Strong to become a visiting fellow.

Strong had been at the Roswell Park Memorial Institute in Buffalo since 1953. Having reached the mandatory retirement age, he had to relinquish his lab. He was looking for a place to continue his work and requested a five-year appointment at the Salk Institute. Although the bylaws specified that a visiting fellow could only be appointed for two years, his mouse colony was so valuable that Salk assured him his appointment would be renewed. Strong planned to bring his large colony and five employees, as well as his entire library of Elizabethan literature, assuring Salk that he would be able to finance his lab almost entirely from federal funds. Salk's assistant, William Glazier, warned that Strong's current and projected grants were insufficient to meet his needs.[41] They would either have to apply for foundation funds or pass on the cost of the mouse colony to those scientists who would use his mice—Lennox, Cohn, Dulbecco, and Salk. Salk hadn't discussed this appointment with the fellows affected, and not all of them needed Strong's colony.

Trouble began the day Strong moved to La Jolla. Many of his data files, records, and several volumes of Elizabethan literature from his library had disappeared. He insisted Salk sue the van line that had transported them. Additionally, although Strong understood he would occupy one of the new labs in the South Building, his precious inbred mouse colony was housed in a metal shed. Strong never did receive the grants he had anticipated, and, faced with supporting his operation for another three years, Salk did not renew his offer at the end of the two-year appointment. When he notified Strong that his budget would be terminated in six months, Strong sued the Institute.

Since they could not agree on a settlement, the case went to trial. *Strong v. Salk Institute* began in June of 1967 and lasted six months. The Institute lawyers considered Strong's case weak: Forced to retire from his previous position, Strong had come to the Salk Institute as a visiting fellow. The Institute bylaws stipulated the maximum stay to be two years. Since Strong had not been able to obtain grant funding to continue his work, Salk offered two of his staff positions in his own lab, and Cohn assumed responsibility for the mouse colony. "When Jonas Salk first appeared on the witness stand," one reporter observed, "the jury acted as if somebody were suing God."[42] Salk testified that their agreement specified that Strong could be terminated at any time. The Institute had supported him for two years, after which they thought it "seemed wiser to channel the resources to other areas."[43] Interrogation of Strong established his failure to obtain grant funding and brought into question his current work's relevance.

Then Strong's lawyers took over. Leonell C. Strong, they said, former director of the Biological Station at Roswell Park, had received an invitation to join the Salk Institute, and Salk had agreed to a five-year commitment. Strong brought his famous inbred mice to the Institute and turned over his research grants to its administrators. During the move, Strong's data and several valuable rare books had vanished. No action was taken to compensate him. He proceeded to breed mice for Institute scientists, and when the needs for his mice grew, his colony was subsumed by the animal lab under the supervision of Dr. Cohn. While Strong was in Japan, one of his original strains died out, representing "irreplaceable work of years."[44] To make matters worse, Salk tried to hire two of his longtime assistants. Meanwhile, Strong had applied to the American Cancer Society for research funds and was told his prospects were good. He had tried to reason with Salk; all he wanted to do was finish his cancer work at the Institute.

Strong's lawyers were building a case of elder abuse by the famous Jonas Salk and his big institute. Most damning was a document they had found outlining a five-year budget for Strong, indicating a commitment. In the end, the jury found that Strong had been employed by the Salk Institute under a five-year contract and was promised reasonable funds to carry out his research. They awarded him $25,000 for lost salary, $24,000 to finance his work, and $11,000 for personal items lost in shipment from New York.[45]

Worse for Salk than losing the suit was the press's scathing reprimand, full of poetic license. "If the case of Strong-Salk had taken place anywhere else," one reporter wrote, "the trial jury would have been in the front pages from coast to coast, but it was in San Diego which is usually the same as not happening at all. Thus, the infamous trial in which Jonas E. Salk's testimony was refuted repeatedly by documents from the Salk Institute's own files remains a well-muffled event to all except the handful of men and women who served on the jury." The reporter went on to say how difficult the trial had been for Strong, given his poor health. "Biting sarcasm, caustic comments, insulting questions and a grueling three-day cross-examination of the elderly scientist," she wrote, "was an ordeal that sent him to the hospital." And Mrs. Strong never recovered from the shock she suffered. The reporter contended that Salk had tried to confiscate Strong's famed colony of inbred mice and that his failure to receive an American Cancer Society grant stemmed from Salk's calling his work "completely outdated." Salk was quoted as saying, "We had to get rid of him." In conclusion, the reporter wrote: "The viciousness of the Salk Institute's attack and the arrogance with which Jonas Salk made statements proven untrue, and the greedy effort not only to destroy the elder scientist's reputation but to strip him of even his colony of mice…added up to a package the jury had no use for."[46]

In the midst of the Strong suit, Kinzel resigned. Publicly, he said he had accomplished his initial purposes and felt his job was done; however, his job was far from done. The Institute continued to teeter on the edge of bankruptcy. The art exhibit fiasco with the fellows' subsequent reproof and Strong's suit surely contributed to his decision.

With surprising generosity, the resident fellows sent the board a memo proposing their estates—the funding guaranteed to them for salaries, travel, equipment, and supplies—be reduced from $115,000 yearly to $70,000 in order to lessen the Institute's precarious financial situation.[47] They were willing to spend more time writing grants. Furthermore, they advised that Salk assume the functions of the president while they searched for Kinzel's replacement. Instead of being pleased, Salk seemed distraught over their memo. He liked Kinzel, and on the last lap of his illustrious career, Institute fellows had berated and harried him. "In the brief time that we worked together," Salk said at Kinzel's memorial service twenty years later, "I learned not only to respect Gus Kinzel but to love him."[48] And, despite his initial desire to control Institute affairs, Salk no longer wanted the administrative burdens.

He begged Warren Weaver to move to La Jolla. "I appreciate more than I can convey your constructive attitude," he wrote. "I could use a large dose of the latter since there has been so much to the contrary expressed in different ways by different people." The recent events had placed an enormous strain on Salk; he wanted to retreat to his lab and let someone else manage the Institute. He especially bemoaned having to once again take the lead in fundraising. "It is a problem with which I can no longer cope personally," he told Weaver. "To what extent enthusiasm, personal pleasure, and high hopes that existed heretofore can be restored, I do not know."[49] At seventy-three, Weaver suffered from heart problems and replied that he would be resigning from the board. The Institute desperately needed a hero to step in and save it.

One arrived in the person of Joseph E. Slater, director of the Ford Foundation's international relations program.[50] At a press conference, Slater said a major consideration in assuming his new position at the Salk Institute was the rapidly increasing importance of the biological sciences in relationship to man and society. Comfortable with complex organizations, well connected, outgoing, and a natural leader, Slater was the perfect man to rescue the Institute—and its founder.

By this point Salk had been pursuing his vision of uniting the two cultures for nine years. Kahn had designed an architectural treasure, and he had collected an astounding group of intellects, promising the ultimate in academic freedom. There was nothing like it. But Salk had paid a price. He rarely saw his family and had not taken a vacation in years. His own research had suffered. And his friendship with Basil O'Connor—which had sustained him through so much—had faded. Although he had envisioned creating a sanctuary where he could work in peace, he had been unable to relinquish control to those with administrative skills. At the same time, he resented having to undertake tasks for which he had no talent. At fifty-three, the sparkle in his eyes and boyish smile from the polio vaccine days had been replaced by deep facial creases and a melancholy gaze. In a moment of despair, he wrote, "I have lost virtually every shred of freedom I ever had."[51]

With the arrival of Joseph Slater, Salk felt liberated. He anticipated more time for his laboratory research and family, both of which were faltering.

A Troubled Marriage

"DIVORCED: DR. JONAS Salk, 53," reported *Time* magazine on May 31, 1968, in its Milestones column, "by Donna Lindsay Salk, 51, on grounds of extreme cruelty, after 28 years of marriage."[1] The circumstances surrounding the divorce were never disclosed.

Salk often described his life as a series of challenges, using the image of a mountain range. Having reached one peak, he sought the next mountain to climb. He hadn't taken his family along on his journey, however. They remained at the periphery of his life. Friends and colleagues recalled few words about his sons, fewer about his wife, and none about his brothers. What they learned about his family came from magazines and newspapers. Even that was minimal and often inaccurate. "Dr. Jonas Salk submits to interviews with about the same frequency as does Howard Hughes," one reporter complained.[2] Even then, Salk remained remote, avoided eye contact, and often spoke in metaphor. Richard Carter's 1966 book on the polio vaccine, *Breakthrough: The Saga of Jonas Salk*, made only brief reference to his family. During his interviews with Salk, when Carter ventured into his private life, Salk changed the subject. His work, not his family, defined him.

Salk rarely saw his brothers, except when necessary—at their father's funeral after he suffered a fatal heart attack in 1959, and at their mother's funeral five years later. "My mother died quite suddenly," Salk wrote an associate on October 12, 1964, "having been fully active although hampered to some extent in recent years. We will, of course, miss her but comfort ourselves knowing that she lived a full and useful life and did not have to be dependent upon others—something she so dreaded."[3] Although she had been difficult, Salk appreciated the influence his mother had had on his life. His sister-in-law Sylvia recalled that Jonas was one of the few who shed a tear at her funeral.[4]

Salk's middle brother, Herman, and Sylvia, his wife, had set up a veterinary practice in Palm Springs, the town where they raised their four children. A gentle, happy man, Herman was beloved by his clients. He wanted a close bond with his two brothers, but neither had the time or inclination. Lee, the youngest, seemed ambivalent toward his siblings, a bit jealous of his oldest brother.[5] A New York child psychologist, he gained renown when he demonstrated that a mother's heartbeat could calm an infant. He later commercialized his concept, developing the Securitone machine, a device that reproduced human heart sounds. It reportedly settled disturbed children and promoted mental health. Lee Salk became a pop psychologist, writing books on children and the family. Lecture tours, talk shows, and three marriages preoccupied him.

Although the press displayed photos of Salk with Peter, Darrell, and Jonathan sailing, swimming, enjoying a barbecue, in reality he spent limited time with his sons. Following the family's grand European tour in 1957, Salk insisted Peter be sent to boarding school at Phillips Exeter Academy in New Hampshire. A shy child, he could not escape notice with the last name Salk. "I was thirteen," Peter recollected, "a young thirteen, a small thirteen, an immature thirteen, and going away from home was challenging."[6] Salk wanted his sons to receive the finest education, and although it went unstated, sending them to elite schools signified his change in social status. Smothered by his mother and living at home until he married, perhaps he wanted his sons to have the autonomy he had craved. Jonathan later thought they may have been sent away because of growing tension in the marriage. Whatever the reason, Donna accepted it. She said she didn't mind missing their adolescent periods, as she would have borne most of the burden. She and Peter were already at odds, and he was just entering his teen years.

Peter graduated near the top of his class and was accepted to Harvard, yet he felt aimless and dropped out of college twice over the next three years. "I was chronically conflicted about what to do with my life," he recalled. Although he enjoyed poetry and languages, as did his mother, he felt a tacit obligation to study the sciences. "I think that it was imbued in me," he said, "that in order to fulfill my role in life, I needed to follow in *his* footsteps."[7] At thirteen, Darrell was sent to Phillips Academy in Andover, Massachusetts, where he thrived. Although a talented actor, when he later entered Stanford University, Darrell, too, chose to study the biological sciences. At thirteen, Jonathan expected to attend boarding school like his brothers, yet his mother kept him home an extra year to spend time with his father. That never happened, and he joined Darrell at Phillips Academy the next year. Thousands of miles from home, Jonathan regretted that his father rarely called, and when he did, the conversation was brief. "He was very involved in his own world and his own life," Jonathan explained. He filled the void with music, composing rhythm and blues, playing piano and harmonica.[8]

Salk encouraged his sons to have a vision, and although he did not pressure them to study medicine, all three received MD degrees. "I suspect there was something imprinted on us," Peter said.[9] If Salk was proud of his children—their sterling academic records, Darrell's acting talent, Jonathan's music—he kept it to himself. Even when he did spend time with them, he set the agenda, usually focusing the conversation on his own preoccupations. "Although we were definitely on his radar," Jonathan said, "it wasn't how he spent his time."[10]

Their father moved to California in December of 1962, leaving Jonathan and his mother in Pittsburgh until school ended the following June. "Mrs. Jonas Salk Happily Anticipates La Jolla Home," a local newspaper reported.[11] Actually, Donna felt despondent about the move; she almost stayed in Pittsburgh. Their marriage was foundering.[12]

❧

To MANY, DONNA and Jonas seemed a mismatch from the start. "I don't know if it was an ideal relationship," his longtime secretary, Lorraine

Friedman, observed. "I think she was the type of person he thought he wanted to be married to, whom he wanted to be the mother of his children."[13] In that regard, Donna proved a fine wife. She relinquished her career with no complaints, raised three sons, and maintained the household. She had anticipated how consuming Jonas's work would be, but not how narrow his world would become. He expressed no interest in the theater, the symphony, the books she read, the music she played. Part of the initial attraction had been his desire to help humankind. An activist at Smith College, Donna had voted for the American Labor Party in the early 1940s and was on the New York Conference for Inalienable Rights' mailing list. A staunch Democrat, she supported the underdog. As Jonas moved more to the right and became increasingly apolitical, civil rights and fair housing laws faded from their conversations.

No one remembers Donna and Jonas laughing together, teasing, holding hands, showing any tenderness. Eschewing a dominating woman like his mother, Jonas ended up with a reserved, reticent wife. The more he withdrew into his lab, the more she retreated into her books and music. Donna continued to play the role of dutiful wife with no apparent resentment, no arguments. "There just wasn't a peep," their son Peter recalled. Beneath the veneer of a happy marriage ran undercurrents of discontent, arising from two prevailing tensions. The first was Jonas's absence from their family life. Not only was he physically absent, he was emotionally absent as well. "He internalized all sorts of things," according to Peter.[14] While still in Ann Arbor, Salk had started his night writings, putting his private thoughts on paper, rather than sharing them with his wife or children.

The second tension centered on lifestyle. Jonas was developing a circle of scientific associates with whom Donna had nothing in common. If out-of-town scientists were visiting his lab, he invited them to dinner, often on the spur of the moment. "That kind of thing would drive my mother bananas," Jonathan recalled. Donna liked her life structured, planned, without surprises. "He doesn't understand," she once complained to her son when his father brought home unexpected guests. "There are only four lamb chops." After Basil O'Connor became his benefactor, Salk felt obliged to attend cocktail parties and dinner dances. Donna hated social affairs. "My mother's idea of a wonderful evening,"

Jonathan said, "was to get into her nightgown and get into bed with a good book."[15]

As difficult as it had been for her, Donna had stood by her husband's side during the polio vaccine extravaganza. Nevertheless, she could not bring herself to play the celebrity wife. The public may have wondered how their hero could be married to this impassive, modest woman who rarely smiled. "He was changed by his fame," his sister-in-law Sylvia said. "She was not."[16] Perhaps Donna thought that once the excitement settled down, her husband would focus on his family. Instead, he was moving on to his next dream. And she was not part of it.

As soon as the boys were in school, Donna began to reconfigure her life. Still liberal in her political beliefs, she overcame her diffidence and became involved in Pittsburgh civic affairs, serving on the board of the Child Guidance Center, on the advisory board of the Anti-Defamation League, on the budget committee of the Community Fund, and as chairman of the Commission on Human Relations. She developed her own network of friends who were interested in her, and not because she was Jonas Salk's wife. In her own quiet way, Donna carved out a life for herself that did not include her husband. There she found fulfillment— and perhaps even affection. There were rumors of affairs.[17] Not that Jonas was innocent. With fame came adoration, and no one adored Salk more than America's women.

When Jonas announced the family was moving to La Jolla, Donna had balked. Jonathan saw the gulf between his parents widening. He detected ambivalence from both about whether his mother should join his father in California. Besides having to leave her friends and civic activities, Donna felt no draw to San Diego. She had been born and raised in New York City; Pittsburgh at least had a symphony and museums. No one would have described San Diego as cosmopolitan at the time. Worse yet, she was expected to play the part of Salk Institute hostess, a role she loathed. In an interview to which Donna reluctantly agreed just before she moved to La Jolla, the reporter described her as a "tall, slender brunette with a friendly, informal manner." She told the reporter that their sons admired their father and were unspoiled by his fame. Calling her husband "a quiet, calm man, very close to family," she said he liked to water ski and sail.[18] "In my family there was a tendency to say everything was fine," Jonathan reflected. "Things weren't nearly as good as people thought they were."[19]

At some point, Donna sensed that she might lose her husband. Her sister-in-law Sylvia recognized that she was shaken by what was happening when Donna bought a hairpiece. "This is a woman who was perfectly content with the low-key way she looked," Sylvia explained. She didn't care about the latest fashions; she didn't visit the beauty parlor regularly. "When I noticed that she was trying to make herself look more attractive, although she was an attractive woman, I realized that this person I thought was solid as a rock was not that self-assured."[20]

Donna still loved Jonas and, despite possible transgressions on both sides, tried to keep their marriage intact. In February of 1963, she wrote to him from Pittsburgh: "It is a considerable effort to put pen to paper for this letter—perhaps because there is too much to say, perhaps too little." A letter was at least a starting point. For a long time, she wrote, her "emotional remarks" had evoked from him a "philosophic, impersonal problem-solving response." She did not want to initiate a philosophical discourse but rather a concrete discussion about their marriage. To begin, there was so much about his current life she didn't know, and she worried he may have compromised his principles. But, she said, "I am prepared to, willing to, and desirous of committing myself to your interests and person physically, socially, emotionally, intellectually." She accepted the probability that she would need to go a large percentage of the way in this. "I am intensely aware...there is much negative feeling you bear toward me and that I would have to face this perhaps repeatedly." She did not understand why he found certain aspects of her life intolerable. Few couples, she argued, live together without some friction. "People don't really split up over the cap on the toothpaste, which can be annoying as hell...if the deep things are secure."[21]

She told Jonas that she intended to work hard on their relationship. In return she needed certain things from him for her comfort and fulfillment. "All of this," she wrote in parenthesis, "has *nothing* to do with the question of my past, my character, my 'deserved punishment.'" She went on to say, "I need a reasonable amount of plain, ordinary, garden variety attention." She understood Jonas's preoccupation with his work, but he also needed to devote some time in his life to her: "To my 'chatter'...to my needs to be 'seen,' acknowledged, complimented on occasion. To go once in a while to a movie or concert…because you want to—because it's pleasurable to be together…because my company can be enjoyable." She wasn't asking for a romantic courtship, just some daily thoughtfulness.[22] She ended the letter by quoting from Milton's *Paradise Lost*, when, after the Fall, Adam says to Eve:

> But rise, let us no more contend, nor blame
> Each other, blam'd enough elsewhere, but strive
> In offices of Love, how we may light'n
> Each others burden in our share of woe. (10.958–61)

In early spring, Donna visited La Jolla, and the couple had a reconciliation of sorts. By April, she was writing about fixing up the house and lake cottage to sell, speaking positively about the move. "People have been asking me how life might shape up in La Jolla," she wrote to Jonas, "many of them (intellectual of course) expressing concern about what there is available….As you know, my whole feeling about the place was a positive one, and the 'Institute excitement' is fairly infectious….Don't know about you, but on the whole I felt the visit was good." At that time, Salk had reached a crisis with Kahn, and the fellows were sending angry letters about the *Life* magazine article, yet he seemed not to have shared any of this with his wife, since she ended her note, "Keep on taking it a little easier. You'll see, it may even feel good! Much love, Donna."[23]

In June of 1963, Donna and their three sons moved to La Jolla. She busied herself with their new home; Jonathan enrolled in the public middle school, presumably to have more time with his father. Yet the Institute continued to consume Salk's attention. "He was only intermittently involved in my life," Jonathan recalled, "when I had science papers." At dinner, his father talked about whatever he was doing. "Although I didn't understand it, I was aware that things were not going well."[24]

For a while, Donna and Jonas maintained a semblance of accord. The next year, Peter returned to Harvard; Jonathan joined Darrell at Andover. Donna immersed herself in local politics and community activism as vice president of the Urban League and southern California chairman for "No on 14," the California fair housing initiative, and serving. on the San Diego County Committee for Governor Edmund "Pat" Brown. She participated in the Family Services Association and the Women's

Advisory Council. Most gratifying was her civil rights work: she was vice president of the Citizens Inter-Racial Committee, a board member of the National Committee against Discrimination in Housing, and a member of the National Advisory Committee on Minority Affairs.[25]

Despite her good intentions, Donna rarely participated in her husband's social life. "She was very shy," one of his friends observed. "It was an enormous burden on her to be the wife of 'the great Dr. Salk.' She seemed to be overwhelmed by the task."[26] If she had to serve as hostess for an Institute function, she performed her duty in a well-mannered yet tepid fashion. Renato Dulbecco's wife, Maureen, recalled feeling uncomfortable in Donna's presence. "She always seemed aloof and judgmental," she said, "as if she were appraising everyone in the room."[27]

Donna was a paradox. An introvert, she was able to overcome her natural reticence on behalf of those in need and those deprived of their rights. She could not summon up the same energy to engage with the high society of San Diego or celebrities from the entertainment world. She could not pretend to be amused, make small talk, proffer a glad hand. She did not preside at the Salk Institute's Women's Association luncheons or buy a gown for a benefit performance. The *San Diego Union* frequently printed pictures of Salk mixing with glamorous movie stars and socialites; none included Donna. Few of the Institute staff or fellows even remembered her. She seemed to be slipping from her husband's life. The gap had grown too wide.

⁂

IN SEPTEMBER OF 1964, Barbara Marx Hubbard, a suburban Connecticut housewife, was lounging by the family swimming pool, watching her five children, when the phone rang. "Mrs. Hubbard, this is Dr. Salk," said the man on the other line. "You have written my vision better than I could have. We are two peas in the same genetic pod. Can I take you to lunch?"[28]

The daughter of millionaire toy manufacturer Louis Marx, Barbara grew up in New York society. She was fifteen when the United States devastated two Japanese cities with the atomic bomb, and she began to question mankind's power and its ultimate outcome. She became engaged in "a philosophical search for greater meaning," she wrote in her memoir. She called it a "hunger."[29] While in Paris during her junior year at Bryn Mawr College, Barbara met an aspiring American artist, Earl Hubbard, whom she married while still a student. She soon found herself pregnant and for the next decade complied with her husband's wishes that she be a good wife and mother. They settled in Lakeville, Connecticut, where her life centered on her five children, housework, the PTA, and the Women's Club. Still she felt unsettled. "That was before the woman's movement," she reflected, "before the futurist movement, before any of those movements."[30] When she read Betty Friedan's 1963 bestseller, *The Feminine Mystique*, she realized how much she wanted something more.

Hubbard thought Western civilization had lost a sense of purpose. She had just begun a quest to find what she called "answers for the future" when she heard that Jonas Salk was building a scientific institute where they were trying to understand mankind. Fascinated, she wrote to Gerald Piel, its first president, about her concept of a "Theater of Humanity" in which they could dramatize the story of "cosmogenesis," adding lessons from biology and social evolution.[31] She thought the Institute could create an atmosphere of hope and possibility. Furthermore, she was sending a grant request to the Deerfield Foundation, through which her father could make a donation to the Institute. Piel gave the letter to Salk, and two weeks later he invited Hubbard to lunch.

This would not be the first socialite from whom Salk was seeking money for the Institute. He probably expected a bejeweled matron, not someone so smart, so young, so attractive. Petite with dark, short curls encircling her face, Hubbard, then thirty-four, had dark eyes that effervesced as she expressed her evolutionary ideas. She later recalled how Salk arrived at her home on a beautiful fall day. Sunlight filtered through the deep red and orange leaves onto her garden, overflowing with marigolds and chrysanthemums, generating a profusion of colors. When she opened the door, the first thing Salk said was, "This looks like the Garden of Eden."[32]

At lunch Hubbard could barely eat as the ideas that had been percolating for years poured out. Salk told her she was a "psychological evolutionary" and reassured her that her nature was good, not wrong or neurotic as she had been led to believe by others. He encouraged her to pursue her vision. "He could see into the essence of my soul," she recalled.[33]

The next week, Salk received a thank-you note from Hubbard. She reminded him to send her a reading list and said, "I want to understand fully the biological metaphors by which you construct all your bridges into the unknown."[34] A series of lengthy letters, filled with philosophical ideas, followed. "Jonas and I became really dear friends," Hubbard later said, "and we spent a good deal of time together with him describing what he understood to be the patterns of evolution that were revealed through our understanding of biology."[35] He called it "metabiological evolution"; she called it "conscious evolution." According to Hubbard, he felt he had been given power for a higher purpose and made her feel that by working with him she was contributing to this lofty goal. "Jonas was warm, seductive, a lover of earth and flesh and life," she wrote in her memoir, "able to make you feel as if you were the most indispensable person in the world to him, that his whole effort would collapse without you."[36]

"It was lovely to hear your voice so clear from so far," she wrote him on October 4.[37] Two weeks later, as she sat in her garden, surveying the beauty around her, she revealed her feelings to him: "I am now doing what is essential to the survival of the human race. That's why I am so full of happiness. I realized this before I met you...but there is a great deal to be said for the word becoming flesh....Although surrounded by warmth and love all my life, I have been at the very center alone...until now."[38] Soon thereafter, Hubbard invited Salk to talk to a local theater group about their ideas and ended the note by saying, "We have a cozy guest cottage."[39]

By now Hubbard was sending weekly, sometimes daily notes. "You'll simply have to brace yourself," she wrote, "for the fact that you are to receive letters from me more frequently than the ordinary decorum of correspondence-intercourse sets for the communication between two people separated by a continent." She told him she had appeared on *Open Mind* and might have the chance to travel across the country giving talks. In this way she could get to California. "Our thoughts are so much together that everything about distance is annihilated but physical separation. I wonder, Jonas, if the special distance between stars will prove as illusionary as the distance between two people who feel an affinity....To end a letter to you is impossible....I am borne along on a tide of feeling that is sometimes more than one person can bear."[40]

Salk's relationship with Hubbard must have been difficult for Lorraine Friedman. She had fallen in love with her boss seventeen years previously when she came to work for him, and she was always there, organizing his life, more of a partner in many ways than Donna.[41] Now when she opened his mail, as she had from the beginning, she read letters on expensive stationery with "Mrs. Earl Hubbard, Lakeville CONN" embossed in gold across the top. From the content, she would have known this woman was more than just a typical donor.

Although Hubbard admitted that the intellectual plane on which she and Salk were attracted had a physical component, she did not consider that the major aspect of their relationship. When asked if Salk had gotten divorced because of her, Hubbard replied, "Oh no. He had lots of women, not just me."[42] Richard Carter, author of *Breakthrough: The Saga of Jonas Salk*, asked a journalist who was writing about Salk how he was going to handle Jonas's skirt-chasing.[43] Although the press hovered, and muckraking—in which heroes were built up to be pilloried—was flourishing, reporters made no mention of the women in his life. The press loved him, and he had friendships with some powerful newsmen. Carter did not intend to be the first to reveal Salk's well-kept secret, especially since O'Connor had preordered a third of the copies of his book. Salk's files, in which Lorraine kept every scrap of correspondence, contain a few suggestive letters, however. "I have been thinking of you almost every day," he had written Mrs. S. B. Goldsmit in December of 1957, "and feel great pain at not having been to see you nor to have talked with you for so long. Each day it becomes worse. Could I ask you to help relieve my aching spirit and telephone me at…my private number…and tell me when I can come to see you."[44] No one recalls who she was, and no other correspondence between them exists. Though Hubbard seemed nonchalant and accepting of Salk's other assignations, one journalist described her feelings for Salk as "a constant torture."[45]

In January of 1965, Hubbard made her first visit to La Jolla, ready to work with Salk. She was disappointed to find him barely cordial and completely preoccupied with setting up the Institute. They had not broken ground on the meeting house, and here she was already planning her Theater of Humanity. To make matters worse, the scientists Salk had recruited, Hubbard soon learned, were more concerned with basic biological questions than with evolution. Nevertheless, she integrated herself into their fundraising, telling Salk that her father would contact General Eisenhower, Omar Bradley, Robert Kennedy, and a host of others he knew. Yet when she sent Salk fundraising materials she had crafted, he replied that she must send all material to the head of their fundraising campaign for clearance. She continued to write regularly to Salk as she sought funds for the Institute. Although she tried to be businesslike, she always inserted a personal note, such as, "I do not know how I am if I do not know how you are."[46]

On Valentine's Day 1966, Hubbard wrote Salk that her children's governess was traveling out west and would like to visit the Institute. "Perhaps she could catch a glimpse of you," she said, "and be able to report back to me of the glorious effect upon your physique with all that exercise."[47] They continued their liaisons in New York City. "I shall take the train to New York Monday and be at the apartment at 11 o'clock," she penciled at the bottom of a note about a seminar she was giving.[48] In time, their relationship became less intense. "Initially it was very hard," she reflected. "I wanted to be a co-creator with him, but he didn't want that."[49]

MEANWHILE, DONNA WAS earning respect for her work with the Urban League and as a trustee of Tuskegee Institute, the historically black university founded by Booker T. Washington. "Donna was brilliant," her niece Jessica Franken said, "fully engaged, accessible in a way that is unique."[50] Salk failed to perceive in his wife what others did. He was too busy with Institute money problems, the art exhibit uproar, the Leonell Strong suit. They used their emotional energy for different purposes. At the end of the day, Donna retreated to her books. And the communication between them all but stopped.

Eventually, Salk came to the conclusion that the marriage had to end. The man who hated confrontation and found it difficult to make decisions asked his wife for a divorce. There seemed to be no precipitating event, just the end of a slow demise. "I don't think even with the discomforts," Peter said, "that she wanted to lose that relationship."[51] Donna suggested they go through therapy. But Salk had made up his mind. Just as when he had decided twenty-eight years earlier that he must have Donna for his wife, now he decided he did not want to remain married to her any longer. Perhaps symbolically, he dropped his middle name, Edward, imposed upon him by Donna's father as a condition of marrying his daughter.

In the summer of 1967, Jonas and Donna separated. They told their sons one at a time, with no explanation. "'Devastating' may be too strong a word," Peter said, describing his reaction. "During childhood something didn't feel always on the level of comfort. [But] to be losing a nuclear family and to have to go through the complexities of relating separately to parents was as stressful for me and my brothers as anyone in that circumstance."[52] Peter felt angry with his father for instigating the breakup. He took a bus to Boston and then on to Woods Hole, where he spent the summer with family friends, trying to get his bearings. Darrell didn't anticipate the divorce either; he had never heard them argue.[53] When he thought more about it, though, he could see they had been drifting apart. Jonathan had just graduated from Andover and spent that summer on a ranch hauling hay. When he returned home to find his father gone, he was not surprised. "My father had been troubled about that relationship for a long time," he said.[54]

On May 31, 1968, the notice in *Time* reported that Donna Salk was divorcing her husband "on grounds of extreme cruelty." Salk's adoring public must have been shocked to see the name of their saint linked to the word "cruel." Yet he was caught in a legal bind. On January 1, 1970, California became the first no-fault divorce state. Prior to that, California law specified seven grounds for divorce: willful desertion, willful neglect, habitual intemperance, felony conviction, insanity, adultery, and extreme cruelty. Since none of the first five were true, and Donna either didn't know or couldn't prove that her husband was an adulterer, her only option was extreme cruelty. Although legally defined as conduct that destroys the peace of mind and happiness of one of the parties to the marriage, "extreme cruelty" was surely embarrassing to such a private man who had effectively hidden his private life from the public eye.

Three months later, Peter returned to Johns Hopkins Medical School, and his brothers left for Stanford University—Darrell as a senior, Jonathan as a freshman. Donna reengaged in her profession as a clinical social worker, and Jonas moved to a Pauma Valley retreat at the base of the Palomar Mountains.

Harnessing the Immune System

"SALK SAYS CURE for crippling multiple sclerosis possible," read the front-page headline in the *Houston Post* on December 4, 1969. "Prevention of a disease similar to multiple sclerosis has been achieved in animals at the Salk Institute," announced the *San Diego Union*.[1] Jonas Salk had co-developed an influenza vaccine, almost eradicated poliomyelitis, tested an anticancer vaccine, and now he was tackling multiple sclerosis. Victims of the debilitating disease prayed for his success; Institute scientists shook their heads. Salk hadn't intended to enter the field of neurology; he had done so via a circuitous route involving a serendipitous discovery and a surprise visit from Harry Weaver, the man who had enticed him into polio research two decades earlier.

∭

FIVE YEARS HAD passed since three large vans moved Salk's laboratory from Pittsburgh to La Jolla.[2] Full of enthusiasm, he had written in his 1963 progress report to the National Foundation that he now had the opportunity to "begin anew, in a new place, on…new, interesting, and significant questions."[3] Many wondered what exactly those questions were. The NF, which still funded his research, intimated that it should be relevant to their main concern, birth defects. The public anticipated cure of another disease. The press didn't care what Salk did as long as it made a good story. "What he wanted to do," Lorraine Friedman said, "was just be a regular guy in the lab and not be known as '*the* Dr. Salk.'"[4] That didn't happen. Journalists hovered, reporting on his every move. Perhaps at some level, he worried that he had already made his one great discovery. And his lack of acceptance by the scientific community still troubled him deeply. "I think that because of this rejection," Peter said, "my father continued to carry the feeling that he had something more to prove."[5] No matter how Salk tried to ignore the expectations, they imposed an enormous burden. "After you've cured a disease like polio, what's the encore?" an associate asked.[6] When Salk gave his answer, it was more opaque than the public or the National Foundation or the press would have liked: he was setting out to harness the immune system.

In the early 1960s, the understanding of the immune system was somewhat simplistic.[7] Its function had long been known—to protect human beings from invasion by foreign organisms. In 430 BC, when the plague decimated Athens, Thucydides observed that those who contracted the disease and survived seemed to be "immune" from another attack, even when nursing those suffering from the sickness. In the late 1800s, scientists discovered that in response to infection, the human body makes antibodies that kill the hostile microorganism. They later found that each microbe has a specific protein on its surface, called an antigen, short for antibody generator, that stimulates the immune system to produce a specific antibody. That antibody matches with and binds to the antigen and, once attached, sets loose a cascade of reactions that eradicate the invader. Vaccination represents the intentional introduction of an antigen, a killed or weakened microorganism such as the poliovirus. Afterward, the body has a prodigious immunological memory, and when it encounters that microbe again, it recognizes it and responds quickly, producing antibodies to prevent full-blown infection. In time, researchers recognized that the immune system has in its arsenal two types of responses: humoral, whereby lymphocytes (lymph cells) produce antibodies, and cell-mediated, whereby lymphocytes sensitized to an antigen kill the invader directly or recruit other killing cells.

For years, physicians sought to gain control of immunity. On the one hand, successful organ transplantation requires preventing the immune system from doing its job—rejecting a foreign substance—in this case the transplanted organ. On the other hand, when the immune system lets down its guard, such as failing to recognize and destroy a malignant cell, cancer results. In approaching immunity, Salk viewed it "through a wide-angle lens," he stated in the *Annals of the New York Academy of Sciences.* "The immunologic system, comprised of many parts in 'proper balance,' provides the natural means for developing and maintaining identity and integrity of self in the immunologic sense. Either too much reactivity or too little reactivity… may lead to disease or death." Rather than focus on a single aspect of the immune system, rather than try to decipher the answer to one scientific question, as did most investigators, Salk chose to attack several major problems simultaneously. He gathered them under the designation "manipulation of the immune system."[8]

To begin, he planned to follow up on the serendipitous discovery he and Elsie Ward had made in 1957 while culturing monkey heart cells for vaccine production.[9] When they injected these self-perpetuating cells into monkeys, benign tumors grew and then spontaneously disappeared in a few weeks as the monkeys developed antitumor antibodies. In the course of their studies, Salk made another curious observation when tuberculosis spread through the monkey colony. It was already known that host defense against TB involves a cell-mediated response, called "delayed hypersensitivity reaction" because it takes several days to be initiated. The infected monkeys appeared to have a deficiency in this part of the immune system. When inoculated with monkey heart cells, the TB-infected animals responded as the others had, making antitumor antibodies. To Salk's surprise, however, these monkeys developed large tumors that did not spontaneously disappear. Something had inhibited the cellular component of their immune systems.

In his 1964 report to the National Foundation, Salk said he was embarking on an investigation of the role of delayed hypersensitivity reaction in tumor rejection.[10] For his model system, he chose experimental allergic encephalomyelitis (EAE) in mice. In 1933, Tom Rivers had shown that injections of brain or spinal cord tissue from one animal into another set up a delayed-type hypersensitivity reaction, which damaged the brain.[11] For years EAE had been used to study this type of immune response. Although initially Salk chose EAE to investigate tumor rejection, he knew the injury seen in EAE—destruction of myelin, the protective tissue that covers nerve fibers—resembled that found in multiple sclerosis. Before long, he was considering the implications of his and Ward's work for treating this debilitating disease.

Salk had learned about multiple sclerosis (MS) in medical school. A neurologic disorder that predominately affects women in their thirties, MS is characterized by a number of different deficits that come and go over twenty to thirty years.[12] Patients often complain of pain and loss of vision in one eye initially; others suffer from double vision. Within a couple of weeks, many recover. Following a period of remission, patients develop numbness in the arms and legs, or a tremor or listing to one side when attempting to walk. With time, involvement of the spinal cord results in incontinence, impotency, or weakness on one side of the body, resembling a stroke. Ultimately, the brain's frontal lobe is affected, causing memory loss, irritation, depression, and finally euphoria, a cheerful lack of concern about the debilities termed *la belle indifférence*. Patients experience periods of remission and exacerbation over the years, with a progressive decline ending in death.

On postmortem, the brain of an MS-afflicted patient appears remarkably normal. But under the microscope, the findings are significant—patchy loss of myelin, the material insulating nerve fibers, throughout the brain and spinal cord. Early in the disease course, infiltration with inflammatory cells is observed, as if a battle is being waged. Later all that can be seen is an empty field of scar tissue, the nerve fibers ravaged. In the 1960s, the only effective therapy was a steroid hormone, ACTH, based on its anti-inflammatory action. Although beneficial for control of acute exacerbations, it did not alter the ultimate progression of the disease.

Most neuroscientists considered multiple sclerosis an autoimmune disease in which the body mounts an immune response against its own nervous tissue. Using the closest animal model system, EAE, several researchers set out to find what it was in the brain that acted as the antigen to incite this response. The first breakthrough came when Elizabeth Roboz Einstein at the University of California, Berkeley, and Marian

Kies at the National Institutes of Health both purified and characterized myelin basic protein (MBP). When injected into animals, it generated EAE. Salk wondered if MBP was the inciting antigen that caused multiple sclerosis. In October of 1965, he paid Einstein a visit, hoping to find the answer.

Elizabeth Roboz had emigrated from Hungary at the start of World War II.[13] Highly regarded for her neurochemistry work, she became a Stanford professor, then married Albert Einstein's son Hans and settled in Berkeley. The first evening Salk spent in their home, he was charmed by the sixty-three-year-old woman, with her jet-black hair, arched eyebrows, and wittiness. As they turned to discussion of her work, she told Salk she had purified five myelin proteins from bovine spinal cords, two of which induced EAE. The next challenge was deciphering what transpired between injection of MBP and the appearance of full-blown EAE. "I am happy that you contacted me," Roboz Einstein wrote Salk afterward. "I have full confidence that our chemical work will become more meaningful if someone with your vision applies a fresh approach to the immunological aspects of the experimental disease."[14] That evening Salk entered the world of neuroscience research, and he could not have had a warmer welcome.

A major stimulus for Salk's interest in multiple sclerosis was his reconnection with Harry Weaver, the unassuming mastermind behind the polio vaccine program. Weaver didn't care about accolades; he just wanted to see diseases eliminated. In 1966, the National Multiple Sclerosis Society (NMSS) asked him to direct their research programs. Weaver's personality hadn't changed much in thirteen years—sharp, exacting, manipulative, and relentless in attacking a disease. He had aged physically, however, with a prominent stoop, resulting from prior tuberculosis and chain smoking. "He reminded me of an old sea captain," Fred Westall, a young Salk Institute scientist, recollected. "He was the toughest guy I've ever known—no crap from Harry at all."[15]

As director of research for the NMSS, Weaver planned to use the same approach that had proved successful with polio. To initiate research on a disease about which little is known, he needed to entice researchers to work on different aspects of the illness, hoping that out of this effort a lead would emerge. The problem was that basic science investigators train in a particular discipline, such as biochemistry or neuroscience, not in a singular disease. To overcome this hurdle, Weaver told the NMSS, "You stimulate a scientist to work toward a specific objective by two means." First, you meet with the scientist and talk about how their work might relate to the disease in question, in this case multiple sclerosis, intimating available money for such. Secondly, you convene people with expertise in one or more facets of the problem. "You sit down for two or three days with them, and you encourage an informal, hard-headed discussion about what we have done, what we haven't done, what we ought to do, and out of such discussions emerge those scientists who have the creativity, the drive, and the imagination to do the job."[16] Once that is accomplished, he added, you hold out the carrot—research funds to support projects that would likely accomplish the initial objective.

Weaver had a cadre of excellent neuroscientists from which to choose. Marian Kies and Elizabeth Roboz Einstein had gained renown in the field for identifying MBP. Philip Paterson at New York University; Ellsworth Alvord, Jr., at the University of Washington; and Murray Bornstein at Albert Einstein College of Medicine had been using EAE to try to decipher the secrets of multiple sclerosis for years. Helene Rauch at Stanford University was attempting to isolate an antibody to MBP. Salk had done no work on multiple sclerosis. Nevertheless, Weaver wanted clinical results, and he knew Salk had no reluctance in moving from basic to applied research. He was smart yet malleable. And he needed Weaver.

Weaver started down the path he had outlined, gathering together scientists interested at least tangentially in multiple sclerosis. He wooed them in Locarno, Switzerland, then at the Westchester Country Club in Rye, New York. There Salk met and began to collaborate with others in the field. Marian Kies made stocks of MBP available to him. Einstein sent Salk serum from MS patients; Salk sent Otto Westphal, director of Germany's Max Planck Institute for Immunobiology, myelin protein his group was purifying. Kies, Einstein, and Westphal talked of forming an investigative unit; Rauch and Kies visited the Salk Institute. Salk addressed Ellsworth Alvord, Jr., by his nickname, "Buster." And he had already bonded with Elizabeth Einstein. For years, letters passed between Berkeley and La Jolla, filled with fond memories and inquiries about each other's lives.

In his 1967 report to the National Foundation, Salk said his group was trying to purify the protein that caused EAE and develop methods to measure antibodies against it in diseased animals. Just as they were beginning to make progress, he became distracted by the art exhibit fiasco, Leonell Strong's lawsuit, Kinzel's resignation, and his separation from Donna. By 1968, when he made a concerted effort to return to his lab, Salk had thirty-one staff members and was receiving more than $300,000 yearly from the NF to support his work. Then in May of that year, Joseph Nee, the NF's senior vice president, wrote him that in view of the government's large-scale support of basic science research, their scientific advisory committee had decided to redirect the Foundation's programmatic efforts. This meant a drastic reduction in their research programs in favor of those with greater importance to the Foundation, such as prenatal care and birth defects. "I am pleased that your grant is one of those that will be continued although, unfortunately, at a reduced rate," Nee informed Salk. "I realize that this will create a hardship for you, Jonas, but I also know you have survived many such problems in the past and will continue to do so in the future."[17] Henceforth, his grants could not exceed $145,000. In the past Salk would have turned to O'Connor to overrule such a decision; however, their personal communication had all but stopped. Besides, Salk was receiving money from Weaver, with whom O'Connor had parted ways just before the initiation of the polio vaccine trial.

Although his funding had been cut in half, Salk continued research on two fronts, cancer and multiple sclerosis, both of which involved manipulating the immune system to control disease. In trying to treat cancer, he injected small amounts of tumor into an animal to act as an antigen and initiate an immune response against the cancer. In MS, however, he needed to inhibit the immune response to an antigen normally found in the body, perhaps MBP. Thus, the object in cancer was to enhance immunity; the object in MS was to suppress it.

Some of Salk's staff worked on cancer. Two phenomena seemed to explain why the immune response to tumors was weak. First, when a malignant cell arose, not enough cancer-killing cells were generated in response. Second, the malignancy itself stimulated blocking antibodies that interfered with the action of these immune cells. Salk and his team planned a two-pronged attack on cancer by augmenting cellular immunity and eliminating blocking antibodies.

Others on his staff worked on EAE. Salk's lead investigator, biochemist Ed Eylar, isolated a fragment of MBP from bovine spinal cord, and, going a step further than Einstein and Kies, he synthesized it. When they injected the man-made MBP fragment into rabbits, it induced EAE.[18] A 1969 press release stated that a portion of a molecule that could incite the animal disease EAE had been isolated at the Salk Institute. The public would not have grasped the significance, except that the reporter said its identification might help figure out multiple sclerosis and mentioned Jonas Salk's name, which left Eylar feeling slighted.

Now that they could induce EAE, Salk set out to curb it. He postulated that MBP in higher doses might suppress EAE through a form of desensitization. To test this hypothesis, Eylar and Salk induced EAE in guinea pigs and rabbits by injecting them with brain tissue.[19] During the incubation period, before the onset of disease, they treated the animals with MBP in high doses for ten days. The animals showed no clinical signs of EAE; autopsies revealed no characteristic pathologic changes. It appeared that just as an animal's immune system was gearing up to attack its myelin, high doses of MBP inhibited the immune response. The incubation phase of EAE, Salk contended, might be comparable to the remission stage just before relapse in an MS patient. These were the results that made headlines.

Salk and Eylar weren't the first to demonstrate this, however. Alvord had already prevented EAE with large doses of MBP.[20] Murray Bornstein had reported that 70 percent of blood samples from patients with MS had demyelinating activity when applied to central nervous system tissue cultures.[21] The public didn't know Bornstein or Alvord, and so headlines stressed Salk's findings, omitting the work of more experienced investigators in the field. Though embarrassed by it, Salk ignored the media and pressed on.

Salk was supported in part by NMSS funds, and, typically, Weaver had strings attached. He asked Salk to speak at a luncheon in Houston about a five-year drive to raise ten million dollars for MS research. He requested that Salk fly to Philadelphia for a televised press conference with the president of the NMSS. Subtly at first, Weaver began to manipulate

Salk's research efforts. Westall recalled that after a Weaver visit Salk would invariably announce, "I've got some new ideas."[22]

Things seemed to be on track, when Salk's relationship with Eylar began to unravel. Those who had worked with Eylar weren't surprised. He often had mood swings, alternating between congeniality and rage. Westall, who initially worked in Eylar's lab, recounted the time Eylar played pool for hours in the recreation room. Late in the afternoon, he came to the lab and demanded of his staff, "Where have you been all day?"[23] Some colleagues suspected he lifted data from other investigators, and he became paranoid about his own work. One scientist with whom he collaborated described their meetings as secretive in nature, like two scientists meeting on a San Diego beach in trench coats.[24] Eylar began to fret that Salk might steal his results, so he started coding all the data in case Salk tried to spy on him. "Everything was coded," Westall recalled, "to the point that half the time he didn't know what the code was."[25] Another junior scientist who worked for Eylar recalled a time that Eylar was scheduled to present his data at a seminar. Before it started, Salk turned to the scientist and quipped, "Maybe I'll find out what's going on in my lab."[26]

In the spring of 1970, Eylar told Salk that he would be receiving a large grant from the Merck Institute and proceeded to buy expensive new equipment and supplies. In the fall, he traveled to Europe and on return announced he was joining Merck. He left behind a $19,000 debt. One evening after dark, a security guard found Eylar and another man with a large dolly, loading boxes into his car. Confronted by the guard, who told him he could not remove anything from the Salk Institute without written permission, Eylar snapped, "This is my own property."[27] When the guard turned to call his superior, Eylar drove away.

Salk didn't seem perturbed by Eylar's leaving. He inherited a superb investigator from Eylar's laboratory, Fred Westall, a chemist who would work with Salk while operating his own research group until the day Salk closed his lab. Besides, multiple sclerosis wasn't the main thing on Salk's mind. He was captivated by his new wife.

22

A Most Unusual Arrangement

THIRTEEN YEARS HAD passed since the success of the polio vaccine
had been announced, yet Salk still retained his celebrity status. A 1968
poll ranked him fourth among heroes after Churchill, Roosevelt, and
Kennedy.[1] If he went to a restaurant, he had barely been seated before
he began to hear murmurs. Soon a heartfelt expression of thanks or an
autograph request would interrupt his meal. On the street, strangers
grabbed his hand and kissed it. Whenever he flew, a stewardess ushered
him onto a plane after everyone else was seated. If the pilot couldn't resist and announced his presence, passengers cheered. "If there were
American saints," one journalist wrote, "Jonas Salk surely would be high
on the list."[2] Beloved by the public, this hero was lonely.

Salk had few close friends. In April 1965, Edward R. Murrow had
died of lung cancer at the age of fifty-seven. No longer would the
American public hear him sign off, "Good night and good luck," and no
longer could Salk seek advice from the man who had been his confidant
ever since his interview on *See It Now*. Murrow had served as a Salk
Institute trustee almost from its inception. Salk had tried to help him
during his final weeks, to no avail.[3] Warren Weaver also had been a
steadying hand throughout the turbulent early years of the Institute.

Salk urged him to move to La Jolla, but Weaver declined due to poor health. First he developed heart problems; then he suffered bouts of confusion from intermittent blockage of an artery to his brain. When Weaver had to resign from the Institute, Salk told him, "One cannot resign from a friendship."[4] Nevertheless, they rarely saw each other after that. Hardest of all, the intimacy Salk shared with Basil O'Connor was waning, and he still did not understand why.

Salk began spending evenings with architects Christine and Russell Forester. Around dinnertime, he often called and asked, "How are you guys doing?" Christine knew Salk couldn't cook and didn't like to eat alone. Sometimes he called and simply said, "I'm hungry." The Foresters provided the companionship Salk was longing for. "We had good food and good wine and talked until the wee hours," Christine recalled, "always very animated conversations about everything and nothing. I think he felt we were a little island he could swim to and not have to be accountable other than to talk of ideas and the world."[5] Although Salk knew lots of people, he felt close to few. Once he told Christine he wished he had a relationship like hers and Russell's. As much as she cherished Jonas, she doubted he could give fully to another.

As always, Lorraine Friedman stood waiting in the wings. "She was in love with Jonas," Fred Westall said, having observed this while working in Salk's lab.[6] She had been ever since he hired her two decades earlier. A head taller than Salk, in her sensible shoes, sweater set, and ever-present strand of pearls, she looked the epitome of the executive secretary. And he never thought of her as more than that.

In May of 1968, Salk became an eligible bachelor, and women started calling. "It was a new thing for him," his sister-in-law Sylvia maintained. "He never was the debonair fellow; he was always a lab rat."[7] Presently he began to pay more attention to his attire, adding modern eyeglass frames and a more stylish haircut. "Now that Dr. Jonas Salk of polio vaccine fame is divorced, doesn't he plan to marry a Hollywood starlet?" a reader asked Walter Scott, whose gossip column was published in *Independent Press-Telegram*. "Dr. Salk has been seeing a good deal of Mrs. J. 'Doakie' Ankenbrandt, divorced wife of Dr. I. M. Ankenbrandt of Pacific Beach," Scott reported six months into Salk's bachelorhood. "She is considered the most likely candidate for Dr. Salk's second marriage."[8]

Unbeknownst to Scott, Salk had already moved into Ankenbrandt's avant-garde La Jolla home. All people remembered about Doakie was that she was quite attractive, younger than Salk, had no profession, and involved herself in charity work and social gatherings.[9] Sylvia Salk referred to her as a "doozy."[10]

Within two months of the *Independent Press-Telegram's* revelation, Salk realized his mistake. "I feel a deep conflict," he confided in his night notes, "between Doakie and myself, my commitment to man and to the world and her commitment to herself." Most fulfilled when devoting himself to some larger cause, he could not do this and satisfy Doakie's needs. As a result, she became angry. Salk worried his relationship with Doakie was beginning to parallel that with Donna. "[It] will repeat itself," he thought, "unless I find someone who is fully accommodating to the strong passion I have for my goals."[11] He concluded his ambitions and marriage were likely incompatible.

✦

THE FIRST TIME they met, French artist Françoise Gilot seemed more interested in her salad than in Jonas Salk—somewhat embarrassing for her friend Chantal Hunt, who had insisted she join them for lunch. Chantal's husband, John Hunt, the executive vice president of the Salk Institute, had invited Salk to their home to discuss "Institute issues." Gilot had warned Chantal that she was tired from completing the lithograph series at the Tamarind Workshop in Los Angeles, and she needed some rest before returning to Paris. "I'm going to go have lunch at a restaurant," she told her friend. "I don't want to see a scientist." Chantal said she didn't need to talk. "Fine," Gilot replied, "I don't talk."[12] Françoise didn't know her friend had described her to Salk as a vital, witty woman. Instead she appeared sullen. Still, her green eyes, thick dark hair which fell to her shoulders, aquiline nose, and sensuality did not escape him.

The next evening, Gilot accompanied the Hunts to a black-tie dinner at the Institute. Seated with other artists, she enjoyed herself. Although she didn't notice Salk, he saw her. Later he told Françoise he found the situation curious. One day she behaved "like a lump," he said. The next day she was "laughing like I don't know what." He wondered, "Who is this person?"[13] So he invited Gilot to the Institute for a private tour.

Once there, this woman who had silently looked at her salad two days before began talking with great animation and sophistication, a mixture of self-confidence and femininity. Salk knew almost nothing about art, and Gilot could not converse about science, but they had one common interest, modern architecture. That was a start.

Jonas became enthralled with Françoise. He didn't know much about her life, except that she was a successful artist, although he had seen none of her paintings, and that she had been Pablo Picasso's mistress, although he likely had not read her best-selling memoir, *Life with Picasso*. The past didn't interest Salk; he was looking to the future.

⚜

MARIE FRANÇOISE GILOT was born on November 26, 1921, in Neuilly-sur-Seine, a suburb of Paris, the only child of a watercolor artist and an agronomical engineer.[14] Françoise had inherited her mother's artistic talent and her father's intellect. From a young age, she spent her free time sketching, trying her hand at watercolors, and visiting museums. Her mother began tutoring her, and at seventeen Gilot set up her first studio in her grandmother's attic. Her father served as her academic mentor, drawing her into discussions about the world. Although rigid and controlling, he was rational. When they disagreed, he made a contract: If she did something to please him, he would do something that pleased her. He ultimately raised a strong-willed, confident, and savvy daughter. After she had earned her BA in philosophy at the Sorbonne, he encouraged her to study law. She aspired to be a painter; he thought she could do both. "If you work eight hours at your school," he instructed her, "you can work eight hours with your paintings, and then you can go horseback riding for an hour, and then you sleep four hours."[15] Her father helped her think sensibly, yet the strength he imbued in her later drove a wedge between them.

The outbreak of World War II marked a tragic time in Gilot's life. Every week she learned of comrades who had died participating in the Resistance and Jewish friends who had been deported. She felt an urgency to contribute in some way. "In 1940, when the defeat of France shattered the pride and hopes of an entire generation of young French people," she recounted in a later book, *Françoise Gilot: An Artist's Journey*,

"I felt that upholding the cultural values we shared was an individual duty and a necessity."[16] The Nazis considered modern art decadent and condemned it. "To choose art at that time was like a testament," she believed.[17] Wanting to express her feelings about the situation in a manner she thought might be unnoticeable to the Nazis who occupied Paris, Gilot embedded symbols in her artwork. *The Hawk* depicted a predatory bird with Paris in the background, the Eiffel Tower rising higher than the hawk's wing. In May of 1943, Françoise had her first exhibition. Around the same time, she met Pablo Picasso. "We were living with a doomsday mentality," she reflected.[18] No one knew how long they would live. "I believe that if I had met Picasso in normal circumstances, nothing would have happened between him and myself."[19]

Alain Cuny, a popular actor, had invited Françoise and her friend the artist Geneviève Aliquot to dine at Le Catalan, a Left Bank restaurant frequented by actors and artists. They had just ordered when Cuny pointed out Pablo Picasso; Yugoslav artist Dora Maar, Picasso's mistress at the time; and an art collector at the next table. Gilot was quite familiar with the Spanish painter who had founded the Cubist movement. His *Demoiselles d'Avignon* and *Guernica* had brought Picasso renown. She also heard rumors of the sixty-two-year-old's charm and notorious behavior. While married to ballerina Olga Khokhlova, with whom he had a son, he began a life-long affair with seventeen-year-old Marie-Thérèse Walter, with whom he had a daughter. Now he had acquired another lover, Dora Maar. Throughout dinner, Gilot noticed Picasso was staring at their table. Afterward, he brought over a bowl of cherries and asked Cuny to introduce his friends. Cuny told him they were artists. Picasso laughed. "Well, I'm a painter, too. You must come to my studio and see some of my paintings."[20] The first visit, amidst a bevy of admirers, seemed innocuous. Picasso invited Gilot back.

In the summer of 1943, Françoise took a 150-mile bike ride with Geneviève, who helped strengthen her resolve to spend her life as an artist. When Françoise informed her father, he threatened to have her committed for insanity, and when she still refused to obey him, he became enraged, slapping and punching her. Gilot moved in with her grandmother, vowing never to see her father again. That winter she revisited Picasso's gallery. Despite their age difference of forty years, a relationship blossomed, first intellectual, later sexual. "One thing stood out very clearly," she wrote, "the ease with which I could communicate with him."[21]

Those were intoxicating times for Gilot. Picasso introduced her to Alice B. Toklas, Gertrude Stein, and Henri Matisse. Françoise delved into her own work, studying at the École des Beaux Arts. A recent movement called New Realities, in which artists created pure abstract paintings, influenced her, and by 1945 she was gaining notice for her art. Busy with her work, Gilot saw less of Picasso. He had become enamored of the young artist and began to pursue her. The next time she visited him and looked at his recent lithographs, she realized most were portraits of her. In May of 1946, Gilot agreed to move in with Picasso. She learned a lot from him, adopting his work habits. At the same time, she found how difficult he could be. "When he wanted, he was the most charming man," she told television talk show host Charlie Rose. Yet he had terrible mood swings.

"Why do you always contradict me?" Picasso used to ask her.

"Because it's a dialogue," Gilot replied. "Otherwise you can speak to yourself."[22]

What followed were years of a tempestuous relationship; two children, Claude and Paloma; and entry into the private world of one of the history's greatest artists. Gilot tried to leave Picasso several times, but he begged her to come back, and she always did. In the end she saw how broken he had left his previous lovers, and she was determined to remain independent and strong. Although he bragged that she would be nothing without him, Gilot was becoming a respected artist.

By 1951, her life with Picasso appeared to be in trouble; his explosive temper and cooling ardor drained her; his Don Juan behavior repelled her. Gilot's work reflected her dismay—stark, somber pictures of objects from her life as a mother and homemaker, called her Kitchen Series. She began to separate emotionally from Picasso, dedicating her energy to her children and her art. Finally she told him she wanted a more equal relationship, and if he remained obdurate, she would leave. "No woman leaves a man like me," Picasso boasted. Even more cutting, he added, "You imagine people will be interested in *you*?... Even if you think people like you, it will only be a kind of curiosity they will have about a person whose life has touched mine so intimately."[23]

Gilot's last painting of this period, *Still Life with Scissors*, contrasts the soft radiance of flowers in front of a window with a pair of open scissors on a table. "Severing a tie that had unified my art and my life in such a powerful way was not easy," she acknowledged, "yet at that point my integrity as an artist and my children's education had to be my chief concern, and I did not hesitate."[24] In the fall of 1953, she took the children and left. Within two years, Gilot married artist Luc Simon, whom she had known since her teens. She returned from her honeymoon to find La Galloise, the Vallauris villa she had shared with Picasso, ransacked and all her books, drawings, and paintings gone.[25] Although he didn't confess to the deed, Gilot never spoke to Picasso again.

At thirty-seven, Gilot felt she had come into her own as an artist. Inspired by London's Kew Gardens, she began the Vegetation Series, gaining recognition for her distinct style. "But as always in life, serenity does not last forever," she wrote. "My relationship with Luc Simon was far from simple."[26] In 1961 they separated, and she took their young daughter, Aurelia, with her. Three years later, Gilot finished writing *Life with Picasso*, which sold more than a million copies the first year. Picasso tried to stop its publication, without success. Her recognition as an artist continued to grow with exhibits in London, Milan, Hamburg, and New York.

In October of 1969, Gilot traveled to Los Angeles to complete some lithographs. It was on that trip that the Hunts introduced her to Salk. When she stopped in New York on her way home, he appeared, as if by chance. After that he followed her to Paris, so she invited him to La Galloise for Christmas. "There was no way to find out who bewitched whom," she told Charlie Rose. "All I can say is that a powerful whirlwind was blowing."[27] Salk found Gilot to be the most alluring and intellectually most engaged woman he had ever known. She had a wonderful laugh, a refreshingly honest way of viewing the world, and the same intensity about her endeavors as he had about his.

Gilot knew Salk's story from news reports and Richard Carter's biography, but none of these captured the man behind the public persona. He did not have a typical scientific mind; rather, he seemed to be an intuitive scientist—"an artist in a different field," she concluded, with a philosophical, almost mystical bent. He cared deeply about his work, not for his own benefit but for mankind's. People described him as aloof, but she perceived his inherent shyness. "He was always alone," Gilot observed. "He never had any people to understand him."[28]

Some thought the attraction had another side. "She was exciting," Sylvia Salk contended, "because she had been Picasso's woman."[29] Beyond any appeal arising from the other's celebrity status or the physical attraction, however, lay the similar way they approached their work—with unflagging zeal. Passionate about her art, Gilot often worked on ten to twelve paintings at the same time. And Salk had written in his night notes: "I seem to want to be on twenty-four-hour call in relation to my basic commitment."[30] It appeared to be an excellent match.

Six months after they met, while the sun was setting over Santa Monica Bay, Salk asked Gilot to marry him. She later recounted the scene to Rose in his television interview. When Jonas proposed, she had replied, "A relationship would be all right, but I don't want to get married."

"Why not?" he asked.

"Because I don't want to live with anybody more than six months a year. That's it. I need my own time to myself, plus I have my children."

Jonas handed her a piece of paper. "Write down everything that you don't want," he directed. "I'll give you an hour." Françoise proceeded to write down those elements that would make the marriage unsuitable for her.

Jonas read it over. "Very good. It fits my life perfectly."

"But we don't know each other," she cautioned, "and it may be disastrous because you're a scientist, and our lives are very far apart."

"No," Jonas countered, in what seemed more like a business transaction than a romantic moment, "even if we're not so happy, at least we'll be like a citadel; we'll be a fortress for each other."

Françoise thought about it. Both felt exhausted by the world and sought a refuge. "In that case, let's try," she replied.[31]

Gilot was forty-eight, an artist, a determined free spirit. Salk was fifty-five, a scientist, averse to conflict. They would live half the year almost six thousand miles apart. "All our friends on both sides predicted impending doom," Gilot recalled.[32]

On June 29, 1970, Françoise Gilot and Jonas Salk married in Neuilly-sur-Seine.[33] Françoise wore a simple, stylish dress, and Jonas a dark suit and tie. Gilot's children, Claude, Paloma, and Aurelia, and Salk's sons, Peter, Darrell, and Jonathan, attended the wedding, as did Chantal and John Hunt, who had introduced them. Their children met for the first time as their parents prepared to say their vows. Twenty-three-year-old Claude Ruiz-Picasso worked in New York as a photographer for Condé Nast; twenty-one-year-old Paloma was studying jewelry design in Paris; and Aurelia Simon, just thirteen, attended boarding school. Of Salk's sons, Jonathan felt the most comfortable, having just spent six months in Paris. Although pleased for their father, whom they had rarely seen so joyous, Salk's sons must have questioned his impetuousness. He had met Madame Gilot only eight months earlier.

"We did not really know each other well when we got married," Gilot admitted. They had been together only a few times. "We were more than middle-aged, and the type of love we shared was an adult love, not passion like when you are eighteen. We understood each other very well, and that was basically the foundation of our union."[34]

In late August, Françoise, Jonas, and Aurelia returned to La Jolla and moved into a house Salk had rented with spectacular views of the coastline. He could barely wait to introduce—some thought show off—his new wife. "He was absolutely thrilled," Christine Forester recalled.[35] At a dinner party at the Foresters' home, Jonas and his new bride danced into the morning hours long after everyone else had collapsed. Forester had never seen him dance more than an occasional waltz. Besides introducing Gilot to friends, Salk also brought her to meet Donna, as if to get her approval. After that, Donna referred to Françoise as her "wife-in-law."[36]

Just as the media continued to equate Salk with the polio vaccine, it forever linked Gilot with Pablo Picasso. The *Harrisburg News*, reporting their marriage, identified Gilot as Picasso's mistress of eleven years. After noting her "discreet wedding" to Salk, the article went on to describe her life with Picasso.[37] A *Philadelphia Enquirer* article about Salk's work on multiple sclerosis mentioned his marriage to Gilot, "an artist who was the mistress of the late Pablo Picasso."[38]

Salk's childhood had centered on studies, his adulthood on work. He never let exercise, the arts, or leisure distract him. Now that changed.[39] On weekends, he and Gilot went to the La Jolla Beach and Tennis Club to swim or hiked in the nearby hills. They bought season tickets to the

Old Globe Theatre. He listened to Schubert and Schumann, enjoyed the opera, even took Aurelia to an occasional musical comedy. He studied French, relaxed at Parisian cafes. As he sailed with Françoise in the Aegean, he learned one could travel for enjoyment. He practiced yoga and meditation, underwent Rolfing, participated in a sensitivity group. Françoise changed his diet, eliminating red meat and lowering the fat and salt content. Within six months, he had lost twenty-five pounds.

Friends, colleagues, and family noticed major changes in Salk's appearance. "He was a man who had no inherent taste," according to Jack MacAllister.[40] In an article entitled "Jonas Salk Unfolding," a journalist described his transformation: "External signs can't be missed. The suit and ties...have been replaced by dapper, almost mod outfits—ascots, turtlenecks, flared pants, bright ties under dark sport jackets. His hair has grown out in attractive waves."[41] Pictures prior to his marriage show a weary-looking Salk, a bit thick about the middle, in a dark suit and thick glasses, with short-clipped hair—an older version of the man whose face millions knew. Now his hair curled down to his collar; he sported sideburns and wore a scarf tied around his neck. For photos, he held his glasses and perfected a thoughtful, peaceful pose. Sylvia Salk called her brother-in-law "Frenchified."[42]

The media now displayed photographs of Salk with a strikingly beautiful woman at his side. She smiled lovingly as he received the All-India Institute of Medical Science Award, or while President Jimmy Carter put the gold Medal of Freedom around his neck. She donned a fashionable gown to attend an Institute fundraiser, accompanied by Governor Ronald Reagan and his wife, Nancy, along with Steve McQueen and Ali McGraw. At home, Gilot proved to be a gracious hostess, welcoming friends and heightening Salk's social standing among the resident fellows. "Françoise brought out the lighter side of Jonas," Maureen Dulbecco observed. "He could be very amusing and enjoy a good laugh."[43] Gilot often invited her European friends for dinner, providing haute cuisine, fine wine, and stimulating conversation. "It was like a Salk clique," Christine Forester remarked.[44]

Although Salk's European colleagues called Gilot "a gracious hostess," some who worked with him expressed less regard for her. "He married the artist's concubine," Don Wegemer sniped. "We used to say,

'Another Jewish guy has fallen victim to a French woman.'"[45] Walter Mack, Salk's friend from Ann Arbor, also disapproved: "All of a sudden he decided Donna wasn't good enough. He divorced her and married some French actress."[46] Friedman, ever protective of her boss, never understood why he chose Gilot. "She wasn't particularly interested in being known as Jonas's wife," she observed. "She had a life of her own."[47] Salk's research associate Fred Westall referred to Gilot as "Picasso's ex"; nevertheless he considered their marriage a good arrangement. "She needed somebody of the stature of Picasso; she can't just marry somebody off the street. And he needed someone who was 'ta-da.'" She snubbed Westall on several occasions. "She is the strongest lady I ever met," he carped.[48] Sylvia Salk thought the newlyweds deserved each other. "She was part of the jet set," she remarked. "It made his life more exciting. But if they had to live together 365 days a year, I'm sure they never would have made it."[49]

Jack MacAllister considered these comments unwarranted. He loved the new Jonas: "He grew up in New York poor, and he never had taste. After he married Françoise, he looked younger and more handsome. She brought out a side he didn't know he had." MacAllister grew fond of Gilot. Although an intellect, she could be giddy and silly. "It was a whole new world for Jonas," MacAllister pointed out. "He'd never lived that way. He had lived in a lab. He was a guy in a white coat."[50] Russell Forester concurred, describing his friend as "1000 percent happier."[51]

His sons noticed the change, too. Jonathan observed that his father seemed delighted to be married. Françoise encouraged his creative side. He started to paint, write poetry; he was living the cosmopolitan life he thought he wanted. "Françoise was more present, involved," Jonathan maintained, "and clearly, there was a bit of a makeover." Darrell, on the other hand, thought his father had lost his roots. "Some of it was a little frou-frou," Jonathan agreed, "but he was happy, and that's great."[52]

According to Gilot, Basil O'Connor was not pleased with the marriage. He had admired Donna and had placed her on the board of the Tuskegee Institute, of which he served as chairman. Gilot sensed his displeasure and thought O'Connor considered her too strong-minded; she had changed his humble, agreeable friend.[53] O'Conner did not attend the wedding, although he may not have been invited. And there is no congratulatory note from him in Salk's files.

Before long, the newly married couple began to live apart. "Jonas was a man of his word," Gilot said. "We were not together year-round." She spent at least six months in Paris or at her New York studio. "I am not the usual wife. Ours was the union of two very busy people who were completely dedicated to their work, and so it was not the typical husband-wife relationship."[54] Most viewed it as an unusual arrangement. "When she was there," one of Gilot's friends noted, "she really had her attention on being there, being with him, entertaining, doing whatever to be part of that community. But when she wasn't there, he retreated into his introverted world."[55] In her absence, Salk resumed his pattern of working incessantly and calling Christine Forester to see what she and Russell planned for dinner.

Although Gilot spent just half the year with her husband, she nonetheless appreciated his diverse facets. "Jonas was many persons in one," she commented in an interview years after his death. In pursuing science, he used his intuition almost more than rational thought. "Things could be evident to him that were not evident to others, creating a lot of misunderstanding about his thinking. Jonas also had a prophetic side in him regarding the evolution of humankind, and in this, as in many other aspects, he was not well understood." She described him as self-possessed, never showing irritation or bad temper, even in trying circumstances. She enjoyed his sense of humor, the way he said funny things with a deadpan mien so people couldn't tell if he was joking. And he was kind. "Many people didn't see that." He often appeared self-absorbed when he was contemplating mankind's future. "He was basically optimistic," Gilot concluded, "even though he had encountered more than his share of opposition." In painting portraits of her husband, what Gilot tried to capture was his spirit of discovery. "We were compatible mainly because, even though we were in different fields, we had that same intrinsic drive, the drive to get into an equation with the unknown. The spirit of discovery allows one to get something known out of the unknown. That's what he had. That's what I loved best in him."[56]

Though many could not fathom their marital arrangement, Salk and Gilot's relationship matured as they grew to know each other better. "We found new discoveries all the time," Gilot recalled.[57] And Salk maintained,

"I have achieved in terms of personal relationships as much with Françoise as I could possibly fantasize."[58] When asked in an interview how she had ended up with two of history's most powerful men, Gilot replied: "Lions mate with lions."[59] That certainly described Pablo Picasso, but hardly Jonas Salk.

23

Salk Unfolding

"THE VOICE OF the intellect is a soft one," Freud wrote in *The Future of an Illusion*, "but it does not rest until it has gained a hearing."[1] The public had expected Jonas Salk to eradicate another disease, cancer or multiple sclerosis. Instead, he began to talk about humankind in evolution. "As we view man at this point in his development," he said in a public lecture, "his critical problem is not his relationship to his natural environment, nor to other living species, animal or microbial. It is found, rather, in man's relationship to man, and in his relationship to himself."[2] In the late 1960s, Salk appeared to have entered a period of philosophical musing. When he gave voice to the concerns upon which he had been reflecting and, because of his fame, "gained a hearing," few understood him; some derided him. "Despite his considerable repute as a scientist," a reporter carped in "Salk's Smear," "his activities outside his special field tend to cancel his contributions."[3]

Although some thought Salk was either experiencing a midlife crisis or exhibiting the effects of Gilot's intellectual influence, neither was the case. Since childhood he believed he had been born for a specific purpose—to perform acts of goodness, which extended from caring for the sick to preventing disease to helping society become more compassionate.

He called this the "immunization and humanization of mankind."[4] In high school, he had been stirred by the essays of Francis Bacon and Ralph Waldo Emerson; as an adult, he favored inspirational and philosophical books: Edwin Burtt's *Man Seeks the Divine*; Jacques Barzun's *The House of Intellect*, a critique of America's attitudes toward the life of the mind; Homer Smith's *Kamongo*, a debate on science and faith; and Robert Jungk's *Brighter Than a Thousand Suns*, an account of the scientists who discovered fission and how they grappled with its implications for humanity.

"He had a very active inner life," his son Peter observed, "processing everything going on around him."[5] Salk awakened several times each night, his mind so stimulated he couldn't sleep. While at the University of Michigan, he had begun psychoanalysis. His therapist suggested he keep a notepad at his bedside and jot down his thoughts when he awoke in the middle of the night, getting them out of his head and onto paper so he could sleep. "With the enormous amount of energy that exists within me and the incredible desire to do things that could be of value for man," he wrote in his night notes, "it is hardly a wonder that I awaken with anxiety when my subconscious mind is aware of all that remains unfinished and undone."[6]

In Pittsburgh, when insomnia drove him up to his third-floor study, he dictated his ruminations for Lorraine Friedman to transcribe the next day. He dated and timed each entry: "3 January 1969 (3:10–4:00 am), 26 January 1969 (2:00–3:05 am)." Initially his night notes served as a means of sorting through his day, his reactions to specific people and events. After the polio vaccine announcement, they focused more on his relationship with the scientific community and his future role. With time they became more abstract, a place for him to expound upon his philosophical views. The day-to-day aspects of his life took on more meaning: "I was in a meeting with so-and-so today, and I saw a tendency of the world to such-and-such. These are the forces that come into play; it's becoming clear to me now how the universe works."[7] Until he met R. Buckminster Fuller, he had kept his deliberations private.

Salk didn't know much about the sixty-year-old man who sat next to him at the University of Michigan, about to receive an honorary degree in 1955. Recounting their first meeting years later, he remarked, "I was preoccupied with the little viruses that I was pursuing." When he asked

Fuller what he did, Fuller had replied that he used scientific principles to solve mankind's problems. "That's what I do," Salk said.[8] Afterward he learned that this great-nephew of transcendentalist Margaret Fuller had been expelled from Harvard for "irresponsible behavior" (Fuller said he preferred to consider himself a "non-conforming misfit in the fraternity environment"); that his early career had been checkered and unproductive; and that when his young daughter died of polio, he had embarked on a quest to help change the world.[9] In his designs and inventions, Fuller sought to produce practical, inexpensive transportation and shelter, the most famous example being his geodesic dome. An early environmental activist, he worried about human survival.

Over dinner, Fuller and Salk continued their discussion: "As Bucky was describing his own feeling of being different from others, [I told him] I had that very distinct feeling myself for a long time."[10] A bond formed between them, and they corresponded for years. Fuller's sentiments in his book *I Seem to Be a Verb* resonated with Salk: "I live on Earth at present, and I don't know what I am. I know that I am not a category. I am not a thing—a noun. I seem to be a verb, an evolutionary process—an integral function of the universe."[11] Fuller spoke and wrote in a unique style seasoned with run-on sentences, such as his famously unpunctuated three-thousand-word single sentence essay, "What I Am Trying to Do," or invented terms, such as "omniwell-informed" and "intertransformative."[12] These may have worked well for Fuller; they sounded forced and phony coming from Salk.

Among Salk's first public remarks on his philosophical views was an address, entitled "Biology in the Future," at the Massachusetts Institute of Technology's 1961 centennial celebration. He mentioned molecular biology, then veered off into bio-philosophy. He characterized scientists as those "whose activities are largely responsible for the direction and the force of change" and humanists as those "who are concerned with the consequences thereof," stressing their need to interrelate. He quoted the British writer Elizabeth Sewell, who wrote of poetry and the natural sciences, "A poem will often tell the thinking mind where to look next," and he ended by saying, "Perhaps it will be from the poets of biology that a vision of the future will come."[13] Two months later at a University of Chicago building dedication, he speculated that biological ideas could "suggest methods to develop means whereby man can control not only his physical disease but diseases of unreasonableness, prejudice, and self-ishness."[14] In lectures throughout the 1960s and early 1970s, Salk often pondered man's place in the metabiological world. Whereas his publications a few years earlier had carried such titles as "Use of Adjuvants in Studies of Influenza Immunization" and "Studies of Poliomyelitis Viruses in Cultures of Monkey Testicular Tissue," now Salk wrote "Awareness of Order" and "The Next Evolutionary Step in the Ascent of Man in the Cosmos." And like Fuller he began to express himself in verse.

On the television show *See It Now*, Salk had charmed the nation. Eight years later, on NBC's *Chet Huntley Reporting*, his demeanor and tone had changed substantially. Instead of the eager young scientist, filling the screen with hope, viewers saw a somber, wary savant who talked of the "biology of the spirit." When Huntley said, "Now it's here, Dr. Salk, that I tend to lose you," trying to nudge Salk, who sat with his arms hugging his chest, his eyes downcast, to reach out to the public as he had done so well in the past, Salk replied, "I do believe that man's view of himself is due for an update."[15] Doubtless many in Huntley's television audience were disappointed. People had tuned in to see a swashbuckling hero, not an inscrutable prophet.

Salk didn't notice the lukewarm responses to his lectures, and no one advised him to temper his divinations. So he overcame his inherent reticence and began to speak more freely. In May of 1969, when he gave the Robert Kennedy Duncan Lecture, entitled "Narcissism and Responsibility in Science and Man," at Carnegie Mellon University, he told the audience, "This afternoon, we are having a happening, and you are in it with me." Attendees from the Mellon Institute, which merged scientific research and industrial technology, had not expected a be-in. Salk proceeded to assert that the major issue facing mankind was a conflict between the need to survive as individuals and the need to survive as a species. To illustrate his points, he used twenty hand-drawn slides, which displayed childlike stick figures. "Nature's game might be called evolution," he said. "The object is survival." With changing values, a whole new social fabric was being woven. He posed a series of questions that sounded as if he had copied them unedited from his night notes: "What do I want?...I don't know and I am in conflict. Why doesn't someone answer? Help? From where? God? Where is He? Parents? Society? If 'no' to all outside myself, then why not myself? Myself? Is that where God is?"[16]

A number of people, in addition to Buckminster Fuller, encouraged him in his speculations, among them Norman Cousins, editor in chief of the *Saturday Review*. Salk admired "A Litany for Modern Man," in which Cousins reflected his own feelings in an elegant way: "I am a single cell in a body of two billion cells. The body is mankind. I glory in the individuality of self, but my individuality does not separate me from my universal self—the oneness of man."[17] They met at a conference in 1969, after which Cousins wrote to Salk: "In Denver you made a very poetic reference to 'sharing the same genetics.'"[18] Salk replied, "We must find a way to be together more closely than has been possible thus far.... I think of you often as I strive to get to the writing that I so much want to do."[19] Although he shared many of Cousins's views and aspired to publish his own, Salk lacked his literary skills. Cousins expressed his thoughts in beautiful, powerful phrases; Salk's seemed to become entangled as they formed in his brain and emerged discombobulated.

Louis Kahn was another figure who had energized him. "When you are with another person who is of this nature," Salk reflected in a 1972 conversation with Kahn, "who makes you feel this way, allows you to feel this way, then you are turned on so to speak."[20] Early on, their familiarity had threatened to scuttle construction of the Institute as Salk got drawn into Kahn's philosophical musings. This taped exchange typified their interactions: "Architecture begins by the making of a room," Kahn explained, "and this room, this place which has its measure, it being small or being large, and the grade to which a person responds, the human response to this enclosure with the world."[21]

"I think the most important thing," Salk responded, "is for people to have the sense and understanding of the nature of things and...to express themselves in whatever metaphor is natural for them....I am interested in seeing how I can discover the convergence in that which has diverged and in that way may I arrive at the source, meaning the nature of the beginning and relationship of it all in a sense, to the cosmos."

"Oh yes, to the cosmos," Kahn shouted.

"To the plan of the cosmos and to the laws of nature," Salk exclaimed.[22]

Yet another influence was Greek architect and engineer C. A. Doxiadis, president of the World Society for Ekistics, a group that aimed to achieve harmony between a community's inhabitants and their natural as well as sociocultural environment. Members included Margaret Mead and Buckminster Fuller. Having befriended Doxiadis, Salk attended several of the yearly Delos Symposia, conducted on a cruise in the Aegean, culminating in a closing ceremony at the amphitheater in Delos.[23] "Thinking of you longingly," he wrote Doxiadis when he could not attend one of the symposia.[24]

Gilot encouraged Salk's prophetic streak as well, although she downplayed her role. "After he got married to me," she recollected, "it was a period in his life when he was more interested in questions of human life in general and culture and not so much of science." She refused to take credit for affecting his content. "We had elaborated our ideas independently, but one might say that our encounter revealed a meeting of minds."[25]

Inspired by Fuller, Cousins, Kahn, and Doxiadis, and emboldened by Gilot, Salk became less self-conscious in sharing his insights. As a result, he gave a number of talks: "Chance, Choice, Change and Challenge" to business leaders at Chicago's Executives' Club, "Man's View of Himself" to the Canadian Public Health Association, "Man, the Trustee of Evolution" at Loyola University, "Responsibility—A Biological Necessity" at the National Conference of Editorial Writers, "Mankind Being BORN—Will It Be Defective or Effective?" to the National Foundation Volunteer Leaders, and "Order-Disorder-Order" at Baltimore's Seton Psychiatric Institute.

In covering his presentations, most journalists avoided critique, given his stature. "Dr. Salk urges restatement of man's aims" began an article in the *Baton Rouge Louisiana Advocate*.[26] Salk had stated that mankind was in the midst of a transition from an epoch of competition and individualism to one of cooperation. He estimated the new era to be three generations away and cited unrest among the youth as a symbol of that transition. One reporter for the *Lynchburg (VA) News* dared to expose the "emperor's new clothes." He quoted Salk as saying, "Each generation during the transition will necessarily be marked by extremeness, the Agnews of the right and the Marcuses of the left" referring to Nixon's vice president and a prominent German Marxist theorist. "Right there the man lost all claim to credibility," the journalist carped. "When Salk recommended that youth follow the 'nonviolent tactics of Martin Luther King'...he exposed himself as a demagogue or fool." In his view, this American hero "displayed the intellectual dishonesty that marks the pseudo-intellectual."[27] Though it lambasted him, Salk kept a copy of the article in his files.

Still rising at dawn, Salk would sit in his living room looking out across the canyon to the ocean and reflect. "I awaken in a sort of dreamlike state," he told Kahn, "and before I am disturbed by anything, I assume my posture and just let things happen, and this is the period of discovery and of work for me. Once I do that, the rest of the day anybody can have; but that part of the day is mine."[28] This contemplative process, he said, was his chance to assess the current weather and coming storms. "He was tapping into something very deep and profound within himself," explained Lisa Longworth, a San Diego psychologist. "He entered a deep state of connectivity to what we might call the creative source of imagination."[29] His night notes provided solace, too. According to his son Jonathan, "Whenever he faced conflict, he would retreat and look at it from a bigger perspective, view the difficulties as a universal conflict. He went to this more philosophical spot, which I think was a psychological way of coping."[30]

Salk didn't dwell on his own problems. More concerned with the world at large, he wanted to share his insights with others and talked of incorporating his night writings into a book. To start, he gave unedited copies to friends and family. Most found them impenetrable and rambling as he expressed in ten words what could have been said in three. "My mother," Jonathan said, "while admiring and supportive of my father, didn't have a lot of patience with all the philosophical stuff."[31] Anthropologist Heather Wood Ion, who would later try to interpret his night writings, described them as "stream-of-consciousness diaries."[32] Jonathan concurred: "Free thought is a good way of describing them. Some passages are quite beautiful, but in terms of pulling together an integrated philosophical whole, it's not there."[33]

Salk sought someone to help organize twenty years of notes into a coherent manuscript. His son Jonathan seemed the most obvious choice;

he had dropped out of Stanford University his senior year. Searching for his own identity, however, Jonathan did not want it to be engulfed by his father's. Arnold Mandell, chairman of the Department of Psychiatry at UCSD, saw how his friend was struggling with hundreds of pages of unconnected thoughts and offered to help. "I took scissors and Scotch tape," he recounted. "I didn't add a single word but cut it up and rearranged it." When he returned the pages to Salk, he seemed pleased and remarked, "Oh, I can write this book."[34]

In 1972, Harper and Row published *Man Unfolding*, and Salk's private thoughts became public. "The purpose of this volume," the book begins, "by bringing together the knowledge we have about human life and about living systems generally, is to suggest a way of thinking about some of the burning issues of our time for which we seek solutions."[35] Through his choices, Salk writes, man could facilitate "evolution or devolution."[36] In the past, human beings coped with disease and deprivation through scientific discoveries and technological developments. "In the course of time," he asserts, "man has so altered his environment, at a rate so far exceeding the development of changes in instinctive behavior...that he is now the victim of stresses upon himself to the point where his intellect, which seems about to overpower him, must be invoked to help save him."[37] Addressing the role of the natural world in evolution, he writes: "By and large, the environment has been looked upon as threatening and unfriendly. I would like to suggest another attitude toward the environment, considering it as a positive evolutionary force which affords opportunity for revealing the undisclosed potential that lies deep within man."[38]

Turning to issues of human conflict, Salk draws an analogy between the immune system and the difficulties in trying to expunge prejudices. He contends that, just as the pattern of prior immunologic experience affects later immunologic response, be it tolerance or intolerance, so are prejudices established by exposure to attitudes early in life. He ponders how their society could launch a man into space but not solve the problems of poverty, starvation, and war. "If man is able to bring under control elements in nature that threaten human life, he should be able to bring under sufficient control their counterparts in the human realm."[39] Mankind should seek means to deal with this disharmony, Salk argues, by applying the biological way of thinking to social, anthropological, and psychological problems. "The thought that man is unfolding, in a developmental and evolutionary sense, provides a measure of hope for those who would work toward a more satisfying life for man on earth."[40]

Most readers found it difficult to get through the book's 192 pages. When one reporter asked about his outline, Salk replied that he didn't have one; he had written down a collection of thoughts over a dozen years. "To have a book with a structure you have to have a plan ahead of time," he said. "That's for an academic book. [This is] more analogous to music or literature in the sense that it writes itself."[41] Perhaps that explains why he included no earlier references to metabiology, such as in John Murry's *God: Being an Introduction to the Science of Metabiology* or George Bernard Shaw's *Back to Methuselah: A Metabiological Pentateuch*. Many believed Salk had coined the term "metabiology," and he apparently did not dispel that notion. To a prospective donor, he described a principle unifying knowledge and human behavior "to which I have given the name metabiology."[42] Perhaps he was unaware of earlier uses of the term. He told a Stanford professor, "As we're beginning to understand sociobiological systems, it occurred to me that the word metabiology could be used for the moment to refer to what I think of as 'the human realm.'"[43]

A book reviewer for the *New York Times* pointed out that Salk's conclusion that one should consider the environment a positive evolutionary force implied man's potential could be more fully realized by a threatening, rather than favorable environment. "It remains unclear," the reviewer wrote, "whether there are any grounds other than perhaps a strain of Puritanism on which to base this conclusion." Although he complimented Salk on his many "illuminating and interesting points," he thought that in striving to make meaningful statements, Salk sounded cavalier, such as his reference to "the life force itself whatever it may be."[44] A reviewer for the *Los Angeles Times* Calendar section addressed Salk's contention that knowledge of immunologic intolerance could be applied to the solution of racial discrimination, stating, "These assertions are not especially provocative." He called Salk's failure to pursue his analogies in enough depth to validate their usefulness a major shortcoming. And he found Salk's examples unconvincing: "It is extraordinarily difficult to discuss being and ego or conscious and unconscious mind in the same paragraph with DNA and viruses."[45]

If his writings were difficult to understand, Salk's verbal communication did not clarify matters. In an interview for San Francisco's Humanistic Psychology Institute, Salk said his book contained "biassociations which have occurred to me as I have observed certain human phenomena in terms of the biological images that are in my mind at all times." He used phrases such as "epistemological contributions," "connections between psychologic and immunologic phenomena," and "the relationship between the genetic-somatic dualism."[46] A writer for *Human Behavior* concluded: "Salk has entered a new phase of his career, his unfolding."[47]

Within a year, Harper and Row published Salk's second book, *The Survival of the Wisest*, described by the press as an extension of Darwin's theory of natural selection.[48] In 124 pages, he warns that accelerating population growth, if unabated, would threaten man's survival on our planet. Learning from the wisdom of nature, man could mitigate this. To illustrate, he shows a figure depicting growth of a fruit fly population in a closed environment. The small colony of flies rapidly expands, then levels off because of limited space and resources. Plotting time on one axis and number of flies on another, he traces a sigmoid growth curve, resembling an "S." He points out that at the midpoint of the curve, there is a change from acceleration to deceleration, and after this inflection point flies by necessity behave differently in order to secure survival of their species. Such a response is encoded in their genes. Since Earth is a closed system, he anticipates population growth of the human species would follow the same curve. He worries that man's individual will and complexity might lead him to react in self-destructive ways.

"Man's ability to act wisely," he posits, "is crucial not only in maintaining and improving the quality of human life on this planet but in determining our very existence." In order for human populations to follow the sigmoid curve, massive changes had to take place "not only in human behavior but also in the deeper attitudes and values that govern behavior."[49] Salk introduces his thesis that to avoid catastrophe humanity must embrace a complete inversion of values: a shift from what he terms Epoch A, based on survival of the fittest, to Epoch B, in which "the welfare of the individual and the welfare of the species are inextricably bound."[50] He talks of the "emergence of being from ego domination"[51] and the need for "'double-win' rather than 'win-lose' resolutions which Man must...develop" in order to survive.[52]

Survival of the Wisest surpassed *Man Unfolding* in clarity. A *Los Angeles Times* book review, entitled "Dr. Salk: Yea-Sayer to the Doomsayers," began: "The doomsters say the climbing population curve is lifting us straight into disaster. Dr. Jonas Salk says it could be elevating us to a higher and better level of human civilization—if we have the wisdom to adapt to a changing world." Although the reviewer called Salk's language "loaded," he considered Salk's central argument "straightforward and compelling" and concluded: "The best hope is that [Salk's] insights into metabiological pathology will be as accurate as his insight into the biological pathology of polio."[53]

In the time between the release of his two books, Salk's image had changed. An interview on *Day and Night* revealed a slim, sleek Salk, his silver curls coiffed, his teeth capped. No longer hidden by glasses, his almost ebony eyes conveyed compassion. Under his cornflower blue suit, he wore a light blue silk shirt, unbuttoned enough to reveal a matching neck scarf. Women described him as chic, urbane, sensual. And he had learned to hone his message, making his statements less opaque.

Salk's books generated some interest among academicians. "Because these books lead in directions that are different from other contemporary analyses and allow some welcome room for optimism," wrote Professor Robert Rosen of the University at Buffalo, "it is imperative that they be widely discussed."[54] Professor Robert Artigiani of the US Naval Academy congratulated Salk on giving him "a deeper appreciation of the spiritual consequences of the evolutionary paradigm and its potential as a control base for post-modern civilization."[55] Several perceived the political implications of his writings. "I know few people whose ideas are so clear and direct as yours in indicating the nature of the current world transformation," maintained Richard Perl, a member of Planetary Citizens, a group devoted to fostering positive change in the world.[56] "Your ideas about Epochs A and B and man's metabiology intertwine with politics," wrote Michael Gough of the US Office of Technology Assessment. "Greater self-reliance, almost analogous with wisdom, is a goal of the new Administration."[57] Michael Flower, a biology professor at Southern Oregon College, wrote: "My bioethical concern began in

1965 over meatball sandwiches and beer." He now offered interdisciplinary courses such as "The Biologist and Social Responsibility."[58] Salk invited him to the Institute to collaborate.

The amount of Salk's mail increased as people sought his opinions. The president of the Wisdom Hall of Fame in Beverly Hills found the scholarship and breadth of *Survival of the Wisest* astounding. "Yours is a rare and brilliant mind," he told Salk. "You possess a literary merit of high rank."[59] A Chicago man tried to interest him in an idea concerning the physics of long-term memory.[60] James Horton wrote about launching a new magazine, *Mind and Body*, which he called an "Epoch B magazine."[61] Notes ranged from the legitimate to the eccentric. "My genetic system is transcending my somatic system," a woman from Long Beach revealed. "It is as if a giant magnet were pulling the pieces of the puzzle together, your theory of metabiological transition being the force and the pieces being some of my own mark as well as yours."[62] Many attached manuscripts or books. Most wanted something, such as a critique of their concepts, help in publishing, funds to pursue an idea, or an opportunity to work with him. Whereas Salk used to respond to every letter, now Friedman often sent a note saying he was unavailable.

Interest in Salk's theories extended across the ocean. Professor Jacques Rueff of the Institut de France complimented him on his books. Salk still enjoyed celebrity status among the French people for his polio vaccine. Gilot introduced him to a number of scholars, and Salk refreshed his French so he could communicate his ideas to the French intellectual community. Their reception, however, was far from welcoming. "There is nothing as arrogant and snooty as a French intellectual," Christine Forester observed. "They are merciless; they never fully accepted him."[63]

Salk's books received mixed reviews from colleagues at the Salk Institute. "I thought they were very superficial and thin," a member of the board of trustees said, "a lot of verbal hand waving, not a lot of substance."[64] Edwin Lennox, one of the original fellows, concurred: "Jonas was neither a good writer nor a good thinker; he operated more at an emotional level than at an intellectual level." He called Salk's analogies of the immune system "phony" and "empty."[65] Neurobiologist Antonio Damasio had a different view: "He was in essence a dreamer and a mystic. The way he approached the problems of humanity was filled with a benevolence that people who cherish objectivity would consider vague."[66] Cancer investigator Walter Eckhart agreed: "I thought Jonas was ahead of his time. His thinking process was different; he would go inward and reflect meditatively, trying to access a different form of thinking rather than the purely rational."[67] This was not common practice for most scientists. "He was much more of an intuitive," said later Salk Institute president Brian Henderson, "but he was working with people who didn't get it."[68] The cruelest comments came from Jacob Bronowski, who referred to Salk derisively as "the prophet."[69] His ridicule permeated the Institute. "The scientific stars he had gathered," Peter Salk said, "were finding themselves embarrassed by his musings about man's place in the cosmos."[70]

Salk cared deeply about mankind and still woke up in the night worrying about its future. Like those ideas expressed in other books of the late 1960s and 1970s, when the politicization of science was becoming an open issue, many of Salk's views were spot on—that man's greatest enemy was now himself, rather than the environment or the diseases that once upon a time had demolished entire populations; that uncontrolled population growth could expunge life on our planet; that the thrill of scientific discovery needed to be tempered by moral clarity lest it provide men even greater means of destruction. Had Salk been able to galvanize people to think about these issues, to incorporate them into their lives, and to take appropriate action, he might have accomplished a great deal. Yet his difficulty expressing his concerns in terms accessible to the general public limited his influence. "Honest to goodness," Mandell said, "I often thought if he was as articulate as he was intuitive... but his verbal communication skills were just terrible."[71] And his innate shyness made him appear aloof and distracted, the very cliché of a pseudo-intellectual.

Salk understood his metabiological concepts would come alive only when applied to actual social issues. He had conceived of his institute as a place to imbue the sciences with the conscience of man—to unite Snow's two cultures—and had selected fellows who espoused this view. He had hoped their interchanges would generate a new school of thinkers he referred to as biophilosophers. Before long, however, he realized that academic and financial freedom proved a more compelling reason for them to accept his offer. Even Francis Crick, although supportive of

his goals, thought the Institute should concentrate on fundamental biological research. "I have little doubt that if this is done," he advised Salk,
"its application will follow."[72] And to Salk's dismay, Bronowski, the humanist of the group, avoided regular discourse with him, treating him
like an intellectual lightweight. As a result, Salk seemed to be trying to
bridge the two cultures within himself.

This changed after Joseph Slater became president of the Institute in
1968. Just before he arrived, Salk had sent Slater a nine-page letter regarding "metascientific areas for the pursuit of knowledge to the solution
of problems of man that remain unsolved."[73] Slater translated the dis-
connected thoughts; he understood what Salk was trying to achieve with
the Institute and did his best to act upon it. In February of 1970, the
scientific journal *Nature* announced: "Salk Institute Goes Public," introducing the Council for Biology in Human Affairs (CBHA), an "instrument for transforming its humanistic concerns into a practical program."[74]
Composed of twenty-five sociologists, law professors, psychologists, and
scientists from the Institut Pasteur, Harvard, and other notable institutions, with funds of two million dollars, the Council would conduct
studies to assess the social and humanistic consequences of biologic discoveries. Bronowski told colleagues that the CBHA would "form public
opinion by informing it."[75] Salk assumed he would be asked to direct the
CBHA, but its advisory committee recommended the chairman be a
leading academician such as Jerome Wiesner, a former president of MIT
and scientific advisor to three presidents, or Nobel Prize–winning scientist George Beadle, who later became president of the University of
Chicago. Meanwhile, Bronowski assumed leadership.

Early on, the Council formed commissions to address population
growth problems such as urban ecology, food supplies, and contraceptive
restrictions, as well as legal and social issues generated by scientific
advances such as genetic engineering. They sponsored seminars for the
media to enhance their understanding of current efforts in the biological
sciences as well as their social and humanistic significance. A conference
with sessions entitled "Chemical Compounds in the Environment, A
Further Perspective on the Environmental Crisis—How Real Is It?" and
"We Master the Gene" drew large audiences. CBHA's workshop on drug
abuse resulted in a congressional report. The group initiated the Voice of

America Forum lecture series, which tackled provocative topics such as using biology wisely and man's place in the universe. Scholars in the social sciences and humanities started visiting the Institute. The Council planned Institute art exhibits and concerts featuring new composers, acquired a collection of rare books, and supported a joint humanities program with UC San Diego.

"[Joe Slater] has rekindled the spirit, lifted the soul, and improved morale in a way that has revived optimism to a new level," Salk wrote in his night notes. "It may be said that he has been responsible for a renaissance in the life and history of the institute."[76] It appeared that Salk's dream—the melding of the two cultures—was finally coming true.

Fall from Grace

FEBRUARY 12, 1970 was a mild, cloudless day in La Jolla. On his way to a meeting of the board of trustees, Salk walked through the Institute's eucalyptus grove, then climbed the steps to take in the panorama that still enthralled him with its magnificence—the expansive plaza, paved with Italian travertine and edged by ten towers, which seemed to fuse with the ocean beyond. He loved how water from the nearside fountain flowed through a channel bisecting the piazza, spilled into a pool at the other end, then cascaded onto the lower terrace. Below, on Black's Beach, surfers waited for the perfect wave. A hang glider's colorful sail caught the wind as he launched from the adjacent Torrey Pines Gliderport. The peaceful morning carried no hint of the turmoil to come.

⁂

A SURGE OF enthusiasm had energized the Institute ever since Joseph Slater had taken the helm as president and CEO on January 24, 1968. Slater had substantial fiscal experience, having assisted West Germany with its post–World War II economic recovery and served as chief economist for Standard Oil Company. He brought superb organizational skills: he had helped form the United Nations, written the blueprint for the Peace Corps, and run the Ford Foundation's international affairs program. Upon arriving in La Jolla, he had set up seven task forces to define where the Institute should go and how it should get there.[1] Five volumes of recommendations resulted. He planned to raise a hundred million dollars to add the exciting new basic science areas of neurobiology and developmental biology and to incorporate the humanities and social sciences under the Council for Biology in Human Affairs. To symbolize the Institute's broadened scope, he suggested changing its name from the Salk Institute for Biological Studies to the Salk Institute.

The fellows applauded their broad-minded, collegial leader. Salk called his appointment an important step in achieving the goals set by the Institute's founders; O'Connor anticipated a new era for the Institute.[2] When Slater began his term, O'Connor gave him a dowry of four new grants totaling $4.1 million over four years, and as a complement to the NF grants the Gildred Foundation pledged another million over four years. Although the National Foundation had contributed almost $25 million to the Institute, it was not yet self-sustaining. Still O'Connor liked Slater and trusted him to secure its financial stability.

Under Slater, the Institute's attraction increased. Robert Holley of Cornell came to La Jolla as a resident fellow six months after Slater. Holley had gained international renown when he determined the structure of transfer RNA, molecules that play a crucial role in protein synthesis. He received the Nobel Prize in Chemistry two months following his arrival. Soon thereafter, Roger Guillemin from Baylor University joined the group.[3] The French-born physician-scientist had discovered that the brain produces hormones that control the thyroid and pituitary glands.

On his first visit to the Institute, Guillemin found himself mesmerized by the building's beauty. He remembered thinking, "Whatever the man has to say, the answer is yes."[4] Salk talked about the Institute's founding premise, "biology with a conscience," then showed Guillemin ten thousand square feet of undeveloped lab space to organize as he wished.[5] When he attended the yearly fellows' meeting, Guillemin could barely believe what he saw: Francis Crick, Jacques Monod, Renato Dulbecco, Robert Holley, Salvador Luria—a host of scientific greats—sitting in one room. He counted seven Nobel Laureates, who seemed to be enjoying each other's company. Guillemin later told a journalist, "It is not an elitist place in a vacuum. It is an elitist place with a purpose."[6] He prepared to move his entire lab from Houston in June of 1970.

"This is the end of the first five-year period," Salk jotted down in a note to himself, "and it is gratifying to see how the Institute has matured. It is now solidly unified."[7] With the fellows thriving and Slater at the helm, he anticipated freeing himself of administrative burdens so he could focus on his research and philosophical endeavors. Slater pressed forward to integrate the biological sciences with the social sciences and humanities, just as Salk had envisaged. That required funding, however, and Slater expected his director to help attract donors. Although Salk preferred to sit in his study tower and think rather than attend affairs where people swooned over him, he complied.

Pictures on the society page of the *San Diego Union* showed Salk in a tuxedo, flanked by Mrs. Joseph Slater and the president of the Institute's Women's Association, inspecting table decorations at the Cuyamaca Club, the setting for a dinner prior to an Andy Williams benefit concert.[8] The *Dallas Morning News* reported that Jonas Salk and actress Jane Wyatt (known for her role in *Father Knows Best*) were in town for a three-day round of fundraising events. Salk wrote thank-you notes to the Lennon Sisters, Bob Hope, Jack Benny, Henry Mancini, Danny Thomas, the Osmond Brothers, Arnold Palmer, and Jack Nicklaus for their participation in fundraising concerts and golf tournaments. A reporter for the *New York Sunday News* once asked Salk if he felt it degrading to "come hat in hand to people, literally begging for donations." Couldn't they obtain research funds through some government monopoly? Salk gave the answer he had learned from O'Connor: "Are you aware that there would have been no polio vaccine if that had been the system that prevailed?"[9]

Salk preferred to pursue wealthy donors who understood his work, such as Armand Hammer.[10] Like Salk, Hammer had grown up in the Bronx, the child of Russian Jewish immigrants. His father, a staunch socialist, named him after the "arm and hammer" symbol of the Socialist Labor Party. Having graduated from Columbia Medical School, Hammer became a successful entrepreneur, exporting drugs to the Soviet Union, and a prosperous investor, controlling Occidental Petroleum. Generous with his fortune, Hammer decided to invest in cancer research.

Salk had come to Hammer's attention in 1968, when he had talked about cancer on Walter Cronkite's *The Twenty-First Century*. Soon after, Hammer visited the Institute and invited Salk to his Beverly Hills home. After an eighteen-month courtship, Salk informed O'Connor that Hammer had proposed funding a cancer research center at a rate of a million dollars a year for five years. Then Salk slipped in one caveat: Hammer had indicated his interest in becoming a trustee and playing an active role in Institute affairs. Salk didn't tell O'Connor that several board members were leery. Hammer had a reputation for being an operator with a propensity to move in and take over. Trustee Edgar Bronfman, CEO of the Seagram Company, said he had known Hammer for sixteen years and didn't consider him a problem; he was interested in the big picture, not the "petty details" with which O'Connor constantly concerned himself.[11] With that endorsement, Slater and the board approved Hammer's appointment as a trustee, and a substantial research grant followed.

Joseph Slater proved to be an effective administrator. Despite his background in economics, however, he struggled with the goal of achieving financial independence for the Institute. "Joe was more of an idea man," comptroller Del Glanz noted. "He didn't really understand finance and fundraising. He was more of a program motivator type of a person."[12] Money problems continued to plague the Institute, and time and again Slater turned to O'Connor to cover the shortfall. As this practice increased, so did resentment from outside scientists when they were told that the National Foundation's financial obligations to the Salk Institute prohibited consideration of their grant applications. And O'Connor did not hide his growing disappointment that Slater had not put the Institute on solid financial footing.

In accepting the presidency, Slater must have understood O'Connor's expectations. Yet he had no idea how difficult O'Connor could be. Still president of the National Foundation, he made not just key decisions but most decisions, taking counsel from only three or four senior people. "He would not countenance any objections to his opinions," stated NF statistician Gabriel Stickle in an oral history, "unless you could substantiate your position."[13]

Now in his late seventies, O'Connor had become more crotchety—"cantankerous," Glanz called him.[14] His vitality was lagging after years of heavy drinking and smoking. He came to board meetings in a wheel-chair. "As things closed in on him," Stickle observed, "he wasn't as crea-tive as in the earlier days."[15] He had run the NFIP as an autocracy, not uncommon in 1950s business culture. The problem was that he kept that mindset into the 1970s, even though radical changes had occurred.

"There was a very clear feeling that I got from Slater," trustee Theodore Gildred divulged, "that he was being oppressed, if not pressed, by O'Connor."[16] Slater wanted a freer hand. A group of Institute trustees tried to persuade the NF trustees to remove O'Connor from the Institute board in order to safeguard their investment in the place. "His role out here is over," they argued.[17] Only no one dared confront the National Foundation's godfather. The situation deteriorated further when Slater revealed that he had been offered directorship of the Aspen Institute, an international think tank, a position more suited to his talents.[18]

⸜⸝

ANYONE READING THE list of trustees who gathered for the February 12–13, 1970, Salk Institute board meeting would have been impressed: an ambassador, a US senator, chief judge for a US Court of Appeals, a member of the board of governors of the Federal Reserve System, the president of the University of Alabama, director of Seton Psychiatric Institute, editor of *Atlantic Monthly*, publisher of *Life* magazine, two Nobel laureates, the presidents and vice presidents of several Fortune 500 companies, and top investment counselors and lawyers.[19] Five served on the NF board of trustees as well. John J. McCloy, assistant secretary of war during World War II, served as chairman of the board. This cre-dential would serve him well in the upcoming skirmish. O'Connor arrived wearing a pinstriped suit with a white carnation on his lapel. Salk wore his white coat, symbolizing the health concerns of mankind—the Institute's raison d'être.

McCloy opened the meeting by welcoming the new trustee, Dr. Armand Hammer. After approval of prior minutes, Slater began his President's Report with remarks that would later sound obsequious: "I would like to express the deepest gratitude...for the past and continuing support of the National Foundation. Without such support our scientific programs would not be at present strength, or, indeed, would not be in existence at all." He hoped the meeting would "see a new forward thrust with the National Foundation on a mutually reinforcing basis." When he became president, his first priority had been to develop sound programs and project a "climate of solidarity" to the outside world. Slater recognized that the Institute's "internal frictions and its rather frantic, unsuccessful attempts to raise private funds" had become common knowledge, their fundraising attempts considered a "bail-out of an essentially bankrupt institution." Yet in just over two years, they had received grants or pledges totaling almost $21 million. Slater said he agreed with Mr. O'Connor's views on the crucial need to raise general funds and build the endowment, although they disagreed on the proposed timing. "This possible difference has not in *any* way diminished *my* high respect for Mr. O'Connor's leadership role in the Salk Institute."[20] Slater told the board his first concern was raising $8 million for resident fellows. O'Connor interrupted to say his first concern should be paying the gas and electricity bill.

Next Slater turned to the Council for Biology in Human Affairs (CBHA), over which he anticipated controversy among the trustees. He reminded the board that from the beginning of his presidency, he had dedicated himself to the Council's development, and it now had full fellow support. Jacques Monod of the Pasteur Institute, currently a nonresident fellow, was considering a permanent Salk Institute appointment in order to devote himself to "philosophical and human implications of the biological revolution."[21] O'Connor asked if other institutions were already doing the work proposed for the Council and suggested the CBHA could participate with them rather than initiate another program. Slater replied that others lacked effective leadership. O'Connor made it clear that no additional funds would be forthcoming; the CBHA had to stand on its own. "I must say, in all candor," retorted Slater, "we must activate these programs or stop claiming we are 'An Institute of Man.'"[22] And with that, he announced that he would assume the presidency of the Aspen Institute for Humanistic Studies on March 1.

Once Slater confirmed what he had intimated for months, the trustees turned to the pressing problem they had been skirting around—a letter sent a week prior to the meeting by Joseph Nee, senior vice president of the National Foundation, to board chairman McCloy. Nee had informed McCloy that in reviewing the $4.1 million special grant given to the Salk Institute, the NF had found several areas of "grave concern": failure to appoint a fundraising chairman and conduct a national campaign, inadequate financial reporting, and development of some programs (i.e., the CBHA) without the board of trustees' consent.[23]

Trying to placate O'Connor and defuse the tension, Salk noted that it had been a decade since the NF had made the decision to support establishment of the Institute, and he had "particularly warm reasons for gratitude to one man in particular."[24] O'Connor did not acknowledge his words. Instead, he informed the group that the NF board was taking a careful look at this commitment; it would take three months to finish their review. When McCloy said this put the Institute in a state of "suspended animation," O'Connor replied he would give them the answer as soon as he could, but he didn't know if the Foundation would continue its current payments.[25] Salk was dumfounded. As he left the meeting, walking back across the travertine plaza and through the eucalyptus grove, he couldn't believe that O'Connor would abandon their dream, or him.

◀╫▶

ON MARCH 1, 1970, Slater assumed presidency of the Aspen Institute; on May 14, O'Connor abruptly withdrew all financial support from the Salk Institute. Attached to the notice were the original conditions of the grant, including the following: "If at any time during the four year period referred to above Mr. Slater shall, for any reason, cease to be president of the Institute, the National Foundation shall have the right on thirty days' notice to the Institute to cancel the payment of any remaining unpaid amounts of the aforesaid grants."[26] Since Slater ceased to be president, the Foundation was giving them thirty days' notice.

In attempts to forestall the pending catastrophe, Slater proposed he stay on as president while starting his job at the Aspen Institute. He recommended that the board create a new position of chancellor and consider the appointment of Dr. Frederic de Hoffmann, a forty-five-year-old physicist and Manhattan Project alumnus who had formed General Atomics to bring nuclear energy to industry. O'Connor countered that if the trustees appointed de Hoffmann as chancellor and hired a head of fundraising, and if Slater had such a competent deputy at the Aspen Institute that he could expend half his time as president of the Salk Institute, "it is rather difficult for one to figure out just what Slater will be doing."[27] Despite this caustic remark, the trustees elected de Hoffmann as chancellor and voted to keep Slater as part-time president. O'Connor, however, did not retract his decision to defund the Institute. The Gildred Foundation, whose grant was tied to the NF grant, threatened to cancel its grant as well. When Salk returned from his wedding in the summer of 1970, the Institute already had a $550,000 deficit. "This has had a profound effect upon the Institute," he wrote in his next Director's Report, "as might be expected when suddenly a severe narrowing occurs in a major artery."[28]

Those involved had different explanations for O'Connor's sudden repudiation. Salk blamed the fellows for failure to embrace the original intent of humanizing the sciences. Some senior staff thought the power broker had become more irascible in his old age. Joseph Nee explained that since the Foundation was providing the Institute with public funds, O'Connor insisted they must assure the public they were spending that money wisely. Yet everyone knew there must be some profound underlying issue; O'Connor had loved the idea of the Salk Institute. "The need to help his fellow man," a journalist had written of him in 1964, "to participate in what Dr. Salk has called 'an assault on the unreasonableness of life,' has become as urgent as hunger."[29] His longtime press secretary, Dorothy Ducas, agreed. "Basil O'Connor is, if anything," she said in an oral history, "even more enthusiastic about the significance of the institute than he was about the conquest of polio."[30] Now he told the trustees he would not compromise; he preferred to see the Institute collapse. In the end, this wasn't about the Institute per se; it was about Basil O'Connor's relationship with Jonas Salk.

As O'Connor's fondness for Salk waned, the thread that tied him to the Institute frayed and eventually broke. Some thought O'Connor was getting pressure from the NF to stop supporting Salk's research after he had lost his scientific luster. Gilot blamed herself for encouraging her husband to stand up to O'Connor. "Basil O'Connor was one of those who always wanted to dominate, not to relate, but to dominate." Gilot disdained personal subjugation, having left Picasso to escape his control.

"Sadly enough," she admitted, "when I got married to Jonas, that dissatisfied [O'Connor] completely. He got furious and broke his relationship with Jonas."[31] She overestimated her role, as O'Connor's coolness antedated not only Salk's marriage to Gilot but also his divorce from Donna.

It had become apparent to Salk in early 1967 that something had come between them. He had sent plaintive notes, which O'Connor left unanswered. He wrote how much he missed talking together: "I hope we can soon see each other."[32] Months passed with no reply. On O'Connor's seventy-seventh birthday, Salk sent a telegram: "I admire you for all the good you've done and for all that you can still do."[33] The two had always exchanged birthday greetings. On Salk's fifty-fifth, however, it was O'Connor's wife who sent him a telegram: "My best wishes to you on your day and every day. Love, Guess Who."[34] Salk tried several times to rekindle their friendship, but O'Connor continued to rebuff him. The distance between them grew. Salk no longer called him "Doc"; he addressed his notes to "Mr. O'Connor," signing them, "Sincerely, Jonas Salk."

Salk thought he understood the source of the problem. "Mr. O'Connor's dissatisfaction," he told Slater and McCloy, "in part at least rests with his impatience and his feeling that we have failed and will not succeed since he believes that we do not *wish* to raise money in the orthodox ways that he believes will be successful."[35] This was a bit of an understatement, thought Charles Massey, who had worked for the Foundation since 1949. "He and Jonas had a father/son relationship," Massey surmised. "O'Connor had given his son unlimited allowance to do what he wanted to do, and his son was not repaying him by helping him raise the money to support the Institute." Overindulged, Salk had come to expect to get whatever he wanted. "I think he believed that he had this privilege," Massey said. When O'Connor committed to the Institute at the height of Salk's celebrity, he had assumed that raising the money would be a cinch. It wasn't. When Massey once asked Salk, "Why won't you help us raise money for your institute?" he had replied, "First of all, I'm not a fundraiser. Secondly, it's not appropriate for me to do that, and thirdly, I have found that fund-receiving is a lot more enjoyable than fundraising." His attitude of entitlement disturbed O'Connor; he told Massey he felt as if he'd been "snookered." At one point O'Connor became so enraged, Massey recalled, he shouted, "I don't give a damn if the whole place slides into the Pacific Ocean."[36]

How far their friendship had slipped since 1951, when O'Connor had met the earnest young physician-scientist on the *Queen Mary*. For a man who had undertaken so many humanitarian efforts—the Red Cross, March of Dimes, National Conference of Christians and Jews, the Tuskegee Institute—O'Connor seemed dispassionate toward individuals, but he seemingly had adopted Jonas Salk. And Salk benefitted greatly from the relationship. He likely would not have developed the polio vaccine had O'Connor not appreciated his talents and supported him. O'Connor had stood by him through the Cutter incident, the scientific community's anti-Salk backlash, Albert Sabin's relentless derogations, and his post–polio vaccine depression. And the Institute would never have been built without O'Connor's patronage. More than that, they had a deep regard for each other. In 1962, O'Connor had sent Salk a note that read: "To Jonas Salk Who Makes All Things Worthwhile."[37] What had started as a mutual admiration had evolved into a bonding of two souls.

Over the years, Salk had accepted the consequences of friendship with such a powerful man. "Jonas was very likely to bow to O'Connor's wishes," Donna recalled. "O'Connor liked it that way. And it made life simpler."[38] He and Harry Weaver had made Salk the March of Dimes poster scientist, creating the hero the public craved, and then had snatched the vaccine trial from him. O'Connor had insisted the Institute bear Salk's name, despite Salk's anticipation of criticism from the scientific community. "We can't raise funds for the Torrey Pines Institute for Biological Studies," O'Connor had told him. "It has to be the Salk Institute or we can't do it."[39] Now, seven years after they had broken ground on this scientific sanctuary, Salk wrote in his night notes, "Sometimes we want something as in the case of the Institute, but it comes at so high a price that even if we get it, the cost is so great that the net effect is lost."[40]

O'Connor had always been domineering, and when several of the people closest to his heart slipped away from him, he became even more possessive. He mourned the loss of his two beloved daughters: Bettyann Culver, a polio survivor and mother of five, had died in 1961 from late complications of the disease. Five years later, his second daughter,

Sheelagh O'Connor, a Seattle psychiatrist, died of pneumonia within hours of being stricken. She was thirty-nine years old. Now his "son" had disappointed him. Fame had altered the humble young visionary. He had divorced Donna, of whom O'Connor was quite fond, and married Picasso's former mistress.

Jack MacAllister referred to their father-son conflict as a Greek tragedy. Salk knew he couldn't have prevented polio or built his scientific Shangri-La without O'Connor. Every time he teetered on a precipice, O'Connor swooped down and saved him. "Those kinds of relationships are always a double-edged sword," MacAllister noted.[41] Over the years, Salk wavered between appreciation and resentment. In his mid-fifties, he began to comprehend the complexity of their bond. "When I lost my anonymity and became public property," he wrote in his night notes, "I was subjected to new sets of desires or demands...never finally rebelling at the point in time at which it was necessary for me fully to take over as master of my own destiny."[42]

Given how different they were, it's amazing the friendship between these two men lasted as long as it did. What had linked them was their concern for humanity, and ultimately, even that wasn't enough. The friction caused by their dissimilar personalities—the optimistic dreamer versus the detached realist—had worn holes in their relationship over the years, culminating in O'Connor's rejection of the Institute—and, it seemed, of Jonas Salk.

᙭

ALTHOUGH SLATER STAYED on as president while commencing his work at the Aspen Institute, the damage had been done, and no further funds came into the Institute coffers from the National Foundation. Many reacted with disbelief; they thought some miscommunication just needed to be cleared up. Frank Rose, who had just assumed a position as chairman for planning and development of the Salk Institute, knew better. When he could not get an appointment to talk with O'Connor, with whom he had worked for fifteen years, he tried to reason with him by mail. He told O'Connor he had received numerous phone calls and letters asking about the disagreement between the two organizations. "I am greatly concerned about what effect this is going to have on our

campaigns," Rose wrote, "and the possible loss to both us and our programs of millions of dollars. I am fearful that we aren't many days away
from the press getting involved, and this is something that neither of us
can afford." The NF had placed one of the world's greatest medical
research centers in a grave financial situation. "Mr. O'Connor," he pleaded,
"we have a great opportunity to do something extremely outstanding for
the health concerns of all people, and whatever personal differences exist,
we must not deny them their hopes and lives." Rose ended by saying that
his discussions with mutual friends "have convinced me that both of our
houses are about to fall. I hope that you will not let this happen."[43]

When another week passed with no word from the National
Foundation, John McCloy contacted the trustees of both organizations.
"We have made every effort," he wrote, "to make a fair and just settlement of the problem with Mr. O'Connor." They needed to take steps to
resolve the issue before it came to public attention. Believing the decision to be unilateral on O'Connor's part, he suggested representatives
from the two boards meet. Then he gave an ultimatum: if payments were
not resumed by July 29, 1970, he planned to send a telegram to the trustees and the national, regional, and state chairmen of the Foundation
informing them that the NF had suspended payments to the Institute.
Did these actions and their serious consequences reflect the intentions of
the National Foundation board? How would the thousands of donors
who gave money to the NF to support the Salk Institute feel? In conclusion, he wrote, "The continued progress of the Institute is sharply imper-
iled, and its highly promising contributions to modern medical and
scientific developments may be frustrated.... It would be really calami-
tous at this stage to jeopardize its existence."[44]

Several days later, McCloy received a telegram from John Nee, senior
vice president of the NF, regarding his "groundless demands." He parried
McCloy's threat: "National will hold Institute and its trustees fully liable
for any damage that may occur to National from such action."[45] Curiously,
Nee served on both boards, as did O'Connor and three others.

When it became clear the NF board stood behind O'Connor and no
funds would be forthcoming, Slater called an urgent executive committee meeting for mid-August. Since Salk was abroad, he sent his views.
Sounding as if prompted by his new forthright wife, he did something

he had never done before—he spoke out against his longtime friend: "The Institute has for some time been on the horns of a dilemma which is diverting and depleting its energies seemingly because of the power and influence of the President of the National Foundation.... It is somewhat paradoxical that it was this same use of power and influence that brought the Institute into existence about a decade ago." The decision as to whether or not they continued a symbiotic relationship rested with their trustees. "Failing an honorable reconciliation with removal of threats, the Institute would have to alter its relationship to the public in respect to fundraising activities; the use of the Institute's name by the National Foundation would have to be re-examined to reflect the new institution; and, in a way, the Institute would become a competitor rather than a collaborator." If the NF trustees stood firm with O'Connor's dictum, the Institute would be seriously damaged and likely destroyed. "I hope that all of the years of anguish and struggle," Salk concluded, "will not have been in vain and that a strong and viable and honorable relationship to and with the National Foundation can be maintained and enlarged."[46] Five months later, the NF cut funding for Salk's laboratory.

Salk was stunned by the action. He informed Nee that Glasser had talked to O'Connor and indicated they would continue to reimburse one-third of his expenses. "I do not think that I would be ungrateful if I interpreted any such action as punitive." Then, unusual for the man who hated controversy, Salk struck back. "I do not intend after the many years of serving the same cause, and with the greatest of difficulties, to be generous in my interpretation or in my behavior," he warned. "I regard the last discussion I had with Mr. Glasser on behalf of Mr. O'Connor as constituting an agreement."[47]

Shock waves rippled through the Institute. In the middle of the siege, Roger Guillemin arrived to set up his program in reproductive biology. No one had warned him of the situation. When he complained that the breach of their commitment made him reconsider the wisdom of his decision, O'Connor told him that if he wasn't happy, he could go back to Houston.[48] "Salk Institute morale is sagging," read an article in the *San Diego Evening Tribune*, "with rumors and confirmed reports of staff departures. It's not announced yet, but Dr. Renato Dulbecco, a star of the Cancer Institute's Cancer Council, will be departing for a London research post."[49]

Nine months had passed since O'Connor's decree, and the situation looked grim. To keep the Institute afloat, Chancellor de Hoffmann froze salaries and recruitments, restricted estate expenditures, made reductions in scientific programs, and curtailed building repairs. McCloy wrote the trustees that they faced the possibility of suspending the Institute's operations. It's hard to fathom why the board of trustees, which contained so much talent and wealth, did not rescue the Salk Institute with a wave of their collective wands. Did O'Connor wield so much power that the chief judge of a US Court of Appeals, a university president, a US senator, the diplomat who brokered the Panama Canal agreement, and the man who helped form the United Nations couldn't negotiate a peace treaty? It would seem so. In September, O'Connor and Nee resigned from the Salk Institute board.[50]

At the last moment, the boards of the two organizations managed to reach agreement, resuscitating the almost defunct Institute. On January 26, 1972, the *Daily Report* announced that the NF pledged to pay off the Institute's mortgage with annual payments of more than $1.4 million through 1975.[51] Salk regretted that the resolution was made without O'Connor's blessing; he had tried to block the move until the end. "It would be nice indeed," Salk wrote Glasser, "if in some way Doc would be willing to see the actual and potential good he has helped to make possible."[52]

The press had been relatively quiet during the entire episode until it was over. "A hiatus between resources and ambitions that became apparent some 2 years ago," wrote a journalist in *Science*, "has left the institute unable to make more than limited progress with its humanist programs." Hopes of establishing large groups in neurobiology and aging had to be shelved. "If the Salk Institute is something of a pauper in rich man's clothing," the article continued, "even to have stayed financially viable is no mean achievement for a pure research organization dependent on public support.... The Institute may not yet have produced anything with the public impact of Salk's polio vaccine but its continued vitality suggests that Salk's second experiment can probably be counted a success."[53]

On February 8, 1972, two years after he had announced his resignation at that fateful board meeting, Slater left for the Aspen Institute, with a sigh of relief.

A month later, on March 9, Basil O'Connor died unexpectedly.[54] He was in Phoenix preparing for the Foundation's scientific advisory committee meeting when he developed heart failure, complicated by pneumonia. He was eighty years old. At his memorial service, Salk read a eulogy he had written in free verse, entitled "An Uncommon Man":[55]

> In eighty years
> His work was done
> To be remembered
> For reasons not trivial.
> An uncommon man—and many men in one.
>
> . . . .
>
> He could see farther than most.
> From where he was, he could see all of which others could see
>   but the parts.
> Nor did many match his lightning, nor his thunder.
> Nor was such generosity easily outdone.
>
> . . . .
>
> Born to be a person—he became an institution.
> To some he was as God.
> He could be believed, but he, himself, was incredible.
> When in his presence, there were none to whom to look
>   higher.
> He will be missed, for greatness comes only now and again.
>
> . . . .
>
> His accomplishments are woven into the fabric of our exist-
>   ence;
> He made history happen. He cajoled and catalyzed.
> His greatest achievement lifted the fears of millions, and for
>   generations to come.
> And, the organizations and institutions he created will bring
>   dividends far into the future.
>
> . . . .
>
> The love he craved he had from but a few and, from all the rest
>   admiration and respect.
>
> . . . .
>
> He was an uncommon man—he will be remembered as a great
>   man.

The poem says nothing about the depth of their friendship. Salk wrote, "He will be missed," not "I will miss him." He said, "The love he craved he had from but a few," not "I loved him." Salk had obscured his feelings about losing his greatest patron and friend. If he cried, he did so in private.

⁂

THE SALK INSTITUTE survived. Besides the basic annual $1 million grant, which would continue in perpetuity, the National Foundation made a special $1 million grant to be paid in four annual installments and forgave the Institute's outstanding notes, totaling $153,500.[56] The Foundation augmented Salk's $100,000 research grant and extended his contract, including his position as director, for five years. Although this entailed administration of all research programs, he obtained relief from these duties, relinquishing them to the president and CEO in order to devote himself to his own research and writings. Salk had won on every point, but he had lost something far more precious.

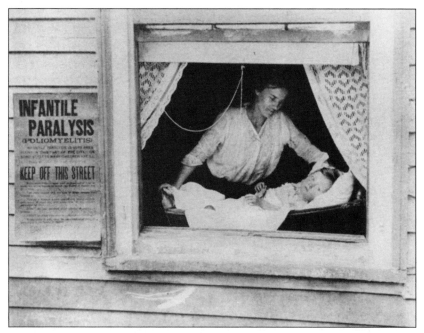

In America's first major polio epidemic, during the summer of 1916, a baby died approximately every two-and-a-half hours. Assuming polio behaved like other contagious diseases, the health commissioner ordered every family bearing a case quarantined. *March of Dimes Foundation*

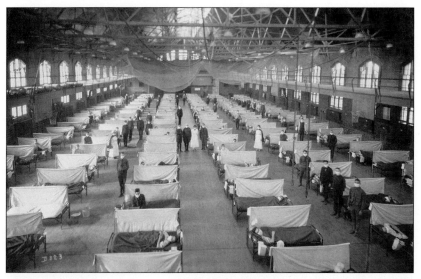

During the great influenza epidemic of 1918, emergency hospitals were set up in auditoriums, gymnasiums, churches, and mansions. The carnage left 850,000 Americans dead, twenty million worldwide. *Courtesy of Special Collections Department, Iowa State University Library*

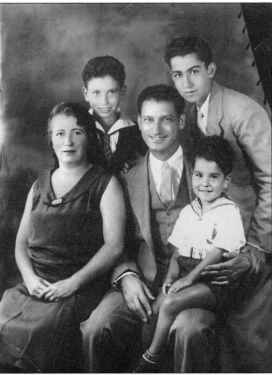

Dora and Daniel Salk with sons Herman, Jonas, and Lee. Dora was a tough taskmaster. Jonas inherited her work ethic and learned how to maneuver around her iron will, a skill that would help him later when confronted by the politics of science. *Courtesy of the Family of Jonas Salk*

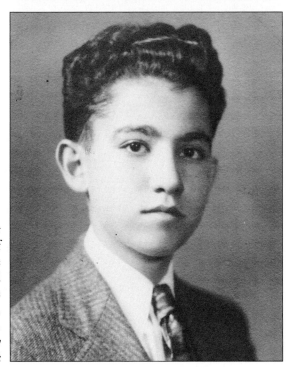

Jonas had few fond memories of childhood. By the time he entered high school, he was a driven, focused, serious individual. *Courtesy of the Family of Jonas Salk*

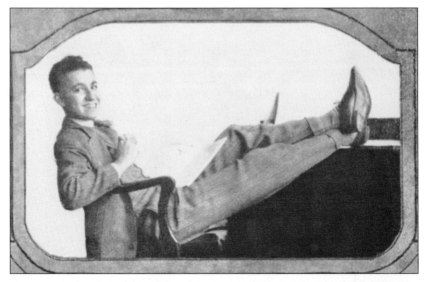

Although Jonas aspired to be a high school "big shot," he was excluded from Arista, the elite student society. "In the society of the chosen few, Jonas should have been chosen, too" read the caption under his yearbook picture. *Seth Poppel Yearbook Library/Townsend Harris High School Archives*

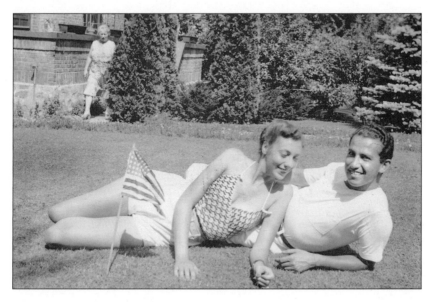

When Jonas Salk spotted Donna Lindsay on the beach in Woods Hole, Massachusetts, he saw much to attract him. Initially Donna was not swept away by Jonas, but he resolved to marry her. She relinquished her career, raised their three sons, and stood by her husband's side during the polio vaccine saga. But she could not play the celebrity wife. *Courtesy of the Family of Jonas Salk*

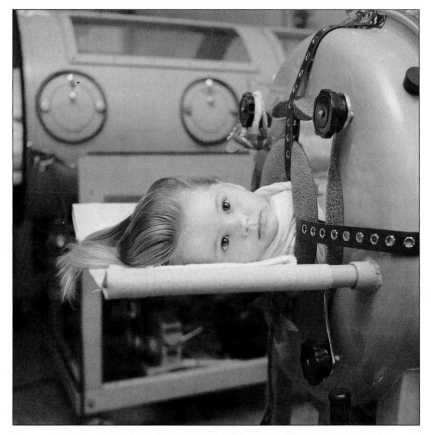

A young girl confined to an iron lung. "For over fifty years, no one could predict where or when the next epidemic would strike. . . . No one knew what it was, or how it spread, or why it had arrived to attack the youngest, most innocent, most precious part of the population. No one had any idea how to prevent its terrible toll." (*A Paralyzing Fear: The Triumph Over Polio in America*, 15). *March of Dimes Foundation*

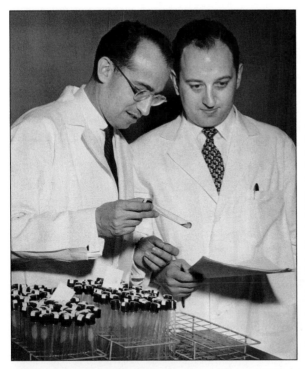

Jonas Salk and Julius Youngner discussing polio vaccine safety test results. Youngner later complained that Salk not only failed to give him proper recognition but also took credit for one of his ideas. *Jonas Salk Papers, Special Collections and Archives, UC San Diego*

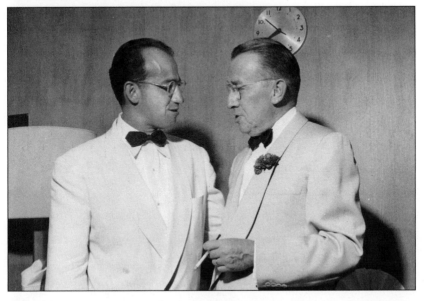

Jonas Salk with Basil O'Connor, the bold, blunt, domineering boss of the National Foundation for Infantile Paralysis (NFIP). In "Doc," Salk said he had found a kindred soul. They would help each other realize their dreams and sustain each other through their darkest hours. *Jonas Salk Papers, Special Collections and Archives, UC San Diego*

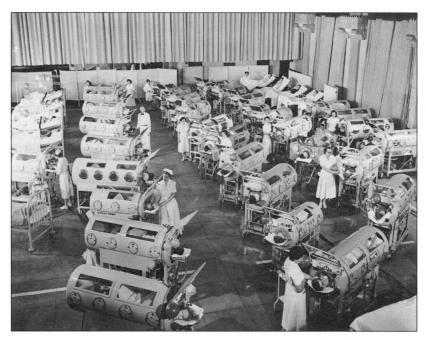

Iron lung respirators and rocking beds at Rancho Los Amigos Rehabilitation Center in Hondo, CA. When epidemiologists forecast that 1952 would be a record year for polio, Jonas Salk told Harry Weaver, research director for the NFIP, that the time had come to test his vaccine in human subjects. *March of Dimes Foundation*

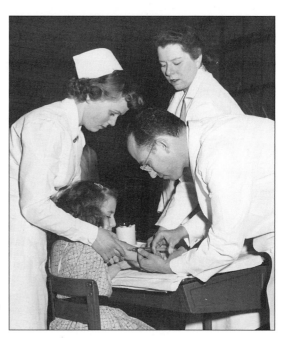

Salk inoculating a child with his polio vaccine. He later told reporter John Troan, "When you inoculate children with a polio vaccine for the first time, you don't sleep well for two or three weeks." *Jonas Salk Papers, Special Collections and Archives, UC San Diego*

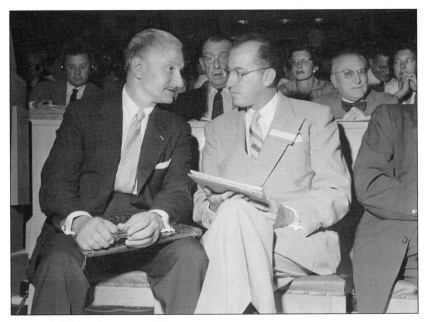

Albert Sabin and Jonas Salk at an international polio conference. For forty years they debated whose vaccine was safer and more effective. The press portrayed them as dueling scientists engaged in a medical feud. Salk told a friend he hoped his biographer would emphasize the difference in their ideas, not trivialize their conduct as "two little Jewish boys from the Bronx fighting it out." *March of Dimes Foundation*

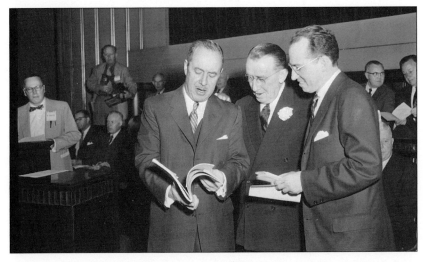

April 12, 1955. Thomas Francis, Jr., Basil O'Connor, and Jonas Salk looking at the field trial results which showed Salk's vaccine to be highly effective in preventing polio. A wave of celebrity followed from which Salk could never extricate himself. *March of Dimes Foundation*

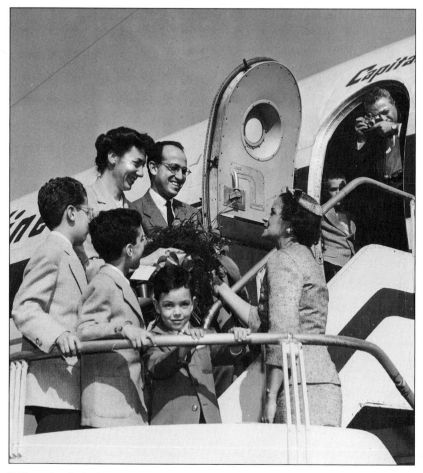

When the Salk family arrived home, a welcoming committee of Pittsburgh city officials met them at the airport. A chauffeur drove them home in the mayor's limousine with police escorts. Donna lamented that their world had changed. *Jonas Salk Papers, Special Collections and Archives, UC San Diego*

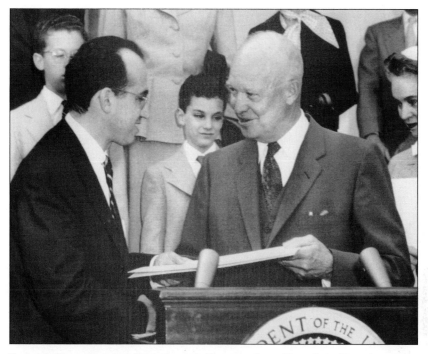

Jonas Salk receiving a Presidential Citation from President Eisenhower in the Rose Garden with sons Peter (11) and Darrell (8) behind him. Perhaps more difficult than having a legendary father was becoming a celebrity by association. *Jonas Salk Papers, Special Collections and Archives, UC San Diego*

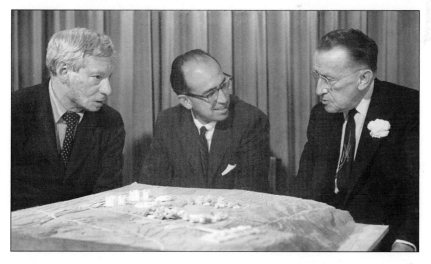

Louis Kahn, Jonas Salk, and Basil O'Connor reviewing the initial concept for the Salk Institute in La Jolla. In Kahn, Salk said he found the perfect architect to give his vision structure. He wouldn't receive the architectural plans for another three years. *March of Dimes Foundation*

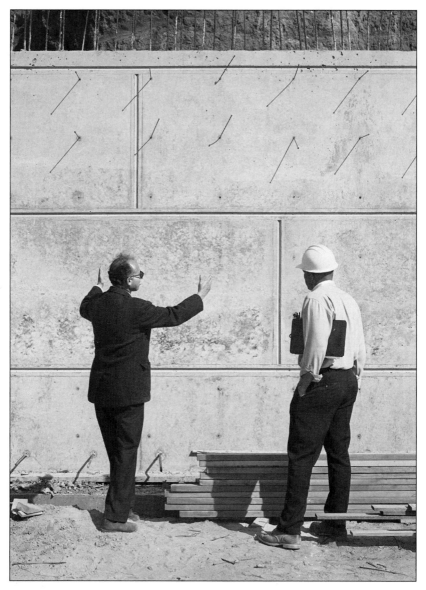

Salk insisted on involving himself in all aspects of the design and construction of his institute. He felt a concrete exterior imparted the monolithic character he and Kahn had envisioned and stood by as twenty-five concrete test slabs were poured on the site. *Courtesy of the Salk Institute for Biological Studies*

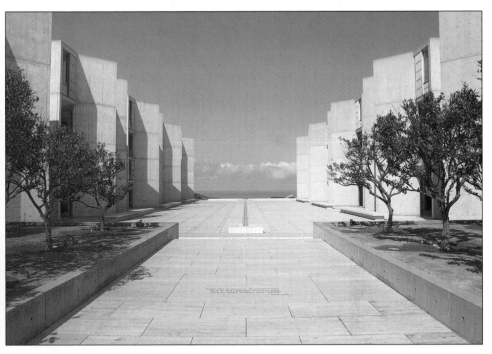

Many consider the Salk Institute Kahn's finest work. "The building is as close to perfection as anything possible," Salk said. *Courtesy of the Salk Institute for Biological Studies*

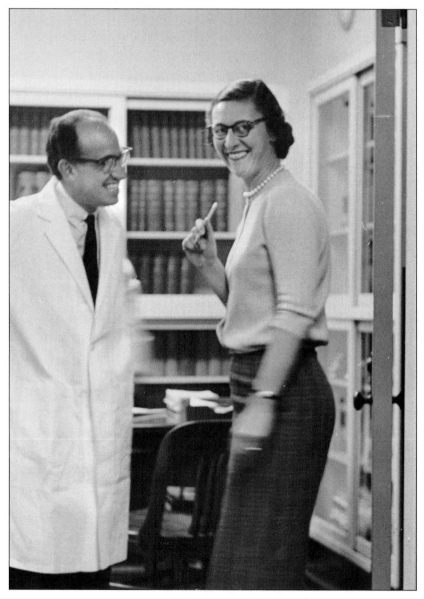

Lorraine Friedman was the epitome of the executive secretary. She provided stability, companionship, and good humor, trying to conceal the fact that she had fallen in love with Salk when he hired her in 1947. She remained unmarried and would one day be buried near him. *Jonas Salk Papers, Special Collections and Archives, UC San Diego*

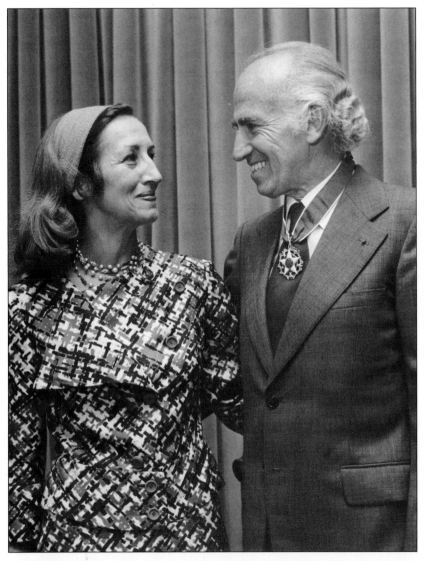

In 1970, Jonas Salk married French artist Françoise Gilot, Picasso's former mistress. When asked how she had ended up with two of history's most powerful men, she replied: "Lions mate with lions." As he received President Carter's Medal of Freedom, the public saw a more fashionable, happier Salk.
Jonas Salk Papers, Special Collections and Archives, UC San Diego

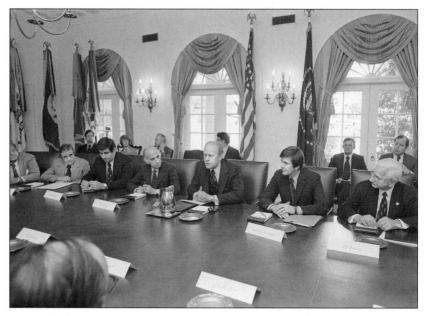

In March of 1976, President Gerald Ford convened a blue-ribbon panel to address a threatening influenza epidemic. Jonas Salk (to his right) and Albert Sabin (left end of table) advised him to immunize the American public in what would be later called the "swine flu snafu." *Courtesy Gerald R. Ford Library*

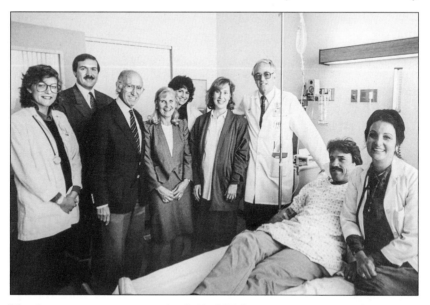

The first patient to receive the Salk AIDS vaccine in 1987. Left to right: Sylvia Hutchinson, Dennis Carlo, Salk, Ruth Dworsky, Susan Groshen, Joan Abrahamson Aronson, Brian Henderson, Patient #1, and Alexandra M. Levine. *Courtesy of Alexandra M. Levine, MD, MACP*

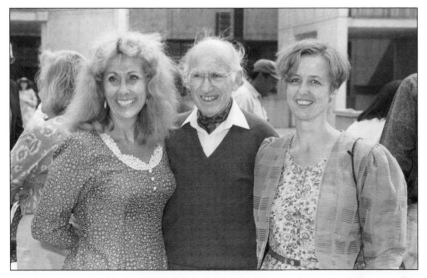

Jonas Salk with Molly Hart Lebherz and Eva Horney Seilitz on his eightieth birthday. *Courtesy of the Salk Institute for Biological Studies*

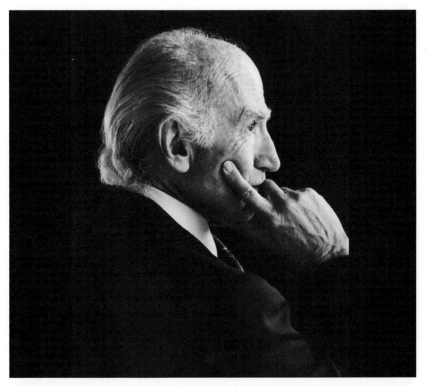

Jonas Salk was a solitary man. In his later years, though still optimistic, he wrestled with a number of unresolved challenges. *Courtesy of the Salk Institute for Biological Studies*

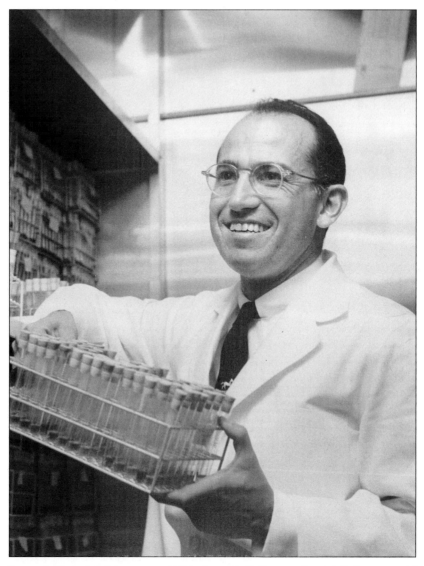

Jonas Salk in his laboratory, 1954. *Jonas Salk Papers, Special Collections and Archives, UC San Diego*

Final Fling

FREDERIC DE HOFFMANN, the new chancellor, seemed capable and earnest. A Harvard physicist who had helped develop the hydrogen bomb, de Hoffmann said his primary emphasis would be to maintain a climate that allowed creativity free rein.[1] Yet he told comptroller Del Glanz that no matter how high the quality of the science, they needed to raise money and balance the budget first. Reserved and unassuming, the forty-eight-year-old was soon working so many hours that his life at home and his life at the Institute seemed to have merged. Before long, they didn't have to worry if they could make the next payroll.

Thanks to de Hoffmann, Salk carried almost no administrative duties and was free to concentrate on his research. Although many resident fellows thought his time as a laboratory scientist was behind him, Salk himself felt that he had more contributions to make. Conducting research on both multiple sclerosis and cancer, he lacked the single-minded focus that had led to the polio vaccine. To some this seemed foolhardy; few scientists investigated two such disparate diseases. At the same time, he was writing another philosophical book and traveling to Paris and New York, where Gilot had her studios.

With regard to cancer, Salk and his senior research associate, Sam Rose, were trying to decipher those parts of the immune system that suppressed tumor growth. "Jonas was enthusiastic about harnessing the immune system to reject tumor cells," explained Walter Eckhart, then a postdoctoral fellow in Dulbecco's lab. Salk and Rose drew blood from animals, concentrated the immune cells, and reinfused them to try to arrest cancers. "Actually, it wasn't a bad idea," Eckhart said, "but they didn't start with mice or rats; they started with cows. We all thought that was crazy."[2] All, that is, except Armand Hammer. Enthused over the prospect of a cure for cancer stemming from Salk's work, the oil tycoon had agreed to fund the Armand Hammer Cancer Research Center, which included Dulbecco, Cohn, Holley, and fifteen other Institute investigators in an integrated approach to cancer. Salk served as cancer council chairman, although he rarely discussed cancer research with Dulbecco, Cohn, or Holley—an omission which would turn out to have serious consequences.

In 1972, Rose took another position, and Salk's son Peter joined his lab. Peter had just finished medical residency training and settled in La Jolla with his wife. Although he had not obtained a PhD or any formal training in immunology or cancer biology, Peter replaced Rose, a senior scientist. "As far as I could tell," a research assistant observed, "Peter *was* the cancer program."[3] A picture in *Human Behavior* shows Salk in a white coat, standing in his lab. "Still primarily a biologist and a physician," the caption reads, "Salk confers with a researcher in the Armand Hammer Laboratory where the search for a cure for cancer is underway." Another portrays him working side by side with his son. "Peter Salk joins his father in research projects that mix precision and daring," it reports.[4] Salk, however, had no NIH grants, no publications in cancer journals; his tumor immunology program languished.

His work on multiple sclerosis was progressing better, due in large part to the addition of two young investigators, Fred Westall and Vanda Lennon. Westall, a straight-talking, scrappy young man, had a PhD in chemistry from the University of California, San Diego, and significant experience in protein synthesis. "Most find complex answers to simple questions," an Institute president said of Westall, "Fred discovers simple answers to complex questions."[5] When Westall sought advice from other researchers about which lab to join, they warned him not to work with Salk. "It will ruin your career," he was told. Nevertheless, Westall found the idea of human application appealing. "I don't think there are too many chemists in the world who have the opportunity to work on a therapy." Harry Weaver, still directing research for the National Multiple Sclerosis Society, arranged for Australian immunologist Vanda Lennon to join them. He considered Lennon and Westall the two young hopes of the MS society, and he wanted them together.

Salk continued to study experimental allergic encephalitis (EAE) in animals since its neurologic damage resembled MS. EAE could be induced by inoculations of myelin basic protein (MBP) derived from the brain or spinal cord. His laboratory, as well as others, had shown that after induction of EAE with small doses of MBP, they could protect the animals from developing full-blown disease by giving high doses of MBP. These high doses induced desensitization in the same way that a series of shots of ragweed pollen extract could desensitize a person suffering from an allergy to ragweed and help prevent attacks of hay fever or asthma.

Salk and his team worked to elucidate the structure and biologic activity of the MBP protein by analyzing samples from the nervous tissue of pigs, cows, and rats, as well as human brains. They investigated the relationship between the source of MBP, dose and schedule of administration, and control of EAE in lab animals. Westall liked working with Salk. Although he was a celebrity, there was no trace of arrogance in his attitude. He didn't spend much time in his laboratory, but enough to set the tone. Every experiment was prewritten; everyone received a copy in advance. "You knew what was going to happen, when it was going to happen, and how it was going to happen," Westall recalled. He considered Salk thorough to the point of punctiliousness. "We looked at how you inject it, where you inject it, the amount you inject, how often you inject. Do you treat for ten days, twenty days? Do you use MBP from humans or guinea pigs or cows? We covered everything."[6] In one experiment, they used one hundred guinea pigs a week.

Westall respected Salk's intellectual honesty; he never overinterpreted data. "We'd do these experiments in every combination and permutation, and whatever the result, that was the result."[7] Yet Salk rarely published those results; he only reported data he considered unique or clinically relevant. All Westall could recall were two abstracts in *Neurology* and three book chapters. Peter Salk concurred: "Much of the EAE work never saw the light of day."[8] As a result, Institute scientists had no idea what Salk had done. "We probably could have written a hundred publications," Westfall speculated, given what they found: MBP extracted from the brains of rabbits, cows, pigs, and humans had similar structures.[9] The suppressive effect of MBP depended on the dose and length of therapy. And it appeared safe; monkeys treated for ninety days showed no signs of toxicity. When he heard these findings, Weaver thought time had come to test MBP in humans.

Conducting research on both cancer and multiple sclerosis required a large laboratory and substantial funds; nevertheless, Salk didn't like to think about money; he never had. In the past, if he overspent, O'Connor had covered it. His grant requests to the NFIP had been pro forma. Now he was treated like any other investigator. Salk tried to convince NF leadership that his research related to their new mission, prevention of birth defects. They did not accept his argument. In 1971 his NF support had been reduced to $50,000 every six months.[10] Once again, Salk faced a financial crisis. He could not squeeze more money from the cancer center; Hammer scrutinized its distribution. And despite Weaver's best efforts, the MS Society had limited research funds. By now, most fellows applied to the National Institutes of Health or National Science Foundation for funding. Salk had submitted an NIH grant that had been rejected. He could not adhere to the NIH's strict guidelines, and at fifty-seven, he could not compete with the brilliant young molecular biologists around the country.

What Salk needed was another Basil O'Connor. He looked over the list of trustees and decided to approach William Bernbach, a legendary figure in American advertising. Salk sent Bernbach a long letter that described his work on multiple sclerosis and cancer, with human trials as the next logical step, and explained that accomplishing this required the generosity of one who displayed true concern for mankind. "Basil O'Connor was such a man," he wrote, "and I have not yet had the good fortune to find another."[11] He requested a million dollars each year beginning as soon as possible. Bernbach declined the request.

So he tried another tack. He wrote to trustee Sol Linowitz, who had made millions when he helped found Xerox, and reminded him of Slater's suggestion that he endow a chair in human creativity to symbolize the Institute's interest in the humanities. Salk said he would be pleased to occupy the position. "The attitude prevails that I am costing the Institute money," he admitted. An endowed chair would "allow me to function as I would like to be able to do without feeling pressured."[12] At the same time, Salk contacted Edgar Bronfman, CEO of the Seagram Company, saying how much he appreciated the Bronfman Foundation's intention to establish an endowed chair with him as the first recipient. No such offer had been made. Neither Linowitz nor Bronfman chose to become his benefactor. Salk had estimated a $600,000 budget for 1972. He was becoming desperate. He requested that the NF send his entire $100,000 up front, rather than in biyearly allotments, citing "cash flow needs."[13]

Then he met Morris Diefenbach. Vice president of the CertainTeed Products Corporation, a building materials supplier in Pennsylvania, Diefenbach had developed multiple sclerosis and hoped that Salk's research might lead to a curative therapy. In 1973, he offered to set up the CertainTeed Jonas Salk Foundation to raise funds for MS research. Salk could not refuse. "Jonas had this habit of big swings of money, no money, money, no money," Westall recollected. "If somebody walked in off the street and handed him a check, he'd take it."[14] Now, however, there had been a procedural change: Salk could no longer accept money outright; he had to go through the Institute's new gatekeeper, Frederic de Hoffmann.

Diefenbach's first meeting with de Hoffmann regarding the CertainTeed Jonas Salk Foundation did not go well. "There is no question," Diefenbach told Salk, "but what his principal concern is that your name would be associated with our foundation.... Although I would not want to repeat them, he made certain statements concerning you and your research work as related to previous financial arrangements which I'm sure you would find most disturbing."[15] Their conversation had become heated; de Hoffmann argued over every point. Nonetheless, he had a problem to solve—Salk was draining money from his coffers—and Diefenbach posed a possible solution.

At the July 12, 1973, executive committee meeting, de Hoffmann presented Diefenbach's proposal to form a foundation that would raise $500,000 annually for Salk's lab.[16] Robert Holley, representing the resident fellows, objected. He warned that the granter should not be misled into believing clinical trials would soon commence, as had been the case with Armand Hammer. Holley insisted Salk's research undergo a thorough review first, as should all the Institute laboratory programs on a regular basis. With those concerns voiced, the executive committee agreed to Diefenbach's proposal in concept only. What Salk did not foresee in pursuing the CertainTeed offer was that it would open Pandora's box, releasing the fellows' pent-up feelings about him as a scientist and his unbridled freedom.

"Salk's enormous staff and space generated irritation," resident fellow Edwin Lennox divulged.[17] Having dispelled the notion of the Institute as a haven exempt from financial concerns, de Hoffmann and Glanz encouraged fellows to apply for federal grants. "I'm not qualified to judge Salk academically," Glanz said. "I'm just an old bookkeeper. But here the fellows are getting government funding, doing their bit to help the Institute, and Jonas is not."[18] Others were less politic. Lennox considered Salk's scientific knowledge somewhat shallow: "Frankly, I think he got in over his head."[19] An undercurrent of antagonism flowed through the Institute. "The scientists who were there, the Nobelists, the pre-Nobelists, really didn't like Jonas," observed a young researcher who had recently come to La Jolla. Salk did not stand in their ranks; "they more or less laughed behind his back."[20] Lennox thought Salk was oblivious to their opinion of him. Psychiatrist Arnold Mandell disagreed. He knew how painful their rejection had become. "Jonas was a common man lost among the geniuses in his own institute."[21] Even so, Salk did not suspect that the resident fellows he had attracted to La Jolla had formed a cabal.

The intrigue centered on the internal review of his laboratory as recommended at the executive committee meeting. On July 22, de Hoffmann received a memo summarizing what the reviewers, comprising the selfsame resident fellows, called "grave misgivings." With regard to Salk's multiple sclerosis research, they noted several excellent laboratories were studying the relationship between EAE and MS; Salk likely would not contribute new insights. Furthermore, the proposed experimentation on MS patients could not be justified. "We think that accepting major support for an expanded activity in this field is ill-advised," they warned, "and could well lead to further damage to the reputation of the Institute." Although the informal evaluation was supposed to encompass only the research Salk proposed to carry out with CertainTeed funds, the group critiqued his cancer program as well. "Nothing in his brief presentation suggested that he had anything original to propose," they reported.[22] They recommended review by an external scientific panel. The memo was signed by Mel Cohn, Edwin Lennox, Robert Holley, Leslie Orgel, and Roger Guillemin.

After that the resident fellows sent a letter to the chairman of the board, John McCloy, that emphasized the imperative for external review of the Institute's scientific programs. Under de Hoffmann's leadership, the financial crisis that had plagued them had almost dissipated, due in large part to their efforts, they wrote. Of the Institute's $6.1 million budget, $4.1 million had come from federal grants they had obtained. "These successes," they argued, "can only continue if our claim to do outstanding scientific work seems credible to the scientific community. It would be tragic to jeopardize our major source of long-term funding through the pursuit of programs of the type the CertainTeed Jonas Salk Foundation wishes to support and intends to bring to public notice in the Institute's name." Lest McCloy minimize their concerns, they advised, "We would gravely regret having to send this letter to the members of the Board of Trustees for it expresses our rather harsh judgments about Dr. Salk's proposed program."[23]

Salk, in the meantime, had signed a letter of agreement with CertainTeed. "You have transformed my life," he wrote the corporation's board chairman. "I did not know how very heavily the problem of funding for our research weighed upon me until you began to lift the burden.... It has kindled new enthusiasm, imagination, and courage."[24] Salk never suspected what would soon ensue.

At the October 12 executive committee meeting, held in advance of the Institute's board meeting, Holley presented the internal review of Salk's laboratory to which they had referred in de Hoffmann's July 22 memo. He reported that the fellows were greatly concerned about the quality of Salk's proposed research with projected expenditures five or ten times the amount justified on scientific grounds. They advised the chancellor not to accept new funds for this program until they obtained an outside review, which might suggest program modifications that would be acceptable with "a minimum of embarrassment." Holley proceeded to recount Salk's reaction when apprised of this recommendation: no one was going to review his program, and he had the votes on the board of trustees to get his way. "I found it absurd for Dr. Salk to suggest that any scientist's program is above criticism," Holley complained. "If the Executive Committee takes the position that Dr. Salk's program does not have to meet any scientific standard, it will make a mockery of any claim that the Institute is a responsible scientific institution."[25]

Holley's vindictive statements seemed out of character for this quiet, modest man who enjoyed taking long walks on the beach to look at tide pools. His warning that the Institute's survival was threatened by the man who had built it surprised some trustees. Likely, he was angered that the allocation of Hammer's annual million-dollar donation included $162,000 to him and Cohen, whereas Salk received $400,000. Perhaps inflamed by his co-conspirators, he thought the time had come for someone to rein in Jonas Salk.

Two weeks later, at the October 24 board meeting, Salk had a chance for rebuttal. Instead of justifying his proposal or contradicting Holley's offensive comments, he suggested the board view CertainTeed's offer not as a danger but as an opportunity. He reminded them of the academic freedom intended in the founding of the Institute; nevertheless, he did not object to an external assessment of all the laboratory programs.[26] Although he maintained his composure, Lorraine Friedman knew it distressed Salk to be rebuffed by his colleagues. Had he not founded the Institute, he told her, he wouldn't have been invited to become a member.[27] Mandell worried about his friend. He was having trouble sleeping, losing weight—symptoms of depression.[28]

The executive committee requested an outside review panel from the Rockefeller Institute, led by Maclyn McCarty. This meant Salk would have to convince the esteemed geneticist who had discovered that DNA carries genetic information that his own research was worthwhile.

The January 30, 1974, annual fellows meeting was quite a contrast to the first Guillemin had attended years earlier, a meeting which radiated collegiality. Guillemin had already begun to regret the part he had played in the showdown he knew was coming. He later wrote a contrite letter to Salk, expressing his regrets at having been pulled into the collusion against him. When they reached the agenda item "Disposition of Review Committee Reports," in accordance with their newly adopted procedures, the external review was presented to the resident and nonresident fellows.[29] For each program, the conclusion read, "Favorable report, no action required." Then they came to Salk's. He turned to face the jury and hear their verdict: tolerance for his unorthodox approaches or condemnation.

No surprise to anyone, except perhaps Salk, the expert panel panned the cancer program. They said his extensive experiments had merely replicated those performed for years by tumor immunologists. Furthermore, Salk's future plans held limited promise. Peter Salk, who had carried out most of the work, had no training in immunobiology. They recommended he seek a postdoctoral fellowship in a prominent laboratory and that Salk recruit a senior scientist trained in tumor immunity. Salk said nothing.

To the resident fellows' astonishment, the panel rated the multiple sclerosis program highly. Neuroscientists nationwide held Salk in high regard. The reviewers found his laboratory group had accomplished a great deal in their approach to EAE, most notably in defining the relationship of structure to biologic activity. Regarding his proposal for human application, working in collaboration with Eli Lilly, the external reviewers considered the steps outlined "well-conceived, with adequate precautions to minimize possible risks."[30] After the meeting, no one congratulated Salk on his MS program, and he did not gloat over its favorable appraisal. Several fellows urged him to terminate the cancer program and concentrate on EAE. He did not defend his cancer work and simply said that he would take their recommendations "under advisement."[31]

Since the CertainTeed Jonas Salk Foundation had been created to support Salk's MS research, and that research had received a positive review, the board of trustees had to allow the collaboration to go forward. On February 8, 1974, Morris Diefenbach announced the establishment of the CertainTeed Jonas Salk Foundation. Its brochure displayed pictures of Salk and noted the Foundation's mission was to encourage the

great scientist to "apply his talents in the pursuit of his present interests."[32] It went on to say the CertainTeed Products Corporation believed
American industry should provide leadership in supporting programs
directed toward improving quality of life. It planned to use corporate
management and personnel to raise $2 million over thirty-six months.
To kick off the fundraising campaign, Françoise Gilot contributed fifty
signed lithographs as gifts for those who contributed $1,000 or more.

Unfortunately, the CertainTeed Jonas Salk Foundation did not live
up to its expectations. Diefenbach blamed the Institute board; with the
eight-month delay, they had lost the opportunity to solicit funds before
the 1973 tax year ended. Salk had assumed the money was forthcoming
and entered January of 1974 with a $165,000 deficit. In April, de
Hoffmann told the trustees that the CertainTeed Jonas Salk Foundation
agreed to pay $205,000 for direct expenses, but two months later
Diefenbach sent a note to the Bank of America placing a hold on further
disbursements to the Salk Institute.[33] Diefenbach's health and authority
within the company were deteriorating; shortly thereafter he resigned
from the Foundation. Instead of reacting with shock or anger, Salk wrote
to the president of the corporation saying he appreciated its generosity; Diefenbach had worked with "great dedication."[34] In the end,
donations from the CertainTeed Jonas Salk Foundation amounted to
$60,000.[35]

Meanwhile, Armand Hammer had become impatient. He expected
a return from his investments and, disillusioned that Salk had not cured
cancer, lost interest in his work. Having spent the anticipated funds, Salk
had overdrawn his account. At the January 1976 board meeting, de
Hoffmann reported all labs as solvent except Salk's. His research costs
totaled more than $300,000; his funding sources remained uncertain.[36]
The National Foundation had notified him that Salk's special grant was
being discontinued on June 30. What an embarrassment to the man who
had founded the Institute. Westall thought the NF leadership was
"brutal" to Salk. "They treated him like crap."[37]

Salk wrote to Sam Ajl, the Foundation's vice president for research,
practically begging to continue his grant without requiring him to go
through their standard review process. Ajl told Salk to complete the usual
application. "Let me assure you," Ajl added, "I have your best interests at

heart."[38] Salk complied. A few months later, the NF's Research Advisory Committee recommended approval of a two-year terminal grant in a reduced amount through June 30, 1978. With diminishing funds and no one to rescue him, Salk had to reduce his staff and relinquish laboratory space. "The institute kept nibbling away at him," Westall said, "taking more and more of his lab. Finally they took half of it away."[39]

⁂

DESPITE THIS FINANCIAL strain, Salk's multiple sclerosis work flourished. With an eye toward human studies, his group was searching for the best source of MBP. Salk did have some doubts about whether EAE was a valid model for multiple sclerosis, the cause of which was still unknown. When he seemed to be procrastinating, Weaver became impatient. He told Salk it was time for human studies or support from NMSS would cease. In response, perhaps justifying his action to himself, Salk wrote to Weaver, "Since the knowledge still lacking to justify a clinical study can be obtained only by doing it, I believe that the time has come to do it."[40]

This would not be the first clinical trial of MBP. Los Angeles neurosurgeon Barry Campbell had carried out a limited study in sixty-four patients using myelin basic protein from human brains, taken at autopsy, which he called BP. Half received a BP shot each week for thirty months; half a placebo for a year, followed by BP for eighteen months. After 4,253 injections of BP, he reported no deleterious effects. Campbell compared neurologic symptoms between the two groups and thought the experimental group showed some improvement.[41] Belgian researchers also conducted a trial using human and bovine BP. They treated thirty-five patients for up to eleven months and found that BP did not reduce the number of relapses.[42] Both trials had their shortcomings: In the former, response had been assessed by patients' self-reports, not neurologic exams. In the latter, the number of subjects was too small to be conclusive. And both had the obvious disadvantage of requiring human brains as the source for BP.

Weaver believed that no one would be better at determining the true potential of MBP for treating MS than Salk. He knew how to conduct a clinical trial, how to work with the pharmaceutical industry and the FDA, how to negotiate the bureaucracy. Although his polio vaccine trials were twenty years in the past, Westall agreed that Salk still had this expertise. "It's like riding a bicycle," he said. "Once you do it, you don't forget."[43] Weaver trusted Salk to make sure the trial was conducted properly and expeditiously. After he made the decision to proceed, Salk seemed energized. Since medicine was not practiced at the Institute, Salk sought collaborators at the University of California, San Diego. He also contacted Eldon Shuey, head of biochemical research at Lilly Research Laboratories. They had developed a method to prepare myelin basic protein from pigs and cows that yielded consistent product, and Shuey thought they could scale up the production. When Salk and a representative from Eli Lilly met with staff at the FDA's Bureau of Biologics, Salk wisely presented this not as a therapeutic trial of MBP but as an exploratory study to clarify whether EAE was a valid model for MS and to establish safety at the dosage level selected. The FDA seemed amenable, and Salk awaited approval to open the trial. Many hopeful patients had signed up to participate. Then, on September, 12, 1977, just as things were falling into place, Harry Weaver died of lung cancer. He had not lived to see the start of the trial he had promoted.

The Study of Myelin Basic Protein as a Possible Therapeutic Agent in Multiple Sclerosis opened in January of 1978 with UCSD professors John Romine and W. C. Wiederholt as collaborators.[44] Eli Lilly agreed to prepare the myelin basic protein. As opposed to poliomyelitis investigators, who had tried to block his every move, or colleagues at the Salk Institute, who had expressed "grave misgivings" about his work, multiple sclerosis researchers were refreshingly supportive. Weaver had fostered those positive relationships early on when he introduced Salk to leaders in the field. Several top neuroscientists offered to analyze immune responses in the trial patients. Campbell sent flow sheets from his earlier BP trial for Salk's use. Others in the field lent moral support. "Let me wish you the best of health, productivity and happiness for the New Year," wrote Bornstein, one of the first to study EAE.[45] When Elizabeth Roboz Einstein learned the FDA had approved his trial, she wrote: "This brought back some cherished memories when some ten years ago you came to my laboratory and later to the house and we discussed the basic

protein.... At this stage of the game, when you embark on treatment
with the basic protein, my sincere wish is that you succeed."[46]

Salk's collaborators may have changed for the better; but the press
had not. "Polio Hero Salk May Be Near Multiple Sclerosis Remedy,"
announced the *Milwaukee Journal*.[47] "Jonas Salk Stalks Another Killer,"
reported the *Philadelphia Enquirer*, displaying a photograph of Salk in his
white coat and ascot standing in front of the Institute, gazing out to the
ocean. "If the experiment proves successful," it read, "Salk...will once
again become a national hero."[48] A UPI story on Salk's trial, featured in
newspapers throughout the country, resulted in a flood of patient letters.

"I heard on the news about the grant you all received for MS research,"
wrote J. Neufeld. "Don't want you to think I got excited but—Whoooeee!
If I can help you in any way...just holler."[49] H. Ousley of San Francisco
wrote: "I am a mess and would like to volunteer my services as a guinea
pig."[50] Some told their own tragic story. A. Mastro of Dunmore,
Pennsylvania, had been diagnosed with MS when her son was a year old.
"To see life pass me by," she wrote, "to watch my family grow and to be
not able to share active experiences with them is truly discouraging to
me."[51] A novelist from Carmichael, California, told Salk: "I write in the
mornings in a slow, narrowing band of energy. I write as if every page
I write will be my last."[52] S. Meyers, a psychiatric social worker and
mother of three, confided, "My secret most fervent wish is to be able to
dance with my husband at our son's Bar Mitzvah."[53]

Others sent sorrowful notes about loved ones. "As a desperate
mother," wrote L. Foster of Calumet City, Illinois, "I am pleading for
help for our daughter...26, married nearly three years. She and her husband are deaf."[54] One mother wrote for her son, a former football star
and president of his school, who could no longer write. Others just
wanted to encourage Salk. "Whether the experiment succeeds or fails,"
wrote a woman plagued by fatigue, "it boosts one's morale to know
someone cares enough to try."[55] V. Bachmann thanked him for his concern, saying, "Up until now, we who are afflicted had nothing to hope for
except hope."[56]

Within a few weeks, Salk received more than a thousand letters. Some
were handwritten, some typed when the fingers had become too weak to
write, some on pink stationery, some decorated with flowers. They arrived

from all over the United States—Titusville, New Jersey; Newburyport, Massachusetts; Mansfield, Ohio. And all were heartfelt. In his earlier years, Salk had written a response to every note. Now he resorted to a standardized letter. Perhaps he was wiser or more tired, or just too sad. Maybe he lacked the conviction that a successful outcome was in sight.

Between January and December of 1978, eleven patients with MS entered Salk's first trial. They ranged in age from twenty-one to fifty-six; five were women; all had relapsing or progressive disease. Romine obtained the clinical histories and performed neurologic exams at study entry and biweekly thereafter. They analyzed blood counts, liver function, and urine on a biweekly basis to assess toxicity and sent hundreds of blood and spinal fluid samples to collaborating scientists for immunologic studies. MBP extracted from pigs was injected daily, starting at 75 mg—one hundred times the dose used by clinical researchers in earlier trials. Salk increased the dose up to 300 mg in some patients. They continued MBP until the disease progressed.[57] Although Romine took responsibility for daily patient care, Salk wanted to meet everyone participating in the trial. "I told him not to see the patients," Westall recalled, "because what better placebo effect than Jonas Salk saying, 'You're going to get well.'"[58]

Romine asked patients to keep diaries of their symptoms and function. Patient B. T. reported that MS affected his legs, eyes, hands, bladder, and speech. "My body was changing so rapidly," he wrote in his diary, "that I didn't have time to adjust to each new problem as it occurred.... Once on myelin basic protein, some of my symptoms were quickly reversed....My speech impediments disappeared. The pain in my left eye stopped....I felt stronger and had more zest for living."[59] Another patient, suffering from MS for fifteen years, wrote: "During 1977, my condition worsened. I became dependent on a wheelchair, more despondent. I experienced extreme weakness, lack of bladder control and fatigue." He spent most days in bed. Then he started MBP. "The level of activity has now increased to the point where I carry on active business affairs, attend frequent evening social and sports events, and put in a normal day from 7:30 am until 11 pm."[60] On New Year's Eve, he attended two parties and left his wheelchair at home. On October 28, 1978, the grateful patients sent Salk a card that read: "Dear Jonas, It is our hope that on your 64th birthday you are feeling as good in body and spirit as we."[61]

That fall, Salk and Romaine conducted an interim analysis for the FDA.[62] Toxicity had been minimal: six patients had transient local reactions at the injection site; two had low-grade fevers. They had discontinued MBP in two patients because of disease progression. Of the nine patients who had received MBP injections for at least two hundred days, four had improved neurologic exams. All but two, however, still had active MS. Salk and Romine presented their preliminary results at an American Academy of Neurology meeting. They concluded that MBP at this dose could be given daily for six months without significant side effects, but they needed a larger, placebo-controlled trial to determine efficacy.[63]

In their next trial, Myelin Basic Protein as a Therapeutic Agent in MS, patients were randomized to receive either MBP or placebo.[64] Within ten months, they enrolled the requisite number of subjects. Before long, however, patients began to complain of itching. Rashes broke out on the chest or back and spread to the arms, legs, and face. Almost every patient was suffering from what Salk knew to be a delayed hypersensitivity reaction to MBP. Eli Lilly could not find any difference between this batch and the MBP produced for the first trail. Salk and Romaine tried changing the dose, the schedule, and the method of injection, giving antihistamines, high-dose steroids, all to no avail. Although they had seen beneficial effects from MBP in some MS patients, the hypersensitivity reaction impeded further study.[65] Salk had ended up in a blind alley. In mid-October 1981, they would give the last injection of MBP. With Weaver gone and no further funding from NMSS, Salk left the field of multiple sclerosis.

Salk had not been able to halt the relentless progression of MS, to aid those countless patients who sought his help as their lives spiraled downward. A cure for multiple sclerosis would have been his grand finale, but he abruptly exited the stage. Years later, when a pathologist wrote inquiring about his MS work, Salk replied, "I have had my fling."[66]

Marginalized

"As a biologist, he believes that his science is on the frontier of tremendous new discoveries; and as a philosopher, he is convinced that humanists and artists have joined the scientists to achieve an understanding of man in all his physical, mental and spiritual complexity." So reported the *New York Times* in a 1966 piece, calling Jonas Salk the "father of biophilosophy."[1] Nine years later, Salk was preparing to attend a board of trustees meeting to hear the fate of humanism at the institute that bore his name.

Salk had struggled to realize his goal of blending the two cultures, the premise on which he and O'Connor had founded the Institute, until Joseph Slater became president and created the Council for Biology in Human Affairs, transforming Salk's abstract social and humanistic concepts into practical programs. Composed of distinguished international scholars and led by Jacob Bronowski, the Council set out to address such crucial questions as: What should society ask scientists to consider? What opportunities and problems arise from biological discoveries? What should political and business leaders know about advances in the sciences in order to be more effective? Slater told the board of trustees he envisioned the Institute's taking a leading role in establishing a network of institutions concerned with mankind.

Resident fellows Salvador Luria, Jacques Monod, and Robert Holley joined the Council. Leslie Orgel, however, expressed the unspoken opinion of other Institute scientists when he warned the trustees that too much emphasis on humanistic issues was "peripheral to the Institute's basic purpose," namely, scientific discovery, and could "dilute the Institute's output in its primary field."[2] Nevertheless, in 1970, the trustees had incorporated the CBHA into the Institute as a permanent program. Two years later, as Slater prepared to leave, he appealed to the fellows that the Council "not be permitted to atrophy."[3] That required an agency or individual who believed enough in its premise to cover its monthly expenses of $4,500. With Slater gone, the CBHA had to justify itself to the new chancellor, Frederic de Hoffmann, who seemed to judge each program's worth by its balance sheet.

Slater didn't know de Hoffmann's stance when he had suggested him for the newly created chancellor position. His credentials looked excellent.[4] Born in Vienna in 1924, de Hoffmann had grown up in Prague, attending a German-speaking high school. He immigrated to the United States in 1941 and attended Harvard, where he earned a PhD in physics. While an undergraduate at Harvard, he had worked on the Manhattan Project and in 1951 became Edward Teller's assistant, performing the mathematical analysis leading to what became the hydrogen bomb. Four years later, he took a position with the General Dynamics Corporation in San Diego. There he helped found General Atomics, which built reactors for nuclear power stations, and served as its president until its acquisition by Gulf Oil. Although moving to the Salk Institute meant a switch from an industrial to a biomedical research environment, he seemed the right man for the position—and he was available.

Few at the Institute knew de Hoffmann. Edwin Lennox had been with him at Los Alamos, where he had a reputation as "an able and shrewd scientific aide of high managerial and political ability."[5] That had been twenty years earlier, however. When Bronowski and Guillemin had had dinner at his home, de Hoffmann had impressed them as both a humanist, driven by concern about social effects of scientific discoveries, and a researcher with fundraising prowess. Guillemin sent a letter on behalf of the fellows to the board recommending they hire de Hoffmann as chancellor. He thought Salk was pleased with the choice; at least he did not pose any objection.[6]

A month later, while in Paris, Salk received an urgent phone call from Jack MacAllister, Louis Kahn's junior architect, who had continued to manage building projects for the Institute. He told Salk he had begun construction on Guillemin's new laboratory when he got a call from a Dr. Frederic de Hoffmann. He had difficulty understanding the man and couldn't place his accent. "I didn't know who the hell he was," MacAllister later recounted.[7] De Hoffmann informed him that he was now in charge of the Salk Institute and invited him to lunch to discuss the laboratory project. The next day, while MacAllister sat on the ocean view terrace of the historic La Valencia Hotel, he looked up to see a short, pudgy man marching toward him. From the cold handshake, MacAllister knew this was not going to be a social event. "He ate his entire lunch with his fingers," MacAllister observed. "He never picked up a fork." Then he leaned across the table, squinted at MacAllister through his thick glasses, and said, "Now that I'm here, we're doing the project my way. That means the engineers work for me. Architects are only good for picking colors. I don't trust them."[8]

MacAllister immediately resigned. Concerned about Salk, he queried people he knew at General Atomics about de Hoffmann and discovered that he had been fired as soon as Gulf had acquired the company. "He was a bastard, very disliked by everybody." Someone at the Salk Institute had not done due diligence in their rush to replace Slater and try to keep O'Connor from pulling the National Foundation grants. De Hoffmann had been on his best behavior during his interviews; no one had witnessed his bad temper. MacAllister called Joe Slater who insisted he fly out to Aspen as soon as possible. The two of them stayed up all night comparing information and trying to decide what to do. By the time they reached Salk in Paris, it was too late. The contract had been signed.

What struck the fellows and staff at first was how hard de Hoffmann worked—around the clock, seven days a week. He required his secretary's constant availability, demanding immediate attention. "There was my regular six o'clock in the morning phone call," comptroller Delbert Glanz recalled. "Fred would say, 'I only have seconds'—his favorite expression—and then he would begin. I was expected to have a tablet at my bedside so I could take notes if I wasn't up yet."[9] He called anybody day or night, weekdays, weekends, holidays as if everyone else was thinking about nothing but the Institute too.

At the time de Hoffmann took over, the endowment totaled a mere $200,000.[10] Glanz had had to approach individual trustees on several occasions for funds to cover the payroll. They considered going down to a four-day work week. Lennox grasped de Hoffmann's predicament; he thought it was a difficult place to administer. "It's too full of baronetcies," he said.[11] De Hoffmann had become the majordomo for a coterie of pre-eminent scientists who wanted larger and larger laboratories and a director who kept dipping into the household coffers.

With Glanz, first the comptroller and later vice president of operations and treasurer, assisting him, de Hoffmann set out to restore the Institute's financial health. First, they redoubled fundraising efforts. He and Glanz attended three or four donor dinners every week, and de Hoffmann always seemed to be rushing off to New York or Europe to solicit funds. Paul Berg, a nonresident fellow during de Hoffmann's tenure, likened him to a rat on a treadwheel. "He was constantly running; he'd come back and deposit the money he raised, and then off he went."[12]

De Hoffmann's second approach was to alter the resident fellows' expectations. Initially Salk had promised them total financial freedom, which turned out to be an idealistic and unsustainable proposition. "I had the feeling by the time Fred came there that we were being a bit self-indulgent with lifetime fellowships," Lennox admitted.[13] Some resident fellows seemed insatiable. Even Salk had become jaded about his all-star cast. "You get gifted people," he confided in Westall, "you give them anything they ever wanted, and either they are thankful for what you did or they want more."[14] In most cases, it was the latter. Salk didn't have the strength to stand up to them anymore. De Hoffmann did. He expected everyone to live off grants, especially the newly hired scientists; no one was entitled. Before long, Glanz wasn't having to ask trustees for handouts; they were running in the black.

Although everybody appreciated this new state of solvency, it came at a price. De Hoffmann ran the Institute like a corporation, apparently more concerned with productivity and the bottom line than with the individuals who populated it. He assumed authority over every decision, down to the color of the tile in the cafeteria. "He was the kind of guy who not only told you how many janitors to hire but how often to clean the floor," Glanz said.[15] He shifted decision-making powers from the fellows to the administration and held meetings to discuss Institute business instead of science. Fellows found his random, odd-hours phone calls irksome. "He was just a busybody who would trouble you for the most trivial kinds of things," Berg complained.[16] Yet de Hoffmann neglected to inform them about important decisions he had made. The fellows lost the participatory democracy they had insisted upon when Salk first established the Institute. To those on the top rung, the fellows and trustees, de Hoffmann feigned congeniality. With those a step down, such as Westall, he did not conceal his temper. Beneath his volatility, Westall detected the chancellor's insecurity: at meetings, de Hoffmann often reminded them he was a scientist, not just an administrator. And he was careful about divulging information. One researcher summed up the feeling of many: "De Hoffmann was a paranoid businessman."[17]

Although on the surface de Hoffmann was courteous to Salk, he considered the Institute director a bit of a prima donna.[18] When MacAllister had recounted his meeting with the chancellor to Salk, it had given him pause; however, he had not witnessed any such behavior himself. De Hoffmann had stood on the sidelines during the laboratory reviews, letting the fellows take the lead. Mostly de Hoffmann ignored Salk—that is, until their diverse views on the Institute made a clash inevitable.

De Hoffmann, a hard-driving, practical businessman; Salk, a dreamer, a Renaissance man—all they had in common was a desire to assure the Institute's future. "De Hoffmann whipped [the Salk Institute] into shape," wrote a journalist, "but it was a shape different from the one Jonas Salk had dreamed of. Gone were plans for studying the interaction between science and society. In their place, de Hoffmann laid plans for a more conventional research institution."[19] Fellows and trustees began to note increasing tension between the two. Busy initiating his MS trial, writing philosophical works, and traveling to Paris, Salk did not realize that de Hoffmann was gradually changing the roster of trustees to reflect his pro-hard-science views. Salk's first indication came when the board, reviewing the Institute's mission, agreed the first priority must be top-notch biological research. Nonlaboratory programs, such as the Council on Biology and Human Affairs, would be maintained only if funding allowed. "Freddie was not a man who lived off visions, off romantic idealism," nonresident fellow Gerald Edelman pointed out. "He was very much a pragmatist, without question."[20] When Salk invited artists and philosophers to the Institute, de Hoffmann thought it "deranged."[21] Salk told friend Al Rosenfeld he considered de Hoffmann a "Neanderthal thinker."[22] For the most part, they simply tried to avoid each other. De Hoffmann awaited the day CBHA would dry up and blow away—and Salk with it. Salk continued to tout its activities as if funds would materialize. "I'd ride up in the elevator with Salk and de Hoffmann," one associate noted, "and they seldom talked."[23]

Although Lennox, Monod, Luria, and others wanted to use science to do something useful for society, their views about how to go about it differed from Salk's. "Left to his own devices," Lennox reflected, "Jonas would have had a much larger contingent of artists, social scientists, and philosophers here. Some of us thought there was some bull in there we didn't wish to have."[24] They considered Bronowski a good compromise, a better synthesizer than Salk, but he had become consumed with making the acclaimed *The Ascent of Man*, a BBC documentary that featured him traveling the world to trace how man's understanding of science changed society. On August 21, 1974, sixty-six-year-old Bronowski died suddenly from a heart attack while visiting friends in East Hampton, New York.[25] "Dr. Bronowski's premature death at the peak of his career is a great loss to mankind," Salk said in a press statement, "at a time when we are in such need of the contributions of the scientist-humanist.... He was an interpreter of life, communicating with artistry the hopes of man as well as the realities with which he must cope."[26] De Hoffmann's response to Bronowski's death was to dismantle the Council for Biology in Human Affairs.[27]

As he did with many actions, de Hoffmann stood in the shadows and let the fellows and trustees steer the Institute in the direction he intended. Five months after Bronowski died, the fellows recommended phasing out the CBHA as soon as funds tapered off at the year's end.[28] Salk knew de Hoffmann could save the Council if he wished to do so.

"It's not something that he wanted to fund in any way, shape, or form," Glanz recollected. "He couldn't see himself out raising money for something so esoteric."[29] The chasm between de Hoffmann and Salk widened. The trustees, many of whom had been handpicked by de Hoffmann, concurred with the fellows at their January 1975 meeting, adding that they hoped the values associated with the Biology in Human Affairs program would remain "a continuing thread in the Institute's work."[30] Salk's dream of creating a fabric weaving scientific inquiry with the conscience of man had been reduced to "a thread."

By the late seventies, it had become clear that the Salk Institute would not merely survive but thrive. Under de Hoffmann's leadership, it had achieved financial stability and gained a reputation as one of the foremost scientific establishments in the world, dominated by a cadre of basic scientists with only a faint humanistic hue. "Under de Hoffmann," wrote science historian Stuart Leslie, summing up the situation, "the Institute all but abandoned the idea of bridging the 'two cultures.'" Salk Institute laboratories seemed almost indistinguishable from those in the research institutes and universities with which they competed. "It was a place of grueling and often tedious work," he contended, "with little time for quiet meditation on the meaning of life. Who had time for philosophical reflections in the midst of a race for a Nobel Prize?"[31] Salk admitted to NF statistician Gabriel Stickle in an oral history that he was disappointed by the shift in the institute's focus. After Bronowski's death they lacked the critical mass to integrate humanism and science. "I kept the idea alive in my own work and my own thinking," he said. "I haven't given up hope that it will manifest itself somewhere, somehow, some way."[32] In an effort to bring about such integration, Salk created a new foundation, not within but outside the Institute.

In *Survival of the Wisest*, Salk had warned that to avoid catastrophe society needed to shift from Epoch A, which he described as based on survival of the fittest, to Epoch B, in which the welfare of the individual and the species was intertwined. That required a gathering of collective wisdom. With that in mind, he brought together architects, artists, lawyers, public officials, and scientists, all dedicated to improving man's welfare through research and education in human values—something that sounded very similar to the now defunct CBHA. Within six months,

Salk launched the Epoch B Foundation, as he called the group. He reported that one member, prominent women's rights activist Perdita Huston, had been commissioned by the United Nations to travel to ten developing countries, where she would study changes in social status and values among rural women who accepted contraception. Journalist Albert Rosenfeld regularly wrote about ethical implications of scientific trends in *Saturday Review*. Gilot, too, became involved in Epoch B; her recent paintings explored the transition from one epoch to another. International journalist Tarzie Vittachi, director of public information for the United Nations Fund for Population Activities, prompted Epoch B members to write a "Bill of Responsibilities" to go along with the Bill of Rights.[33]

One person Salk did not invite to join Epoch B was Barbara Hubbard, the Connecticut housewife with whom he had had a liaison in the late fifties. Now engaged with the Committee of the Future, Inc., which she had founded in 1970, she was examining goals for the millennium, based on her concept of conscious evolution. She had developed a social conferencing process called SYNCON (synergistic convergence), in which she brought together groups of diverse people from different fields to find common goals and match needs with resources in order to solve community problems.[34]

When Rosenfeld told her about Epoch B, she was livid. "I was *amazed* at my recent phone conversation with Al Rosenfeld," she wrote Jonas. Rosenfeld had told her he could not participate in the Committee of the Future because Salk had persuaded him to join the Epoch B Foundation. "He outlined your plans," she continued, "which are, of course, similar to mine." She had revealed her agenda to Jonas, yet he had said nothing about his. "I had this sinking feeling that you would view them as competitive rather than cooperative.... Then I *reviewed* our relationship and realized that although I had done everything in my power to help you, you had literally never lifted a finger to cooperate with any effort of mine. Your behavior is more Epoch A than Epoch B." She considered it unpropitious for society's transition that "leading evolutionaries should still be so dominated by ego that they cannot share their efforts."[35] Salk penciled a note onto her letter: "I talked with her by phone. All is well." Hubbard had good reason to be concerned. At the time, Epoch B had $20,000 in liabilities with no liquid assets, and she and Salk were contacting the same potential funding sources for their organizations.

One of Epoch B's most successful endeavors was the so-called Mohonk Meeting. Forty journalists from around the world gathered at the Mohonk Mountain House in the Catskills to contemplate a controversial issue in journalism—the applicability of professional and moral journalistic standards developed in Western democracies to developing countries. "What I found so intriguing," wrote a journalist for the BBC, "was to watch Jonas Salk constructing what is virtually a theology-view of the coming and present kingdom—without the use of 'God.'"[36] A reporter for Associated Press called it "a charismatic experience" and Salk "a beautiful human being."[37] At week's end, participants expressed enthusiasm for creating new media values which, according to Salk, epochal change demanded.

⬧

NOW THAT DE HOFFMANN had forced Salk's humanistic activities off campus, he set out to reduce Salk's power as director. "The Bylaws language regarding the Director has been modified in practice," the minutes of the January 1974 board of trustees meeting had read, "and the resulting uncertainties may have caused strains in relationships between the Director and other elements of the Institute." The board suggested a subcommittee "to examine what Dr. Salk's responsibilities and obligations should be so as to give him a role which will assure him both the dignity to which he is entitled and which will contribute to a harmonious relationship with the Salk Institute."[38] The bargaining or coercion that ensued was not documented, but a year later Salk announced: "As part of the changes in academic structure and organization being contemplated, consideration is to be given . . . to my desire to relinquish the responsibilities of Director."[39] Trying to avoid humiliation, Salk said he looked forward to devoting more time to his laboratory research and writing, but those close to him knew he was devastated.[40] Mandell, chairman of the UCSD Department of Psychiatry, worried about how despondent Salk seemed.[41]

On January 22, 1976, the Salk Institute bylaws changed, officially eliminating the positions of director and chancellor. Frederic de Hoffmann became president and CEO, and Salk was given the title of founding director. In his new position, Salk retained a lifetime guaranteed salary of $57,000, a $1,000 monthly housing allowance, and life and health insurance. He kept his resident-fellow status with an office and an estate of $110,000 per year to cover his salary, secretary, and other expenses, as well as some laboratory space until retirement or until his research program reached completion. Now relieved of all directorial responsibilities, he became an ex officio member of the board of trustees and executive committee, meaning he had no vote, which meant he had no authority, no power. In four years, at age sixty-five, he would have to relinquish his office, his laboratory, his estate, his position on the board, and his status as a resident fellow. At that time, he would be left with a fixed salary and the otherwise empty title of founding director. Salk had been marginalized in the Institute he had created.

The Swine Flu Snafu

THE THOUSANDS OF new recruits who arrived at Fort Dix shortly after New Year's Day in 1976 faced frigid weather with windchills between 0° and −43°F.[1] Located sixteen miles south of Trenton, New Jersey, Fort Dix served as a major infantry training center. In mid-January, an acute respiratory illness broke out among inductees; seventy-two required hospitalization. Colonel Joseph Bartley reported the cases to the local health department, whose director suspected influenza. Dangerous for the elderly and infirm, the flu does not normally pose a threat to healthy young men, so he did nothing. The men recovered in a few days.

On February 3, nineteen-year-old Private David Lewis of Ashley Falls, Massachusetts, went to the dispensary complaining of cough, fever, and muscle aches. The medical officer diagnosed influenza and confined him to his quarters for forty-eight hours. The next night, however, he joined his platoon on a five-mile training march. Partway through, Lewis collapsed and was transported to the emergency room, where medics pronounced him dead. On postmortem examination, the pathologist found Lewis's lungs weighed almost twice normal. When he sectioned them, bloody fluid drained into the pan. Microscopic exam revealed widespread hemorrhage in both lungs. The alveoli, the thin-walled air sacs where oxygenation takes place, had ruptured. An infiltration of lymphocytic cells throughout the trachea, bronchial tubes, and lung indicated Lewis's body had put up a valiant fight against some microbe. The pathologist's preliminary diagnosis was overwhelming viral pneumonia.

More cases followed. Colonel Bartley sent the New Jersey public health laboratory throat washings from nineteen patients admitted to the Fort Dix hospital as well as swabs from Private Lewis's trachea. The lab reported Type A/Victoria, the influenza strain anticipated that winter, in most. But the virus in five patients, including Private Lewis, could not be classified, and specimens were shipped to the Center for Disease Control (CDC) in Atlanta. On February 12, CDC virologists identified a novel strain of influenza A in all five. They labeled it Type A/New Jersey/76.

Not much progress in influenza immunization had been made since Salk left the field twenty-two years earlier. He and Thomas Francis, Jr., had developed an influenza vaccine, and Salk, fresh out of medical training, had conducted large field trials to prove it reduced the incidence of influenza by 92 percent. The United States had not instituted a nationwide vaccination program, though some strains proved virulent. In 1957, Asian flu, which had originated in Kweichow Province in southwestern China, killed seventy thousand Americans. Eleven years later, the Hong Kong flu infected almost a quarter of the US population, causing thirty-three thousand deaths and an estimated $3.9 billion in medical costs and lost income. In both cases, vaccine had been produced too late and in insufficient quantity. Microbiologists found the causative agent in each pandemic to be a new subtype of influenza A.[2] Viruses were thought to become dormant, in some cases residing in an animal reservoir, and reawaken periodically, sometimes as a variant of the original virus. Virologists predicted an epidemic approximately every two years and a pandemic every ten, when a new mutated virus emerged. Despite this, Salk found the public attitude toward influenza apathetic—they saw it as an inconvenience rather than a mortal danger. "Courage and boldness are needed," he had written in 1970, "to overcome the recurrent feeling of failure and helplessness with each recurrent epidemic in spite of all the knowledge and understanding we possess."[3]

Although vaccine preparation had become more sophisticated, resulting in enhanced strength and purity, the inoculate still contained killed virus of the type expected that year. An advisory committee reported annually to the surgeon general which viral strain it predicted to emerge the following winter. Vaccine production generally started in February, to be ready for fall inoculations in anticipation of the first outbreaks in December. A handful of drug companies produced enough vaccine to immunize senior citizens and people with chronic illnesses, the only groups for whom vaccination was recommended. In early 1975, the advisory committee had predicted Type A/Victoria, a somewhat weak strain from Australia, would strike the next winter, and that was the strain isolated from a number of Fort Dix recruits in February of 1976. What was alarming was the presence in other recruits, including Lewis, of A/New Jersey/76, which resembled the subtype that had killed twenty million people, mostly young adults, worldwide during the 1918 pandemic. The virus had remained a mystery until the 1930s, when those who had survived the scourge were discovered to have antibodies against a Type A virus found in pigs; hence the illness it caused was termed "Swine Flu." That strain had lain dormant, probably residing in livestock. Now it had resurfaced—a virus that was a fraternal, if not identical, twin to the 1918 influenza virus.[4]

On February 14, CDC director David Sencer called an emergency meeting of public health experts. Having led the CDC for ten years, Sencer lived in the fast-paced world of infectious disease, where a day's delay could mean major loss of lives. He presented the facts to the group. Influenza Type A/New Jersey/76—Type A/Swine for short—had been isolated from soldiers at Fort Dix; one had died. The group had a crucial decision to make: alert the public and advise widespread immunization or wait to gather more evidence and risk an uncontrolled outbreak. They decided not to publicize the situation yet but to start preparing vaccine against this new virus. Six days later, the Bureau of Biologics (BoB) of the US Food and Drug Administration met with virologists from academia and industry to prepare them for rapid development and production of a new vaccine. "A feeling of urgency gripped the session," recounted Philip Boffey, a reporter for *Science*.[5] A go or no-go decision had to be made by April 1 for vaccine for an entire nation to be ready by the start of flu season. Four companies that manufactured vaccine, Merck, Sharp and Dohme; Parke, Davis; Wyeth; and Richardson Merrell, were sent samples of the Type A/Swine virus in preparation.

On March 10, Sencer reconvened his group. By then five hundred at Fort Dix had tested positive for Type A/Swine infection; to date only fourteen cases of full-blown influenza and one death had been reported. The flu season had passed, with the last case documented on February 9. The question was whether the virus had gone back into hibernation or was spreading through the population subclinically, without causing symptoms, waiting to emerge the next winter. The group worried about a subsequent pandemic and, given the high stakes, concluded they had no choice but to act.

Three days later, Sencer prepared a memorandum entitled "Swine Influenza—ACTION" for his boss, Theodore Cooper, assistant secretary for health in the Department of Health, Education, and Welfare (HEW).[6] In it he stated that the "ingredients for a pandemic" during the 1976–77 winter had materialized.[7] Although he outlined four possible courses of action, Sencer advised the government to purchase 200 million doses of vaccine and inoculate the entire population. He estimated the cost for such a program to be $134 million; the cost for a pandemic could be in the billions. "The Administration can tolerate unnecessary health expenditures," he argued, "better than unnecessary death and illness."[8] President Gerald Ford's advisors urged him to accept the recommendations. Some feared the worst. Cooper, extrapolating from the 1918 pandemic, projected one million deaths. One staffer, who declined to be named, told the president they could not ignore Sencer's appeal, which would without a doubt leak to the press. "That memo's a gun to our head," he warned.[9]

Before making his decision, the president assembled a blue-ribbon panel of experienced virologists, epidemiologists, and pharmaceutical experts to advise him and to lend weight to his decision. A call from the White House drew Salk back into the struggle against influenza. Also invited were Albert Sabin; Edwin Kilbourne, the leading influenza virologist at the time; and representatives from the AMA. When the new virus had been identified at Fort Dix, Kilbourne had told a *New York Times* reporter that "those concerned with public health had best plan without further delay for an imminent natural disaster."[10]

On March 24, the meeting convened at 3:30 p.m. in the Cabinet Room. Sencer briefed the group on the Fort Dix outbreak. No further cases had been reported, which was not unexpected since the influenza virus usually disappeared in the spring and summer. President Ford first called on Salk, whom he had seated to his right. Salk stated that he supported nationwide immunization; he had been advocating this for years. The president then turned to Sabin. He agreed with Salk. "We were damned if we did and damned if we didn't," he later admitted at House hearings.[11] No one around the table could assure the president that an epidemic would not strike the following winter. If they were unprepared, the toll could be enormous. The president asked for a show of hands in support of vaccination. Unanimously the panel advised an all-out assault on swine flu.

That evening Ford, flanked by Salk and Sabin, addressed the public on prime time television. He informed them that a soldier at Fort Dix, New Jersey, had died from the same type of influenza that had killed more than half a million Americans in 1918–19. After consultation with top scientists and public health officials, he had become convinced of the likelihood of a similar epidemic. He planned to initiate the National Influenza Immunization Program and was asking Congress to appropriate $135 million to vaccinate every American man, woman, and child. The president ended by boldly stating, "We cannot afford to take a chance with the health of our nation."[12]

"Warning: The Virus is Present and Active" read the headline in the *Los Angeles Times*. The paper quoted Salk as saying, "We have long needed to be prepared to close the barn door before rather than after the horse has been stolen. How would we do it? By isolation and quarantine? By the use of facemasks? By wearing camphor? These were the only methods available when I was a child in 1918." He applauded the decision to commence a nationwide immunization program; sixty-four cents per person was a small price for preventing an epidemic. Salk went on to deliver his recurring message: until they had a vaccine that included all influenza strains, health officials would have to resort to changing the vaccine yearly, based on surveillance findings. "If ever we are to lighten the economic burden of illness and reduce the tragedy and waste of death at all ages, we are going to do so by practicing preventive medicine." Ancient Chinese physicians were paid only as long as the patient remained well, he pointed out. Whether or not this virus turned out to be as deadly as it had been in 1918, Salk concluded, "it seems to me prudent to develop the habit of safeguarding our health."[13]

Two weeks after President Ford addressed the nation, and with minimal debate, Congress passed an emergency appropriations bill, which the president signed on April 15. Not everyone approved of the decision, however. Walter Cronkite led off the CBS evening news with a White House correspondent who described the president's decision as "premature and unwise."[14] The *New York Times* printed a series of editorials criticizing the absence of public debate, suggesting Ford had used the influenza scare as a political gimmick for the upcoming election. His advisors had panicked, one editorial insisted; they had used the direst interpretation of the meager data in reaching their decision. Following the media's lead, academic and public health naysayers called the predictions unjustified scientifically. Some opposed vaccine production altogether, concerned that vaccination itself could be dangerous. Others, including Sabin, who now took issue with the executive decision he had supported, suggested that the government store vaccine and use it only if an outbreak occurred. Sencer argued that influenza spread with such rapidity it would overtake last-minute efforts, since vaccination took two weeks to provide immunity. Salk agreed with Sencer. They should store doses "in people, not warehouses," he told a CDC advisory committee.[15] From then on, the CDC and HEW turned to Salk for advice.

After the 1968 Hong Kong flu outbreak, Salk had written in his night notes that the threat of another influenza epidemic had reawakened "the highly-charged feelings" he had had to suppress fifteen or sixteen years earlier. He felt he had "awakened from a long sleep like Rip Van Winkle as if I returned after I had been banished to Siberia." He sensed the urge to pick up the influenza story where he had left it in 1953. "I shall not be ashamed or afraid nor a shrinking violet," he added defiantly.[16] At the time he had written that note, however, the Salk Institute, his multiple sclerosis research, metabiology, and his private life consumed him. Now he had the opportunity to champion a universal vaccine as a means to eliminate influenza forever. When a reporter for the *Medical Post* started interrogating him about the wisdom of mass immunization, Salk chastised the journalist for attempting to turn public opinion against the influenza program.[17]

On April 21, 1976, the first swine flu vaccines were tested in limited field trials. Two months into the assessment, Parke, Davis disclosed a major blunder. It had produced two million doses of vaccine against the wrong viral strain. Then, the four pharmaceutical manufacturers reported that they could not achieve suitable antibody levels following inoculations in children and young adults, the group most lacking in immunity to the Type A/Swine virus. To add to the immunization program's problems, no casualty insurance company would insure the swine flu vaccine manufacturers. They were still smarting from the 1974 case of *Reyes v. Wyeth* in which a jury had awarded $200,000 to an infant who contracted poliomyelitis after receiving Sabin's live-virus vaccine. The liability issue threatened to scuttle nationwide vaccination against swine flu. A preventive medicine expert estimated 2,300 people would suffer strokes and seven thousand heart attacks within two days of inoculation. This was the same number expected to occur even without vaccination, yet the vaccine would be blamed. Consequently, insurers refused to underwrite coverage for the four drug companies. Although they had prepared more than a hundred million doses of swine flu vaccine, the companies would not release them without protection. Time was running short; to prevent a winter epidemic, vaccine distribution needed to begin soon. On June 16, Paul Rogers, chairman of the House Health Subcommittee, submitted HR 14409, which would indemnify manufacturers against claims arising from inoculation of the vaccine.

On June 28, Salk testified before the House Subcommittee on Health and Environment. Soft-spoken and magisterial, he gave committee members a tutorial on influenza immunization, reassuring them that results had been good in the past when the virus used to make the vaccine matched the one causing the outbreak. Sudden, periodic changes in strain resulted in epidemics, as had happened in 1957 with Asian influenza and in 1968 with the Hong Kong flu. The majority of the world's population didn't have antibodies against these strains.[18] When asked by a journalist, "How much credence do you give to the possibility of a massive malpractice suit?" Salk replied that it was "grossly exaggerated."[19] He could not imagine any such damage claims from the influenza vaccine, because it was a killed vaccine which carried no risk.

By this point, Salk had become a major influenza spokesperson, encouraging the public to get vaccinated. No one under fifty, he said in a television interview, had antibodies to the swine flu virus. During an epidemic, up to 80 percent of the population could become infected. When asked about Sabin's proposal to wait for an outbreak before vaccinating everyone, Salk replied that that approach was "completely impractical."He called it"Russian roulette."[20]The press loved these comments. The *Washington Post* reported this as "Sabin, Salk Split over Flu Shot Plan"—a bit of hyperbole; at this point Sabin mostly ignored Salk.[21] His polio vaccine was firmly entrenched worldwide, and although Salk persisted in attacking the live-virus vaccine, he drew few to his cause. It would be a year before Salk persuaded the National Academy of Sciences to reexamine polio vaccine policy, once again pitting the two men against each other.

Nationwide vaccination continued to provide fodder for the press. "President Ford may not know it," read an article in the *New York Times* in late June, "but with each passing day the government's 135-million dollar emergency swine flu immunization program appears less necessary and more unwise."[22] An editorial entitled "Right On Swine Flu" pointed out that five months had passed since the Fort Dix outbreak, and no new cases had appeared. "It may be that the politically charged atmosphere of this presidential election year and the dependence of most researchers here on federal dollars—explain the relative paucity of... plain-speaking expert voices in the country." The editorial called Ford's vaccination program "an inflated response to a minimal danger."[23] *Newsweek* dubbed it the "Swine Flu Snafu."[24] Congress meanwhile got bogged down in hearings. It appeared the manufacturers would not make the October 1 deadline, if they made any deadline at all. Then, on August 1, 1976, just as the tide of opinion was turning against the vaccination program, the public saw firsthand the havoc an uncontrolled infectious disease could wreak.[25]

⁂

IN LATE JULY, a Navy veteran from a small Pennsylvania town had just returned home from an American Legion convention in Philadelphia when he started coughing. As his condition worsened, he coughed up blood and suffocated. Soon thereafter, another veteran from suburban Pittsburgh developed a high fever and cough. He died in a matter of days. Across the state reports started coming in of veterans with high fevers, up to 107°, some with diarrhea, some delirious, all coughing, then gasping, followed in many cases by rapid death from pneumonia, despite intensive care units, respirators, and antibiotics. All the victims had one thing in common: they had attended the 58th American Legion Convention held July 21–24 at the historic Bellevue-Stratford Hotel in Philadelphia, as had thousands of veterans and their spouses. The similarity of this disease to the 1918 Spanish influenza, with its rapid onset, fever, and respiratory death within hours, led many to fear the unthinkable: the swine flu had arrived earlier than anticipated. "20 Flu-like Deaths in Pennsylvania, 115 Ill, A Mystery" reported the *New York Times* on August 4.[26] "Six Days, 25 Deaths, and Still No Answer" read the headline in the *Pittsburgh Tribune-Review* the next day.[27]

The media covered the outbreak in grim detail, printing photos that contrasted the elegant hotel where the disease had originated with people wearing facemasks, veterans on respirators, and funerals. The CDC sent twenty epidemiologists to Philadelphia to determine the cause of the illness. On August 5, they announced their results. To the surprise of many, the infectious agent was not the swine flu virus. Just what it was remained a mystery, however. By the time the disease had run its course, 221 veterans and their spouses had become ill; thirty-four died. Although the virulent infection acquired a name, Legionnaire's disease, it took five months to identify the previously unknown bacteria, subsequently named *Legionella*. Legionnaire's disease had nothing in common with swine influenza except its high mortality, yet the incident goaded legislators to act promptly. On August 10, Congress passed a tort claims bill under which the government would assume liability for injuries resulting from the influenza vaccine.

⸎

WHEN THE NATIONWIDE immunization program began on October 1, many, including some proponents, felt apprehensive. Not Salk. Influenza vaccines had been used for decades; nothing was different about this vaccine except the number of people to be inoculated. In the first ten days, more than a million Americans lined up for their shots. The program seemed to be going as planned. Then, on October 11, three Pittsburgh septuagenarians died suddenly after vaccination.

The press beat the CDC to Pittsburgh, where the coroner told CBS News he suspected that a bad batch of vaccine was the culprit, since the three had been inoculated at the same clinic. The Allegheny County Health Department suspended vaccinations as did nine states. Although autopsies revealed heart failure in two, the coroner still implied that there had been negligence. At an emergency press conference, Sencer pointed out that the three elderly men had underlying health problems. In this age group, they expected ten to twelve deaths per 100,000 daily. Thus, these were probably coincidental. Still, sensationalism trumped statistics. The press kept a vaccination deathwatch. HEW Assistant Secretary Cooper complained about the media's "body count mentality."[28] President Ford tried to calm the public by getting vaccinated in front of television cameras. Although polls indicated more Americans were declining immunization, a third of the adult population proceeded to get vaccinated.

The program seemed to be running smoothly again until November 19, when a Minnesota family practitioner called the local health agency to report a patient who had become paralyzed shortly after vaccination. He thought the patient had Guillain-Barré syndrome (GBS).[29] Named after the physicians who first described it, GBS is a rare disorder in which the immune system attacks one's own nerves and destroys myelin, the protective sheath around nerve fibers. Three to six thousand cases are reported yearly in the United States, mainly in older adults. Patients experience a sudden onset of paralysis, which starts in the toes and moves upward over the next few days, paralyzing the hands and the face, affecting breathing and swallowing in some cases. Rarely fatal, GBS usually resolves or at least improves within several weeks. In 1976, the clinical course was well-defined; its cause was not. About half the cases followed an infection.

The relationship to vaccination seemed remote; review of the medical literature turned up just one report. Then three more Minnesota cases, one fatal, were reported to the CDC, along with three from Alabama and one from New Jersey. With no specific diagnostic test, physicians could not be certain these represented GBS; other neurologic diseases began with acute paralysis, such as poliomyelitis, botulism, and multiple sclerosis. Neurologists joined the CDC virologists, epidemiologists, and statisticians in an extensive investigation.

By mid-December, health officials had registered fifty-one cases and eleven deaths. According to national statistics, this represented only a small increase from the average yearly number of GBS cases. But the press focused on the eleven who had died so far. Sencer argued that death or debility from GBS might strike one person among one to two million of those vaccinated, whereas the death rate from influenza reached tens of thousands even in a nonepidemic year. Still, the CDC received daily calls about new victims. Sencer called experts at the FDA and National Institutes of Health, who advised a one-month suspension while the investigation continued. Then a young Wisconsin hog farmer developed swine flu. After several more unnerving days, the CDC identified his virus as a nonvirulent subtype and traced its source to a pen of sick hogs.

Sencer contacted Cooper about the proposed suspension, and he promptly called Salk in Paris. Salk concurred they had no other choice. On December 16, 1976, the HEW suspended the National Influenza Immunization Program. It was never restarted. More than forty million Americans had received a swine flu vaccine. The CDC investigation uncovered 1,098 patients who developed GBS between October 1, 1976, and January 31, 1977. They found that 532 had been vaccinated at least five weeks prior to onset of paralysis; thirty-two of those died. Overall, the vaccinated population had a GBS incidence five to six times higher than the unvaccinated population. "The markedly increased attack rates observed among recipients of A/New Jersey vaccine," the report concluded, "provided strong support for the hypothesis that vaccination was etiologically linked to GBS."[30] Scientists could never determine why.

An epidemic did not materialize that winter. The Type A/Swine virus once again went into hiding. And the press had a field day. So did the lawyers. Blame was directed at the CDC, HEW, the scientists involved, and the president. The *Washington Post* called the vaccination program a "fiasco"; the *New York Times* called it a "sorry debacle." Ralph Nader's group demanded that Sencer resign.[31] Sencer stood by their original recommendation. "Better to have an immunization program without an epidemic," he insisted, "than an epidemic without an immunization program."[32] What the critics failed to acknowledge was that Ford's decision to proceed with mass immunization was supported by the FDA, Public Health Service, state health departments, Congress, AMA representatives, and virology experts.

In the end, four thousand suits were filed for damages suffered from vaccination. Many, such as ones involving impotency and recurrent fainting spells, were dismissed. Guillain-Barré posed the biggest problem. It remains a puzzle. According to distinguished virologist Samuel Katz, "We still don't know much about Guillain-Barré Syndrome other than it is an unusual immunological response that some people may have to various stimuli."[33] During the 1977–78 flu season, no cases of GBS were reported following vaccination.

In a testimony before the Senate Committee on Labor and Public Welfare, Salk cautioned that the recent government effort should not become "a platform for ridicule." He further emphasized: "Rather than berate those who are accused of 'crying wolf,' we should direct our attention to protection against the influenza viruses which are certain to continue to cause epidemics in the future."[34] The failure of an epidemic to occur in 1976 didn't erase that threat. "The fact that it left a calling card last winter is an indication that it intends to go into business because there is a large susceptible population." Salk hoped the swine flu saga would provide a "shot in the arm" for influenza research.[35] And once again Salk stressed the need for an influenza vaccine against all known subtypes as well as mass vaccination if they were ever to eradicate this disease that killed up to twenty thousand Americans even in nonepidemic years.

Return to the Polio Vaccine Controversy

BERNARD REIS GRADUATED summa cum laude from Cornell, attended graduate school at Harvard, and taught English at Vassar. His comfortable life started to unravel in February of 1967 after his infant son received Sabin's oral polio vaccine. Though his son was fine, Reis began to complain of severe muscle aches, which he thought to be influenza. Then he collapsed; his legs, he said, felt wooden. Paralysis set in with such rapidity that he required intravenous feedings and an iron lung. He had contracted poliomyelitis from the live, presumably weakened, poliovirus his son had been given in a sugar cube. After eleven months in the hospital, Reis returned home in a wheelchair. His health never recovered, and his marriage did not survive the strain. By the time he tried to sue Pfizer, the vaccine manufacturer, the statute of limitations had passed. "My life has been little more than hell in slow motion," he wrote in a 1981 *Washington Star* article. At that point, he was living on Social Security in a New York City welfare hotel. "My life is solitary, aimless, impoverished." He had contacted government officials; no one expressed sympathy or interest in his story. "When I consider the ways in which the Sabin oral polio vaccine has totally destroyed my life, two questions occur to me: How many more tragedies such as mine must there be before the scientific community in this country comes to its senses? And why did this supposedly compassionate nation so icily turn its back on the sad victims of this lethal product?"[1]

⁂

TWENTY YEARS HAD passed since Salk called the American Medical Association's recommendation to change over to Sabin's oral, live-virus vaccine an unwise, risky, politically driven decision. Despite Salk's warning that live virus, although attenuated, could revert to its virulent form and cause polio, Sabin's preparation had prevailed as the vaccine of choice for America's children. In his almost single-handed efforts to have Sabin's vaccine delicensed, Salk had been overruled by the American Medical Association, American Academy of Pediatrics, surgeon general, and Center for Disease Control. By 1968, US pharmaceutical companies had stopped manufacturing Salk's killed virus vaccine.

In the meantime, Salk had become engrossed in other activities: he built the Salk Institute and tried to keep it afloat, sought cures for multiple sclerosis and cancer, engaged in philosophical speculations, dissolved his first marriage, and married again. Then in 1973, he had suddenly reentered the poliomyelitis arena. Salk attributed his reawakening to eight-month-old Anita Reyes.[2] On May 8, 1970, a public health nurse had given the baby the oral polio vaccine during a community-wide vaccination drive in Hidalgo County, Texas.[3] Two weeks later, Reyes's arm and leg dangled lifeless at her side. Her parents, migrant workers from Mexico, sued Wyeth Laboratories, saying they had not been warned the vaccine could cause polio. The jury heard just one witness for the plaintiff, the local general practitioner. The defense lawyer called expert witnesses from the Center for Disease Control, Federal Drug Administration, and academia who estimated the chances that Reyes had contracted polio from the vaccine one in 5.88 million. Nevertheless, a federal jury in Brownsville, Texas, awarded the infant $200,000. Wyeth appealed the ruling, but the Fifth Circuit Court of Appeals upheld the decision, stating that if informed, the parents might have declined vaccination.

The American Academy of Pediatrics called upon the scientific community to help persuade the Supreme Court to overturn the ruling.

At that, Salk jumped back into the fray. The *San Diego Union* published "Poliomyelitis: Reflections after Twenty Years," in which Salk described how a thirty-year-old man, not previously immunized, had contracted polio from his five-month-old daughter after she received the Sabin vaccine. While the public distinguished between the two vaccines as one being oral and one an injection, Salk wrote, the real difference was that the oral vaccine contained live virus. He used the analogy of fighting fire with fire versus insulating against fire. "Using fire to fight fire occasionally backfires."[4]

Next, he sent a piece to the *New York Times* entitled "Polio: The Cure for the New Controversy," in which he stated that, at the twentieth anniversary of the polio vaccine's development, poliovirus still crippled. "The reasons for this are clear," Salk argued. "So is the remedy. Why then do the authorities, who are aware of the problem, seem to be looking the other way?" The only advantage he could see for the Sabin vaccine was its ease of delivery, which was not worth the cost. He also pointed out that Americans had no freedom of choice, as did the French and Canadians. "It's not too late to change back," he submitted. "In the absence of other voices, I feel a responsibility to inform the public that they can justifiably demand that if nothing else, the killed virus vaccine at least be made available in the United States."[5]

Determined to reverse the 1961 recommendation, Salk targeted those who set national vaccination policy. In the years since he had withdrawn from the polio vaccine controversy, many of his allies had retired or died, as had the vaccine issue. He was determined to reengage in battle, even if as a sole crusader. He started with the American Academy of Pediatrics (AAP), a powerful organization dedicated to the health and well-being of children. When its leaders asked pediatricians nationwide to petition the Supreme Court to overrule the *Reyes v. Wyeth* decision, Salk sent a letter to be published in the academy's *News Plus Comment*. "It seems to me that the consequences of the court's action to which the Academy draws attention could be obviated by requesting reconsideration of the decision made not by the courts but rather by those organizations which have recommended the exclusive use of the live over the inactivated polio virus vaccine."[6] Samuel Katz, chief of pediatrics at Duke University and chairman of the AAP's Committee on Infectious

Diseases, posted a rebuttal: "A court decision regarding liability for a case of paralytic polio cannot form the basis for a medical or scientific decision regarding the safety and efficacy of a vaccine."[7] Between 1961 and 1972, 550 million doses of oral vaccine had been given in the United States. Fifty-one recipients or their contacts had developed paralytic polio—one per ten million doses distributed, he calculated. Many of these had an immune deficiency disease, which put them at high risk. Thus, the AAP had no basis on which to alter its recommendation.

Salk called attention to errors in Katz's statements. Between 1961 and 1972, 120 vaccine-associated cases had been recorded, not fifty-one, and Katz had used the wrong denominator in calculating risk. "Such calculations in biostatics of that sophistication are beyond me," Katz replied. "The major concern at this point is that continued debate in the lay press, medical newsletters and other such forms do not resolve the issues nor do they help the readers other than to confuse them."[8] Salk requested their interchange be published in *News Plus Comment.* When an AAP staff member told him Katz thought the subject had received adequate attention, Salk accused the AAP of minimizing the live vaccine's safety, even to its own membership.[9]

Undeterred, Salk wrote to the American Medical Association, raising the same concerns he had with the AAP. To his request that his letter be published in *American Medical News*, the editor replied that they considered the vaccine risk exceedingly small. Salk then turned to the Center for Disease Control, which he believed might be more responsive, given that it had just reviewed all polio cases connected to vaccine since 1961. its published conclusion was noncommittal: defects in the surveillance program had obscured an accurate determination of risk. He had no better success with the Bureau of Biologics (BoB) of the Federal Drug Administration. When he learned the BoB had convened an expert panel to review the oral vaccine, he sent pages of comments. Four days later, Katz contacted him to say he had just attended a BoB meeting and was pleased to report the oral polio vaccine's success and safety had been reconfirmed.[10]

Salk had reached an impasse with the AAP, AMA, CDC, and FDA. Every major organization involved in vaccine decision-making had disregarded his advice. "He was certainly a popular hero," one senior researcher explained, "but he was not popular in the scientific community."[11] Salk knew his persistence had become grating. "I went against the tide," he reflected years later. "I went against the stream; I went against tradition; I went against the establishment. And so they treat you appropriately. They either ignore you or castigate you."[12] When in June of 1975 he read about *Givens v. Lederle* in the *San Diego Union*, however, he knew he could not yield.

Sherry Givens, a twenty-five-year old from Tampa, had contracted polio in 1972 when she changed her infant son's diaper soon after he had received the oral polio vaccine.[13] She sued Lederle Laboratories for $12.5 million. From her wheelchair, she listened to Sabin testify that the oral vaccine could not have given her polio. When the court found Lederle not guilty, Givens appealed. This time, the jury concluded that Lederle had not provided adequate warning and awarded Givens $262,000—minimal compensation for a young mother who would never walk again.

As *Givens v. Lederle* was making headlines, Salk detected an opening in the blockade he had encountered. Katz asked him to meet with the AAP's Committee on Infectious Diseases, and the BoB invited him to present to their expert panel, as did the US Public Health Service (USPHS) Advisory Committee on Immunization. In a lengthy, detailed document, Salk crafted his arguments for reinstating the killed vaccine.[14] By this time, the vaccines were no longer identified by their developers, Salk and Sabin, but by their formulations: inactivated poliovirus vaccine (IPV) and oral poliovirus vaccine (OPV). Ironically, much of the public thought the sugar cube contained the Salk vaccine.

The rationale for changing to OPV in the early 1960s had been based on its presumed advantages: less cost (no needles and syringes); ease of delivery (in a sugar cube); herd immunity, in the case of OPV meaning that the spread of the weakened virus in the community effectively vaccinated the unvaccinated; and induction of lifelong immunity. These beliefs Salk would have to refute. The last would be the most difficult, since most of the scientific community still maintained that inactivated virus generated only partial immunity, whereas live virus vaccines, such as smallpox and yellow fever, induced enduring immunity.

Salk began with the latter, elucidating why scientists thought IPV generated incomplete immunity. In 1955, the FDA's Division of Biologic

Standards had lowered his vaccine's potency. Once manufacturers returned it to its original strength, antibodies could be measured in recipients six years after inoculation (he later detected antibodies at twenty-five years). He pointed out that polio had been eradicated in Finland and Sweden, where IPV had been used exclusively.

Next he addressed the downside of the herd immunity. With OPV, the recipient swallowed live, attenuated virus, infecting the intestines and generating an immune response. Subsequently, he excreted live virus in fecal material and spread weakened poliovirus to the community, thus immunizing others. That may have sounded advantageous, but Salk emphasized two problems. Although attenuated, the virus in OPV could still cause polio in people with suppressed immune systems. Even worse, as it multiplied in the intestines, the virus could mutate back to its original strength—revert to virulence—and infect those with normal immunity.

Then Salk attempted to refute the assumption that the simplicity of OPV delivery in a sugar cube increased vaccination rates. Recent data showed that more children received three injections of DPT— diphtheria, pertussis (whooping cough), and tetanus—than three OPV doses. Although the oral vaccine cost less, Salk calculated these cost savings would be offset by compensation to those who developed paralysis. That led to Salk's main reason for condemnation: OPV crippled not only recipients but also innocent bystanders. The last poliomyelitis case in the United States from the naturally occurring ("wild-type") poliovirus had been reported in 1972. After that, as one of Salk's colleagues heard him say, "There were only two ways you got polio in the United States. Either you walked in from another country with an infection or you got the Sabin vaccine."[15] Although OPV advocates estimated the risk of paralysis to be only one per three to four million distributed doses, Salk reminded them that each case involved a person whose life had been altered forever—or who died. Finally, Salk raised an ethical question. Upon receiving the MD degree, physicians recite the Hippocratic oath: "I will use those dietary regimens [later modernized to 'prescribe regimens'] which will benefit my patients according to my greatest ability and judgment, and I will do no harm or injustice to them."[16] Stressing "do no harm," he suggested this was a breach of their solemn vow.

When Salk presented these arguments at the AAP meeting, Katz found him to be surprisingly "affable, bright and not at all aggressive, quite in contrast to Albert."[17] Afterward he wrote Salk, "There is no doubt that your presentation made a very convincing case for re-examination of current attitudes and recommendations regarding inactivated poliovirus vaccine and its availability."[18] A year and a half later, Salk received the AAP's formal statement. It advocated inactivated polio vaccine for children with immune deficiency diseases and their siblings, and for adults with no prior immunization who planned travel to countries where polio remained endemic. For healthy children, however, the oral polio vaccine remained the recommended choice. Salk was incredulous; no one appeared to have listened to the other points he had made.

Salk presented similar arguments to an expert panel convened by the FDA. When he requested a copy of the panel's deliberations, a staff member replied it was not "legal" for him to see them prior to their submission to the commissioner.[19] Eventually the FDA panel expressed concern about OPV yet noted that if they did change national policy, there was no available IPV in the United States. At least they had used the word "if."

Given the seeming indifference of organizations with regard to polio, Salk sought allies among elected officials. On June 28, 1976, he was asked to testify before Edward Kennedy's Senate Subcommittee on Health, which had been convened to address vaccine shortage. Because of liability concerns, both Pfizer and Wyeth Laboratories had stopped manufacturing OPV. Salk started his testimony with an as yet unanswered question: Where did responsibility and liability lie in the event of polio caused by vaccine—with the government, physician, clinic, or patients? He reminded the subcommittee that there was an alternative, the inactivated vaccine. Further along in his testimony, Salk pulled out his trump card. "Implied in this discussion," he said, "is the fundamental ethical question: Who has the right to decide which vaccine will be used when it has been established scientifically that one carries an inherent risk of causing paralytic polio and the other does not?"[20]

That night on *NBC Nightly News*, David Brinkley reported that the Senate Health Subcommittee was trying to understand the reasons for a polio vaccine shortage.[21] He turned to his guest, Jonas Salk, who warned

Americans about the risk of acquiring polio from the live virus vaccine. Knowing the press's power, he proceeded to outline the public's dilemma in the *San Diego Union*: if manufacturers were warning about the vaccine's dangers, as dictated by the courts, and the public health department was urging the public to use it, what should people do?[22] He sent Pittsburgh reporter John Troan his subcommittee testimony and offered copies of his correspondence with the AAP and USPHS. "The matter of live and killed poliovirus vaccines has now become a public issue," he told Troan.[23] When later asked to comment by a writer for *Science*, Sabin snapped, "Didn't the world settle that 25 years ago?"[24]

Just as Salk was becoming discouraged, a letter from David Bodian, the Johns Hopkins scientist who had laid much of the foundation for the killed vaccine, lifted Salk's spirits. Bodian agreed that the OPV strain responsible for most vaccine-associated paralysis should be withdrawn. "I suppose that the feeling in the USPHS," he wrote, "is that one does not rock the boat when the incidence of polio is as low as it has been in the recent years. Yet the medico-legal cases are doing some rocking, I understand."[25]

Heartened by Bodian, Salk took a new tack with the policy-making groups, stressing potential legal ramifications. He sent the AAP a note asking if it knew the liability implications for their position. "The Academy is a quasi-official body," he noted. "It possesses authority, and with authority goes responsibility."[26] He wondered whether the academy fully appreciated its responsibility to physicians and the public to provide a basis for an unbiased and enlightened choice. Surely the organization's legal counsel had advised them. An AAP official replied to Salk that they would consider his concerns. When he heard nothing, Salk persevered. "I can now see the nature of the struggle between myself and others," he wrote in his night notes, "and why I am behaving in a manner that suggests obsession."[27] Perhaps some did think him obsessed; he preferred to view himself as tenacious in battle.

At a National Institutes of Health immunization conference, Salk reiterated the points he had made with the AAP. "At present," he said, "it appears as if the authority for making polio vaccination policy resides with scientific advisory committees; however, the responsibility for liability as a consequence of such policy has remained unspecified. When authority

and responsibility are separated this way, the courts will intervene." In conclusion he said, "It would seem to me that the scientist can best serve as a
resource... not as the policy maker. I am reminded of an old saying that
may be apt here, 'an expert should be on tap and not on top.'"[28]

Increasingly frustrated, Salk showed his research associate, Fred
Westall, a letter from the AAP president. "It essentially said, 'Who cares
if a few people get sick with the Sabin vaccine?'" Westall recalled. "Well
I know one person," he told Salk. "The lawyer for these people."[29] Salk
recognized the truth behind Westall's words. Soon thereafter, he began
to work covertly with attorneys of OPV victims, starting with the lawyer
for Daniel Sheehan, the first polio patient in Pima County, Arizona, in
sixteen years.[30] On January 16, 1977, the thirty-seven-year-old had contracted the most virulent form of polio from his infant daughter after she
had received the oral vaccine. Paralyzed from the upper chest down, he
required a respirator to breathe. He and his wife sought $4.5 million from
Pima County and the vaccine manufacturer.[31] The suit contended that the
defendants knew the vaccine carried certain risks but had failed to warn
the Sheehans when their daughter was immunized. Nine months later,
Sheehan had a respiratory arrest and died, turning the case into a wrongful
death claim. The Arizona Court of Appeals determined that the unavail-
ability of an alternate vaccine contradicted the presumption that the
plaintiff would have heeded the warning and selected another vaccine.

Jurors from other trials sided with the injured. Although courts
agreed on the basic legal principles, interpretation in individual cases
gave rise to inconsistent verdicts. The number of suits escalated, though
there weren't many large settlements for the plaintiffs. Salk continued to
give advice pro bono, including to Lawrence Katkowsky, legal counsel
for nine-month-old Karl Schindler.[32] A few months after he had been
given the oral polio vaccine in Marine City, Michigan, Schindler developed a high fever; his arms and legs became paralyzed. He never recovered. Doctors found the baby had an immune deficiency that rendered
him unable to produce antibodies against the live virus, even though
weakened. Cultures from his throat, stool, and spinal fluid grew poliovirus. With Salk's advice, Katkowsky filed a suit against the United
States for improper licensure of an unsafe vaccine, failure to withdraw it
once found unsafe, and failure to provide the public a supply of killed

vaccine. They asked for $4.5 million to cover a lifetime of debility and extended the suit to include the AAP and Lederle. The case dragged on for eight years, at which time Katkowsky wrote Salk, "We received an opinion granting us everything except the victory."[33] Salk found each story heartbreaking. As for Sabin, he told a *Science* writer that he considered litigation "a plague upon American society."[34]

Finally, in 1977, Salk had his first breakthrough when the Institute of Medicine (IOM) decided to reexamine polio vaccination policy. This nonprofit organization of elite academicians, a branch of the National Academy of Sciences, gives authoritative advice to officials about major health issues. When the IOM chairman asked Salk to submit a written statement, he included his letters, presentations, congressional testimonies, and publications recounting the entire polio vaccine saga. In just a few months, the IOM submitted its report. To Salk's gratification, it concluded that since OPV carried a risk of paralysis, IPV should be made available as an alternative for use in special cases. Although the IOM did not advocate widespread substitution of the killed virus vaccine, *Medical World News* called the decision "a vindication of sorts for Dr. Salk."[35]

Three months later, on July 4, 1977, President Jimmy Carter awarded the Presidential Medal of Freedom to Martin Luther King, Jr., posthumously, and to Jonas Salk. Salk's citation read: "Because of Dr. Jonas E. Salk, our country is free of the cruel epidemics of poliomyelitis that once struck almost yearly. Because of his tireless work, untold hundreds of thousands who might have been crippled are sound in body today."[36] The medal provided Salk an opportunity to petition the president about the oral vaccine. He suggested that the secretary of health, education, and welfare had been swayed with regard to vaccine policy by "misleading and incomplete information."[37] Carter declined to become involved, perhaps reflecting on the criticism his predecessor had encountered during the swine influenza debate.

❧

ALBERT SABIN, MEANWHILE, had been relatively quiet on the polio vaccine issue. In 1973, when Salk reopened the debate, Sabin was struggling. His personal life lay in shambles.[38] On his sixtieth birthday,

Sylvia, his wife of thirty years, had locked her bedroom door, lain down on her couch, taken an overdose of phenobarbital and sleeping pills mixed with alcohol, and tied a plastic bag around her head. Their teenage daughter Debbe discovered her mother's body. Although horrified, friends and family weren't surprised; the marriage had been rocky for years, and Sylvia had long been unhappy. Sabin spent far more time in his laboratory, on planes, or in Russia and Mexico than he did at home. Those were the peaceful times. When he returned, the house echoed with screaming and yelling. Sylvia numbed herself with alcohol and sedatives.

Nine months after Sylvia's funeral, Sabin married Jane Warner, formerly the wife of financier Marvin Warner, who was later imprisoned for the Home State Savings Bank scandal. Debbe described her new stepmother as a "southern belle" who was attracted to the celebrity of being Albert Sabin's wife.[39] They had to marry in the hospital, as a few days before the wedding, Sabin had kicked his deceased wife's dachshund, who bit into his calf, tearing the Achilles tendon. Before long, similar high-decibel bickering erupted between Sabin and Warner. In 1970, Sabin moved to Israel to become president of the Weizmann Institute of Science, leaving Jane behind to care for her son and his second daughter, Amy.

After two years, Sabin was relieved of his Weizmann Institute position. According to the official statement, he had departed due to his health; he had undergone coronary bypass surgery. Insiders said Israeli scientists found his domineering personality intolerable. His second wife found him intolerable, too. They divorced in 1971, and soon thereafter he married Heloisa Dunshee de Abranches, a Brazilian socialite. In 1973, while studying cancer-generating viruses at the NIH, Sabin reported that the herpes simplex virus caused cancer—a major scientific breakthrough. A year later, just after he had accepted a position as distinguished research professor at the Medical University of South Carolina, he published an embarrassing retraction. Subsequent experiments revealed his initial conclusion about the herpes virus to be mistaken.

When Sabin finally did strike back, decrying Salk's contention about the danger of his vaccine, he argued that other viruses could cause diseases with clinical findings similar to those seen in polio, and the vaccine could not be incriminated in individual cases because of a temporal association between the disease and the vaccination. These persons likely had contracted the wild virus in the community prior to receiving the vaccine. He cited the Russian and Japanese experiences where suspected infections, when tested for virus type, were not found to have been caused by the vaccine. "Albert would never, ever admit there was a vaccine-associated polio," Katz recalled years later.[40]

Once again newsmen began to portray Salk and Sabin's debate as a medical feud. The *New York Daily News* called it a "long and bitter quarrel";[41] The *Chicago Reader* dubbed it the "tale of two egos."[42] The two adversaries differed in combat style, however. Mild-mannered and courteous, Salk abhorred altercations. Most who worked with him can't recall an unkind word from him about Sabin. Yet Salk never let up in denouncing his vaccine. "He kept fanning the flames," Neal Nathanson, a distinguished microbiologist, recalled.[43] Sabin fluctuated between being aloof and off-putting one moment, bombastic and accusatory the next. "He could be somewhere with Dr. Salk and be quasi-civilized," Debbe Sabin recollected, "but if he didn't like what Salk was saying, he would shut him down in a heartbeat."[44] Sabin demeaned Salk with regularity, promulgating the impression of Salk as a super technician who took someone else's techniques and concocted a vaccine. When a reporter, interviewing Sabin later in life, noted all the awards and citations covering his walls, he boasted, "It makes me feel good because it says, contrary to what's been written in some newspapers, that I developed *the* vaccine, not *a* vaccine, that has eliminated polio as a major threat to human health."[45]

Although Salk insisted he did not consider Sabin a rival, several witnessed his exasperation. Nathanson recalled the backbiting at scientific meetings as Salk and Sabin engaged in a "battle royal." "They both had big egos and were real stump thumpers," he observed, "in a way not considered seemly in the scientific community."[46] A young professor recounted the time Salk gave grand rounds at the University of California, Davis. She was disappointed when her hero spent an hour excoriating Sabin in what she described as a "bitter, angry diatribe."[47] Yet Salk told a reporter, "It was as if there was a vaccine war.... That I could never understand. I was not the perpetrator of it."[48]

In debate, the more articulate Sabin had an edge over Salk. His status among elite researchers provided a strong advantage as well. "Sabin was accepted by the scientific community," a Salk Institute neuropharmacologist

observed, "and so his views were held to be right. Jonas wasn't well accepted by anyone except the March of Dimes Foundation, and so his
views were judged to be wrong."[49] Yet the media favored Salk. In an
article entitled "The Polio Pioneers Are Still Busy," a *Newsweek* reporter
quoted Salk as saying that, although lab research still enthralled him, he
found time to write a book about evolution and to travel with his wife
(identified by the reporter as Picasso's former mistress). "My life is not
boring. It's like driving in the fast lane." An accompanying picture
showed a youthful-appearing Salk with his hair styled and his teeth
straightened and whitened. In contrast, Sabin looked haggard. The caption under his photo read: "Sabin: Keeping an Old Man Going." The
article quoted Salk as saying it was "unfortunate that an air of competition exists. I can assure you that I do not share any such feeling."[50] Salk
told his friend Arnold Mandell he hoped his future biographer would
emphasize the difference in their ideas, not trivialize their conduct as
"two little Jewish boys from the Bronx fighting it out."[51]

Undoubtedly Sabin did consider Salk a rival, driven not just by a
clash of scientific ideas but also by jealousy over Salk's public acclaim.
In 1955 Basil O'Connor had accused Sabin of having public temper
tantrums out of envy.[52] Debbe Sabin recalled her father's antipathy
toward Salk: "He was in the 'I don't like you, and anything I can do to
obstruct you, I'm going to do' category." For years her father had told her
he was driven by his great love for humanity; it wasn't about the fame.
"But oh, it was about the fame," she observed. "When the fame dwin-
dled, he didn't like that. I think he was very much driven by his own
celebrity."[53]

In his efforts to eliminate polio while safeguarding the public's
health, Salk saw himself as a lone voice in the scientific wilderness, at
least in the United States. "The idea of a return to the Salk vaccine in this
country has remained alive in one mind," Peter Salk observed, "that of
my father."[54] Basil O'Connor, Thomas Francis, Jr., and Tom Rivers had
died, as had many of his original advocates. His only supporter appeared
to be his middle son, Darrell. Most people remembered Darrell as the
adorable eight-year-old who, after the presentation of his father's presidential citation, had asked President Eisenhower what he did besides
play golf. Like Peter, Darrell had studied medicine. While still in pediatric

training, he and his father had coauthored a provocative paper in *Science* in which they outlined the requirements for inducing lasting immunity against an infectious disease, applying them to poliomyelitis control. As an assistant professor at the University of Washington, Darrell began to write and speak about IPV as the only means to eradicate polio worldwide. He soon learned the Salk name carried burdens as well as advantages. He recalled a conference discussion period during which he asked his father a question to help him bring up a point he had omitted. "Did your father put you up to that?" a prominent scientist asked Darrell.[55]

Although he considered himself a collaborator, Darrell found his father reluctant to relinquish control. Once, when the two disagreed about how to proceed with a new vaccine project, Darrell said, "Only one person can take the lead. Who will it be, you or me?" He expected his father to say, "You." Instead he replied, "I'll get back to you."[56] Two days later, he told Darrell he planned to direct the project himself. Although Salk may have had difficulty sharing responsibility, he may also have been trying to protect his son from Sabin. "Darrell Salk doesn't know what the hell he's talking about," Sabin once carped. "[His work is] completely out of focus, distorted information, erroneous information—just a chip off the old block."[57]

By 1980, Salk had made minimal headway in getting OPV delicensed. No longer a covert legal advisor, he began to serve as an expert witness in personal injury litigation "Vaccine Alternative Available When Man Died," the *Tucson Daily Citizen* reported Salk as testifying in Superior Court for plaintiff Mary Sheehan.[58] His rhetoric became more accusatory: "Salk Says Sabin Vaccine Caused Death," read the *Arizona Daily Star*.[59] And he used the media to incite public outrage. "How Many More Must We Cripple?" asked the *Pittsburgh Press*.[60]

Salk had exhausted almost every avenue. He had petitioned the Center for Disease Control, American Medical Association, and World Health Organization, and hounded the American Academy of Pediatrics, Bureau of Biologics, US Public Health Service, and the surgeon general. He had submitted articles and letters to the editors of major medical journals and had spoken at scientific conferences. He had testified before two congressional committees, even appealed to the president. He had worked surreptitiously, then openly, with victims and their lawyers and prompted the media to come to their aid. When the major decision-makers barely budged, he had attacked OPV as an agent of paralysis and death, posed ethical questions, and finally made freedom of choice, an American ideal, the central issue. But after nearly a decade of such efforts, polio vaccine policy had not substantially changed.

Salk knew inertia to be one problem. Manufacturing processes and immunization programs for OPV were in place; changing them to accommodate IPV would be costly. As well, many worried the change might shake the public's confidence in immunization. "The limiting factor," Salk wrote in *JAMA*, "is in part developmental and economic and in part the need for political will. This reveals, once again, that all of the problems of man cannot be solved in the laboratory."[61] Others thought Salk's reputation in the scientific community biased vaccine decision-makers. "I think it typifies how egos and issues get in the way of science," one researcher reflected. "There is no question about it that politics and egos played a role in keeping his polio vaccine out. Ultimately, hopefully, science prevails."[62] Salk reached the same conclusion. For science to prevail, he needed to design a low-priced, more effective, safer vaccine, substantiated by data the scientific community couldn't ignore.

WHILE TRYING TO change American polio vaccine policy, Salk had pursued a collaborative effort to improve his vaccine in France, where scientists still revered him. In the early 1970s he had contacted Dr. Charles Mérieux, president of the Institut Mérieux, which produced both OPV and a variation of Salk's IPV. Informing Mérieux that the United States would need an IPV source to meet demand once Americans could choose their vaccine, Salk added that he hoped Mérieux's company would become the major supplier. Marcel Mérieux, Charles's father, had founded the company in 1897, after which the Mérieux family became a dynasty in the biological and pharmaceutical industry.[63] Under the direction of Charles, an enterprising physician, the Institut Mérieux mass-produced vaccines against meningitis, rabies, measles, diphtheria, and tetanus. Charles Mérieux had even found a way to combine four childhood vaccines—diphtheria, tetanus, whooping cough, and IPV—into one shot, called Tetracoq.

In late 1975, Salk visited Mérieux, intent on persuading him and his son, Alain, to adopt two new techniques to facilitate large-scale IPV production. First, Salk suggested they begin using microcarriers, designed by engineer Toon van Wezel of the Netherlands' National Institute of Public Health and Environment. Van Wezel had increased the number of cells grown in each flask of tissue culture by adding microbeads to the medium. Secondly, Salk proposed that instead of cultivating poliovirus in monkey kidney cells, which divided just a few times before dying, Mérieux should use cell lines that grow indefinitely. Fascinated, Charles Mérieux began collaborating with Salk on what he called "the rehabilitation of the Salk vaccine."[64]

Salk's first scheme would be easy to implement, the second more problematic. Mérieux estimated his company had sacrificed twenty thousand monkeys over a twenty-five-year period, so he found the idea of perpetually propagating cell lines intriguing.[65] Salk had caused an outcry among American researchers years earlier when he had proposed growing poliovirus in the immortal HeLa cells. They warned that if a cell line divided indefinitely, it might cause cancer. In time, nontumorigenic continually propagating cell lines, such as Vero cells, isolated from kidneys of green monkeys, became available. Microcarriers and Vero cells yielded high viral titers in cell culture. With these two innovations, Mérieux, Salk, and van Wezel developed a more immunogenic vaccine, the new enhanced inactivated polio vaccine (eIPV).[66]

Linked by their passion to rid the world of infectious diseases, Mérieux and Salk became close friends. The Frenchman addressed Salk as "mon cher Jonas et grand ami."[67] In 1977, the two joined Hans Cohen, director of the Netherlands' National Institute of Public Health and Environment, to create the Forum for the Advancement of Immunization Research (FAIR), under which they conducted clinical trials, mostly in developing countries. Within months, Salk had urged French epidemiologist Phillipe Stoeckel to initiate a study in Mali to find the lowest eIPV dose that could produce immunity in a two-shot schedule, thus reducing cost.[68] Their work progressed without delay, which was a change for Salk, who had become accustomed to obstructive scientists, heel-dragging organizations, and cautious pharmaceutical companies in the United States. FAIR soon established that after two eIPV doses, all recipients developed high antibody titers. In 1978, French prime minister Raymond Barre presided over the opening of Mérieux's new plant for eIPV production.[69]

Three years later, Salk notified Stoeckel that the WHO had revised its recommendation to read: "The pressing need is to make more generally available inactivated poliomyelitis vaccines that have uniformly high potency and that will reliably give the immunogenic response in children after one or two doses. Such vaccines will be useful particularly in the developing countries where poliomyelitis is largely uncontrolled."[70] He sent Alain Mérieux, who had succeeded his father as president of the Institut Mérieux, a telegram saying interest in the new generation of IPV was increasing: he expected French licensure by the end of 1981, and the US Bureau of Biologics welcomed an application for a US license.

In March of 1983, the National Institutes of Health hosted an international symposium on poliomyelitis control to consider how to immunize the world's children. Attendees concluded OPV didn't work in tropical and subtropical regions of Africa and Asia due to some interfering factor, likely bacterial infestation in the human gut. Thousands had been paralyzed despite multiple OPV doses. Thus the eIPV data generated a great deal of interest. Even the AMA, which had snubbed Salk for years, published his history of polio, labeled "Landmark Perspective," in their journal. "The story of poliomyelitis," Salk concluded in the article, "will reveal the way in which preconceptions about the cause of the disease and about the requirements for immunization were tested, refuted, or disproved by careful observation and experimentation. There remains now to test, refute, or disprove the prediction that poliomyelitis can be eradicated and the viruses extinguished from the human population."[71]

Recounting the NIH symposium, one reporter observed, "The old rivals were there." He depicted Sabin as agitated, his twenty-year vaccine dominance slipping; he described Salk as wearing "a cool and elegant armor of composure."[72] When Alan Hinman from the CDC tallied ninety-nine vaccine-related polio cases in the past fourteen years, Sabin challenged him. "What's the proof?" he asked. "Everyone," Salk said, "all but one man, believes the evidence. It is remarkable, simply remarkable that he casts doubt upon it." With that, the recurring debate flared up.

The two would never settle their argument, Salk told a *Los Angeles Times* reporter. "It will be up to the world to decide what the reality is."[73]

◈

IN MAY OF 1983, while he was a visiting professor at Georgetown University, Sabin's legs buckled, and he fell down a stairway.[74] On examination, neurologists found impaired muscle strength and absent reflexes. They thought the seventy-six-year-old had arthritis in his neck vertebrae and prescribed a cervical collar. Over the next month he worsened, resorting to using a cane to walk. In mid-June, Sabin suffered unbearable neck pain. Johns Hopkins specialists diagnosed ossification of the posterior longitudinal ligament. In this rare disease, found mostly in Japan, patients develop calcification of the ligaments in the back of the neck, which compress the spinal cord, causing pain and neurologic complications.

Immobilized with a metal brace, Sabin didn't improve. Heloisa, his wife of twelve years, had to feed him. After four months in a brace, with no relief, neurosurgeons performed a decompression laminectomy to relieve the tension on his spinal cord. At first, his pain abated. Then it recurred with a vengeance. "I had the most excruciating pain of my life," he told *People* magazine. "I couldn't bear it." He wanted to die. Ten days later, his condition worsened. "Just like a bolt, I became paralyzed from the waist down. My feet, legs, hips felt just like wood." His physicians lowered the pain medication, concerned it might impair his respirations, "I was beyond myself," he recounted, "yelling 'Get me the hell out of here.'"[75]

Nine days later, as Heloisa sat at her husband's bedside, his eyes rolled back and he stopped breathing. An attendant ran to the door and shouted, "Dr. Sabin is dead!"[76] A medical team rushed in and managed to resuscitate him. Eleven days later, Sabin could breathe on his own and was taken off the ventilator. His ascending paralysis continued to baffle everyone. They called it polyneuritis, an inflammation of the nerves seen in several diseases, among them Guillain-Barré.

For months, this man who used to control every aspect of his environment and the people around him was imprisoned in his own body. "He was just driving everyone nuts in the hospital," said his daughter Debbe. "He refused to deal with the loss of independence and was verbally abusive."[77] After intense rehabilitation, Sabin began to regain use of his hands and arms and could pull himself up into a sitting position. One might wonder if it ever occurred to him during those hellish months, "This is how polio victims feel." If so, it didn't seem to make much difference; he still maintained that his vaccine had not caused one case of polio. As soon as he could sit up, he began to harangue Salk from his wheelchair. Paralyzed or not, he refused to concede.

A Trojan Horse

WHEN PRESIDENT FREDERIC DE HOFFMANN opened the annual Salk Institute board of trustees meeting on January 15, 1980, he no longer appeared the defensive outsider, blunt to the point of being rude.[1] Ten years of fundraising dinners with the well-heeled had refined his expressions and manners. But he had not changed in one regard—his insistence upon total control. The Institute's success had boosted his confidence, and as the board met on this occasion he had a lot to boast about. Three prominent neuroscientists, Maxwell Cowan, Floyd Bloom, and Helen Neville, had joined the Institute. Cancer researcher Renato Dulbecco and his wife, Maureen, also a scientist, had returned from England, and Francis Crick of DNA fame planned to spend the rest of his career at the Institute. Roger Guillemin had received a Nobel Prize, and yet another Institute scientist had been elected into the National Academy of Sciences—"probably the largest proportion of members from any institution anywhere," noted trustee Floyd Bloom.[2] With respect to their fiscal affairs, de Hoffmann reported increased revenues of $14.5 million.[3] A shrewd businessman, he had attracted foundation dollars, negotiated government contracts, and set up a for-profit corporation. The Institute's net worth had reached an all-time high, as had the number of grants and awards garnered by its cadre of elite scientists. "It just got better and better," recalled Nobel Laureate Paul Berg.[4]

Pleased that the Salk Institute now ranked with the Pasteur and Rockefeller Institutes, Salk still hoped that one day scientists and humanists would work side by side within its walls, that one day they would build the meeting house Kahn had designed for collective reflection. As the Institute's prestige had grown, so had its personnel, now consisting of 128 scientists and 162 supporting staff. Salk reminisced about the early days when he knew everyone's name, when the entire group of fellows could fit into one photograph. Asked to describe the Institute, he used to say it was like a poem, brilliant minds gathered among idyllic beauty and tranquility. Now the scientists had become politicians and entrepreneurs, using their studies, initially intended as sites for quiet contemplation, to debate overhead, academic appointments, and square footage. "It seemed like everyone was bickering," Salk later told a close associate.[5]

Salk's relationship with de Hoffmann had mellowed a bit in the decade since de Hoffmann had taken the helm. Or so it seemed. "The Board of Trustees," de Hoffmann said, concluding the January 15, 1980, meeting, "want to be recorded as thanking Dr. Salk for his continued efforts on behalf of the Institute and his deep interest in the advancement of science and mankind."[6] Long overdue, the tribute sounded a bit formal and forced, particularly to those who knew de Hoffman's true sentiments. A year later, he told the trustees that Salk's great vision in founding the Institute had been realized. At the 1982 board meeting, Salk in kind commended de Hoffmann for having achieved financial security. "We are no longer dependent as a minor on the parents from which it sprung," he said.[7] In response, de Hoffmann again thanked Salk for his great foresight and vision in creating the Institute. Finally, when Salk had reached his sixty-fifth birthday, at which time according to the bylaws he was to give up his laboratory, the board, with de Hoffmann's assent, extended Salk's appointment to age seventy.

De Hoffmann could afford to be generous. Although the board included an impressive slate with executives from the advertising world, the leader of Metropolitan Insurance, and a top Bank of America executive, he now had total authority over the Institute. He had filled vacant trustee positions with candidates of his choosing. Floyd Bloom, a newly recruited neuroscientist who represented the fellows on the board, noted that "no real business would ever be conducted at the board of trustees meetings that had not been agreed upon by private meetings beforehand. I got to vote, but the votes were all prearranged."[8] And as Maureen Dulbecco observed, "De Hoffmann had made the board a rubber stamp. Nobody ever said boo. One or two people may have argued with him, but they were soon gone."[9] No one complained, however, when de Hoffmann secured a $26 million government contract or ended the fiscal year with a $12 million surplus.

Despite all their mutually laudatory words, Salk and de Hoffmann detested one another. De Hoffmann considered Salk a burden and an embarrassment. Salk thought of de Hoffmann as his bête noire. The adulation spouted at board meetings didn't fool anyone. "You could sense the friction," Bloom noted, "but it was always politely administered. Yet you could see these mind games being played out."[10] De Hoffmann's passive-aggressive behavior irritated Salk. He held Institute events and did not invite the founding director. "How can they just ignore me?" he asked a friend. "He probably wishes I were dead. He didn't think I'd live this long."[11] Some wondered why de Hoffmann supported extending Salk's retirement until age seventy. Others thought that it was because Dulbecco and Crick, two Institute stars, would soon turn seventy too, and he didn't want to lose them.

Salk understood neither the source of the hostility nor how to handle it. He questioned whether or not their relationship could be salvaged and if there was any point in trying. At 6:30 one morning, he wrote in his night notes: "There are wide differences between FdeH and myself. I can now see...how important it is to see this, to know it, to acknowledge it and to know what to do about it when our paths cross."[12] He concluded that the issue between them was ideological. According to Salk's office administrator, Kathleen Murray, de Hoffmann scoffed at his "crucible for creativity."[13]

They may have had ideological differences, but most believed that their antagonism centered on control, and the crux of their hostility involved the depth of each man's feelings about the Institute. They behaved like two rivals fighting for the affections of a lover. De Hoffmann had almost no family; he had devoted himself to making the Institute a success. "He identified with the place," treasurer Delbert Glanz explained. "It was his passion; it was his life."[14] Salk noticed that de Hoffmann referred to it as "*his* institute," acting as if he were just "a subsidiary of the FdeH Institute."[15] Salk loved the Institute, too. "The building," he once rhapsodized, "is as close to perfection as anything possible." He vowed never to be separated from it.[16]

De Hoffmann considered Salk a drain on resources, complaining to Bloom that Salk occupied space that could be converted into grant-producing laboratories and that he didn't help in fundraising to recruit new scientists or to support those already on staff. "If Jonas were dead," de Hoffmann told Bloom in frustration, "he could bring in more money than if he were alive."[17] Intent upon closing down Salk's lab, recapturing the space, and ending its constant financial drain, he crafted a plan.

In August of 1983, de Hoffmann sent Salk a draft aide-mémoire—a proposed arrangement for Salk upon his retirement, now slated for 1984.[18] In it de Hoffmann acknowledged the original dual charge of the Institute to attain scientific excellence and to explore the fulfillment of man's biological potential. He recognized that so far the Institute had accomplished only the first goal and that Salk had expressed interest in devoting the next five years of his career to examining the latter. Thus, de Hoffmann proposed to Salk that he form his own foundation for this purpose and mentioned a grant of a million dollars over eight years. Salk appreciated de Hoffmann's generous gesture. De Hoffmann, however, was taking no chances that Salk would try to keep his lab and likely assumed Salk would die before the entire eight million was dispensed. Throughout the memorandum, he referred to the proposed organization as the "'N' Foundation." Tucked inside Appendix 8 was a statement that read, "It would seem best if the 'N' foundation did not contain the word 'Salk.'"[19] Somewhat casually, the memo mentioned the "wind-down" of Salk's scientific research. "In as much as Dr. Jonas Salk devotes himself very extensively to the buildup of the 'N' Foundation," the aide-mémoire concluded, "it is understood that Dr. Salk will not have the time to continue his autoimmune and neoplastic laboratory work with the Salk Institute effective Oct 28, 1984."[20]

Salk responded to the plan with enthusiasm. He prepared to seek an agreement with the city of San Diego that would allow his new foundation to occupy lands currently being used by the Institute. Since the foundation's goal was to prevent "crippling of the mind," he talked of finally building Louis Kahn's meeting house for collective reflection on the site.[21] Regarding the new foundation's name, he told de Hoffmann, "While Salk has been the Institute's name now for twenty-two years, it has been mine for sixty-nine years, and I have grown quite attached to it. I am not prepared to deny my own identification with the 'N' foundation."[22] Knowing full well what the trustees' reaction would be, de Hoffmann suggested Salk present the aide-mémoire at the next board meeting.

At this point, there seemed to be two camps among Institute scientists and trustees. One felt that since Salk had created the Institute and devoted much of his life to what was now recognized as an elite research organization, he was entitled to whatever he wanted. The other felt that although he had founded the Institute, he had been a poor administrator and mediocre scientist, and that on the whole the board had been more than generous with him. The time had come for him to leave. By 1984, many more were in the latter camp.

On January 2, 1984, yet another cloudless day in La Jolla, Salk once again passed through the eucalyptus grove, crossed the travertine plaza, looked out to the sea, and prepared to face the board of trustees. This was an important meeting for him—a discussion of his proposed retirement plan. He did not anticipate any dissent; the aide-mémoire had been de Hoffmann's idea, and he usually vetted issues beforehand. De Hoffmann began the meeting with another positive financial account, after which he turned to Salk for the founding director's report.

"The Institute was begun with strong representation of the biological sciences," Salk began, "and the intention to explore realms of broader human concern. In time, the biological base became stronger and the activities related to broader human interest ceased." He was referring to events in 1975, when the board eliminated the Council for Biology in Human Affairs. "I would like to accept the challenge to develop aspects of the Institute's charter that still remain unexpressed."[23] He laid out his plan, including the construction of Kahn's meeting center, for which he requested the board make available undeveloped land. Two resolutions were proposed: "RESOLVED that Dr. Jonas Salk's position as a resident

Fellow of the Salk Institute…will terminate effective 31 December, 1984, that he will continue to occupy the position of Founding Director." He would, on a reasonable schedule, agreed upon between him and the Institute, turn over occupancy of his laboratory. "RESOLVED that a new nonprofit, tax-exempt foundation, 'The Salk Foundation'…be formed complimentary to the Institute to undertake substantive work on the fulfillment of man's biological potential."[24] The Salk Institute would grant to the foundation a million dollars over an eight-year period to carry out its work.

Max Cowan, a neurobiologist and vice president of the Institute, spoke first. No one wanted to prevent Salk from engaging in any field he chose, Cowan said; nonetheless he felt that he had to express the "deep concern" of the senior scientific staff at the dissipation of the Institute's efforts and assets in any endeavor that was not a part of the field in which the Institute had established its "enviable position."[25] Even Renato Dulbecco, who twenty years earlier had told Salk he found the concept beautiful, cautioned de Hoffmann that an institute dedicated to this field might attract people who were neither biologists nor philosophers, who dabbled in both but were unlikely to make a serious contribution, let alone a synthesis between the two fields. "I am afraid that it will be populated by has-beens," he told de Hoffmann, "by people who throughout their lives have been searching in vain for a focus, and let's be frank, by charlatans."[26]

The trustees cloaked their concerns with talk of the board's duties and guiding principles. Trustee Frank Dupar, a prominent businessman and son of the founder of Western Hotels (later renamed Westin Hotels and Resorts), said he was "deeply troubled by the founding director's proposals because of what appeared to be a proposition that the trustees give away valuable assets to another organization," something which appeared "to violate the fiduciary responsibilities of the Board."[27] Having sought an opinion from a legal expert on nonprofit corporation law, he learned the action would likely breach the established statutory obligations of trustees.

Chen Ning "Frank" Yang, a physicist and recent Nobel Laureate, who had been a professor at Princeton's Institute for Advanced Study for seventeen years and a trustee at Rockefeller University for six, spoke next. "Decisions to expand into new disciplines," he said, "taken by these institutes in the sixties, generated tremendously dangerous problems for them." Those at the Rockefeller University had to be "phased out." The Princeton institute was "torn apart and almost went down the drain."[28] Given these experiences, he warned the board to be wary.

Stunned by the board's response, Salk sat stony-faced, offering no rebuttal. He waited for de Hoffmann to come to his defense; after all, he had proposed the aide-mémoire in the first place. Instead, when asked if the aide-mémoire had been, as Salk intimated, a proposal generated by the Salk Institute, de Hoffmann explained that a board member had suggested the memorandum. Although he gave no name, this was probably Senator Jacob Javits, the liberal Republican from New York, who, unable to attend this meeting, had asserted his full support for anything submitted by the founding director. Acting upon his suggestion, de Hoffmann said he had proceeded to write the aide-mémoire with the understanding that it was to serve only as a paper for discussion with Dr. Salk. Hence, it should be clearly understood that it had no formal standing.

Somehow Salk maintained his equanimity and complimented the trustees on the quality of their remarks. He said they had given him new "insights and food for thought." He would rethink the whole matter. But that wasn't the end of it. As a final blow, Frank Yang proposed a resolution reasserting the Institute's "sole dedication to basic science research." They did not put his resolution to a vote, the meeting minutes reflected, "because it appeared to be redundant and merely a statement of the longstanding policy of the Institute."[29]

Salk had been duped into believing the memo was a fait accompli rather than a "paper for discussion," as de Hoffmann had put it. Now it appeared that all he would have left was an office and the empty title of founding director. Few knew how crushed he felt. "He was quite resilient," Roger Guillemin recalled.[30] Salk tried to reassure his son Peter, telling him that the episode just represented an experiment that was playing itself out. But Peter knew that Part C of the Institute's original articles of incorporation included the stated purpose of studying the factors and circumstances conducive to the fulfillment of man's full potential. De Hoffmann had excised it from the official statement of the

Institute's intention. And his father's demotion to founding director and nothing more seemed "like being put out to pasture." Although Salk was certainly disappointed, he told Peter, "Reality is reality."[31]

To only a few did he express his dismay. Salk told his assistant Barbara Robinson that in founding the Institute he had wanted to give the fellows as much freedom as possible. "That's how discoveries are made." He had created a place where scientists had carte blanche, yet when he wanted to bring about a union between the arts and sciences, they denied him. "Why should they have the freedom to do what they want, but I don't have the freedom to do what I want?" he asked her.[32] "The very disdain," scientist Gerald Edelman said, "that these people had while they were at the trough, benefiting from this man's particular vision, is an interesting paradox."[33]

De Hoffmann may have stabbed Salk in the back, but the wound was not fatal. When Salk responded to the board calmly, saying they had given him new insights and he planned to reconsider the whole matter, de Hoffmann might have guessed that he had a fight on his hands. Salk would not go away, even with the board positioned against him. He told one trustee he felt entitled to ongoing compensation, and so he enlisted the help of his friend Bayless Manning, a former Stanford Law School dean and one of America's leading authorities on corporate law. The move provoked de Hoffmann, who didn't hide his contempt for Salk. "De Hoffmann couldn't stand the sight of him," Maureen Dulbecco acknowledged. "He didn't want him on the campus."[34] Salk wrote in his night notes: "The truth of the matter, simply stated, is that FdeH wants me *out* of the Institute, and, if possible, *off* the premises. He can possibly have the first but not the second."[35] Trustee Samuel Stewart, a corporate attorney and Bank of America executive, began to work with the board's executive committee to reach an agreement.

On October 28, 1984, his seventieth birthday, Salk signed an agreement with de Hoffmann. Instead of the original arrangement—a $57,000 salary and an emeritus title—Salk would receive $70,000 per year; a waiver of the $7,900 balance owed on his housing loan; two secretaries; a suite of offices on the top floor of the Institute; $10,000 each year for telephone, postage, and supplies; $10,000 for travel; and $10,000 for scholarly interests. In return, "Dr. Salk shall promptly surrender and release the laboratory space," the agreement read. And the Institute would have the exclusive right to the use of Dr. Jonas Salk's name in perpetuity.[36]

Salk could no longer procrastinate; he had to give up his lab. "He was very sad about that," a later companion, Joan Abrahamson, recalled.[37] Despite his forays into administration and metabiology, Salk considered himself a physician-scientist foremost, destined to help mankind in order to fulfill his duty of *tikkun olam*. When he closed his laboratory door behind him, he knew that part of his life was over. To make matters worse, his dream of melding the two cultures, of bridging the gulf between the sciences and humanities, had been dealt a fatal blow. "The whole thing was a disaster," he told Westall.[38] "To Jonas, that was the central idea of the place," Jack MacAllister reflected. "The driving force was the notion of this dialogue between the sciences and the humanities. He didn't want to build just another science mill. This needed to be special."[39]

Most disturbing of all was the affront to Salk's dignity. He told a close associate he felt savaged by the scientists and trustees, and especially by de Hoffmann. "I gave my life to this place. They wouldn't be here except for me."[40] He had become a pariah. Arnold Mandell worried that Salk was so distraught he might do himself harm. "Some nights I didn't think he would make it," he disclosed.[41] The Salk Institute was meant to be his refuge. He savored its beauty every time he entered the courtyard and looked out to see the tower colonnades in relief against the sea and sky or the display of sunlight and shadows across the walls. It was his magnum opus; it stirred his soul. Salk may have retained a salary, two secretaries, and an office suite, but he effectively had been shut out of the institute he had created.

Disciples, Sycophants, and Lovers

JONAS SALK HAD been forced to terminate his laboratory research, and he no longer served as the Salk Institute director. Science had trumped humanism; the Institute appeared to have only one culture. Epoch B, an alternate organization through which he hoped to infuse biological studies with the conscience of man, had run out of funds. Although he had struggled with his scientific endeavors and Institute affairs for forty years, Salk did not choose to relax at his Palomar retreat or travel someplace where he didn't need to deliver a lecture or ask for money, or simply watch the sun set over the Pacific Ocean. He still felt driven to improve the welfare of mankind, albeit in the role of an elder statesman.

Salk served on the board of the MacArthur Foundation from its inception. Established to produce positive changes in society, it offered substantial fellowship awards to exceptionally creative individuals who worked to improve the world. His long list of board positions included such diverse groups as the International Society of Child Ecology and the Sino-American Center for International Scientific Study; he promoted the Native American Rights Fund, allowing the group to use his name for fundraising purposes. A member of Physicians for Social Responsibility's advisory board, he spoke out against the proliferation of atomic weapons. President Carter invited his comments on a strategic arms limitation agreement at a breakfast briefing and asked for his support for SALT II. Salk endorsed the 1982 Bilateral Nuclear Weapons Initiative and served on the national advisory board for the Nuclear Weapons Freeze Campaign. The president of the International Physicians for the Prevention of Nuclear War, which won the 1985 Noble Peace Prize, thanked Salk for his "many seminal contributions to the growth of our movement."[1]

Salk expressed particular concerns about future generations, asking, "Are we being good ancestors?"[2] As a member of Save the Children's advisory board, he gave the introductory talk at their 1983 meeting. He engaged Robert McNamara, then president of the World Bank, in efforts to reduce infant mortality, starting with the five million vaccine-preventable deaths worldwide. Together they helped organize the Task Force for Child Survival, in which the WHO and UNICEF agreed to lead a "planned miracle"—immunization of all the world's children by 1990—a task Salk called a "moral commitment."[3] In 1984, he gave the opening remarks at their first international meeting, the Bellagio Conference to Protect the World's Children.

For a man used to reaching a goal through his own industry, Salk found working with large organizations frustrating. When asked by the Rockefeller Foundation director how to translate its mandate of effecting well-being throughout the world into specific programs, Salk had no advice. "You can see the mood that I am in at the moment," he replied, "not discouraged, simply the wiser as a result of the experiences I've had as I continue to try to make progress in the developing countries.... Nature is yielding, human nature less so."[4] He found solace in his night writings, however, and once again decided to put his thoughts into a book.

Thanks mainly to his son Jonathan, Salk's third book, *World Population and Human Values: A New Reality*, was released in 1981.[5] Salk had been asked to write a brief commentary for the United Nations on trends in world populations, and Harper and Row expressed interest in publishing it as a book. Jonathan became involved when his father asked for suggestions regarding the introduction and conclusions. Peter Salk had engaged in his father's cancer research; Darrell collaborated on his later polio work. Now Jonathan's turn had come. As usual, his father rambled

in his writing. Jonathan rewrote the manuscript to make it more accessible to the general public. When Salk read the edited version, he said
the length and tone were "not in harmony with the original concept."
Jonathan had made it too academic; Salk wanted free expression. "After
a delay of several months," Jonathan recalled, "at least on my part for the
dispersion of ego, we sat down and resolved many of the conflicts in
ideas and styles."[6] The book's central premise was that "the world is at a
fateful point of transition both in population growth and in human
values, attitudes, and behaviors."[7] The current generation holds mankind's future in its hands; life for their progeny depends on how they deal
with consumption of natural resources and relationships with each other.

World Population and Human Values received a better reception than
either *Man Unfolding* or *The Survival of the Wisest*. "Taking one single
element from *The Survival of the Wisest*," read one review, "they turned
what was originally a lofty, scholarly work into a visually and aestheti-
cally-appealing presentation."[8] The editor of the *Journal of Social and
Biological Structures* described the effect created by the "soothing, almost
dreamlike text," combined with "simple visual images," as "astonishing."[9]
Salk's next book, *Anatomy of Reality*, released two years later, stressed the
importance of being good ancestors.[10]

Now seventy, Salk had reached yet another fork in his path: whether
to operate in a world of power and authority—serving on boards, building institutions, effecting policy—or to opt for a more reflective life as
a writer and thinker. For the most part, he chose the latter, believing it
to be the way he could be most influential. When he asked Jonathan to
help him write another book, based on his night notes, Jonathan hesitated. "Delving into the enormity of those night writings felt like a
swamp that I might not get out of."[11] Besides, he had been accepted to
Albert Einstein College of Medicine.

Those who had similar concerns about mankind contacted Salk. He
received numerous requests to read and comment upon manuscripts,
serve as a consultant, or participate in various projects, most of which
arose from his writings about man's future. Yet he no longer felt compelled to acquiesce to every appeal. "I've had to come to the conclusion
that I cannot go on adding and adding commitments indefinitely," he
wrote to the president of San Francisco's Institute of Noetic Sciences.

"I have had to declare a time bankruptcy, and until I once again can become solvent, I must suffer the consequences of my past indiscretions."[12]

Salk was seeking intellectual intimacy. Those with whom he had felt comfortable expressing his innermost feelings—Basil O'Connor, Edward R. Murrow, Buckminster Fuller—had died. And at age seventy-three, Louis Kahn, having just returned from Bangladesh, was found dead in the men's room at Pennsylvania Station.[13] His address had been crossed out on his passport, and he lay in a New York City morgue for three days before anyone identified him. An autopsy revealed that Kahn had died from a heart attack. Hundreds of thousands of dollars in debt, he left nothing to his wife, mistresses, or children.

In the early 1980s, a colleague introduced Salk to neuroscientist Antonio Damasio. As they talked about science, philosophy, and architecture, a friendship bloomed despite the almost thirty years' age difference. Damasio understood why those who cherished objectivity found Salk's writings vague. Yet he considered them primers for his *Descartes' Error: Emotion, Reason, and the Human Brain*, which was published to acclaim in 1994. He later founded the Brain and Creativity Institute at the University of Southern California, which he described as a variation on Salk's dream of uniting the two cultures.[14] At the time they met, Damasio worked at the University of Iowa, too far away to fulfill Salk's yearning for an intellectual bond.

In the early 1990s, Salk began to have monthly dinners with psychiatrist Edward Mohns. As they talked for hours at San Diego's Marine Room, Salk's favorite restaurant on the beach, the pounding surf created a dramatic backdrop to their conversations. "We had a splendid time intellectually and unspoken emotionally," Mohns recounted.[15] One recurring theme was how mankind's noncognitive sophistication and behavior had not matched its technical virtuosity. They discussed political systems, struggles for dominance, even paranormal communication, but rarely their private lives. Once Salk did shift from the philosophical to the personal and asked Mohns if he, as a psychiatrist, considered him neurotic. Mohns replied he did not psychoanalyze friends. In their evenings together, however, he sensed Salk's vulnerability and unmet need. "My response to him emotionally was often one of unspoken compassion."[16] Although Salk shared volumes of his night notes with both Damasio

and Mohns, neither accepted the daunting task of reading and responding to them.

Salk continued to search for somebody to help clarify the thoughts
expressed in his night writings, a torchbearer to help actualize his metabiological visions. In his quest, he began to gravitate toward women,
especially young, attractive, intelligent women. His administrative assistant, Barbara Robinson, thought that a number of them flattered Salk
for their own advancement. She tried to shield him. "But if somebody
thought that his writing was wonderful," she recalled, "he wanted to talk
with them, correspond with them, hear more about what they thought of
his work."[17] Kathleen Murray, another of his assistants, found the situation annoying. These women took up her time, not to mention Salk's. Yet
he never discouraged them. "Each one thought she was *the* special
person," Murray explained, "*the* interpreter of his metaphysical work."[18]
Some became disciples; others appeared to be sycophants.

Many interactions followed a similar pattern: He would meet a
charming and seemingly perceptive woman whom he engaged in discussion about metabiological evolution. "I've been waiting for you my whole
life," he would say. "No one has been able to understand the breadth of
my thinking." Nightly calls, walks on the beach, meaningful dialogue,
and in several cases outright affairs followed. "I think he enjoyed the
conversations," recalled Murray, "but some became very attached to him,
and then it became a burden, a burden created by his own participation
in the attachment."[19]

The situation proved harder for Lorraine Friedman. She and Salk had
worked together for more than forty years. Always professional, always
protective, referred to by some as Salk's majordomo, she provided stability,
companionship, and good humor. In time, Lorraine became too protective, almost possessive in her behavior as more young women sought his
advice. Salk began to chafe under her vigilance. "I was miserable," she
later confessed. "I didn't like feeling unnecessary."[20] With some prompting,
she eventually retired. Friedman would survive her beloved boss by ten
years and be buried in a cemetery plot near his. "Jonas has got his right-
hand person helping him out," Fred Westall noted after her funeral.[21]

Salk's first disciple had been Barbara Hubbard, the Connecticut
housewife with whom he had had a liaison in the 1960s. Over the years

they had stayed in touch. Hubbard founded the Committee for the Future as well as the Foundation for Conscious Evolution, wrote several books, and became a sought-after public speaker. Some Democrats considered her a potential vice presidential ticket mate for Walter Mondale in 1984, although the party eventually selected Geraldine Ferraro. Hubbard considered Salk her liberator. "In the past year I produced a surprising new baby—an evolutionary interpretation of the New Testament," she wrote him in 1981. "Please note the dedication to you."[22]

Another longstanding disciple was Eva Seilitz Horney. In 1974, the year after high school, she had moved from Sweden to Santa Barbara to work. While there, she took courses at Santa Barbara City College. One day, a circular from the Center for Democratic Institutions caught her attention. Twenty-two, she had never heard of Dr. Jonas Salk, but was searching for meaning in her life and thought that his talk on a new epoch sounded fascinating. "It was an almost mystical experience," she recalled, "a celestial collision of light which overwhelmed me completely."[23] She approached Salk about his ideas, and he suggested that she read his books. Afterward she wrote to him of their profound effect; she was committing her life to metabiology. Two weeks later, they met again at the Center for Democratic Institutions, where Salk told Eva, "If I have written my book for only one person, that's enough for me."[24] And following yet another chance encounter, he wrote, "The forces of ESP must have been powerfully at work for our paths to have crossed as they did not only last April but again the other day. I am very pleased to see how clear-minded you are and what you are planning to do. It shows in your eyes and in your whole being."[25]

Two months after they first met, Salk invited Eva to his home. "That opened up even a deeper understanding [between us]," she reflected. "We met each other on a soul level."[26] With that began an attachment that lasted decades. They corresponded regularly; soon she called him Jonas. She sent drawings and photos. One showed a petite blonde, young enough to be his granddaughter, under a Christmas tree.

Horney returned to Sweden, got married, enjoyed motherhood, and continued to write to Salk. He always replied. Almost every year, he invited her to spend a few weeks at the Institute, where he provided a studio. They discussed her efforts to initiate an Epoch B group in Sweden and her interpretation of his night notes. Gilot was rude to the young Swede. "She thought I was after her husband," Horney supposed. "I don't blame her, because she was about the same age as me when she met Picasso. I probably would have been disturbed too if I was his wife and saw the radiation flowing in between us, especially at the beginning."[27]

With academic degrees in English and interfaith studies, Horney worked to promote public existential health. Among many pursuits, she directed a national yoga program to reduce aggression and encourage social transformation in the Swedish prison system. She coordinated development of a unique housing project, attempting to create an environment that eliminated community alienation. Through the years, she had always been able to turn to Salk for advice. But in his seventies, he became more remote. Horney thought his vibrancy had dampened. "It was obvious that his personal life was blocking his more subtle energies. The spiritual connection that we used to have wasn't as strong."[28] At one point, she sent him a postcard with a picture of a lone elk. It read, "The thought of not being able to see you this year makes me so sad. I guess it is the realization that you are getting older, too, that is hard for me to accept. I miss you more than ever."[29]

Of all the women with whom Salk had relationships later in life, Joan Abrahamson provided the most balanced, productive one. Their friendship had started out in the same way as had many others. In March of 1981, she attended an anniversary party for her fiancé's parents.[30] She knew Françoise Gilot had an apartment in the same building, and as an artist herself, Abrahamson hoped to meet her. Partway through the evening, in walked Gilot with Jonas Salk. Gilot briefly said hello, but it was Salk who began to engage the twenty-nine-year-old in conversation.

Abrahamson came from an established San Francisco family. A member of Yale's first class of women undergraduates, she went on to receive a Master of Arts from Stanford, a doctorate in learning environments from Harvard, and a law degree from Berkeley.[31] She had worked with the United Nations Human Rights Commission in Geneva and UNESCO's Division of Human Rights and Peace. At the time she met Salk, she was serving as a White House Fellow, having been special assistant and associate counsel to Vice Presidents Walter Mondale and George H. W. Bush.

As the evening wore on, Salk continued to monopolize Abrahamson. He told her he found transitions fascinating and asked about the shift from the Carter to Reagan administrations. He talked about how living systems solve problems, postulating the same principles could be applied to politics and human affairs. Throughout the party, he never took his eyes off her. At the end of the night, when Abrahamson said she had hoped to talk with his wife, Salk invited her to breakfast. Gilot could have felt threatened by this stunning, highly educated young woman with whom her husband seemed captivated; however, Abrahamson charmed her as well.

By the time Abrahamson departed, Salk had determined to work with her as an advisor, a collaborator, or perhaps a muse. Instead she accepted a position as Vice President Bush's assistant chief of staff, accompanying him around the world. After that, she married Jonathan Aronson, a professor of communications at the University of Southern California's Annenberg School. Salk was patient; he knew in time he would find a way to collaborate with her.

On their first meeting, when he had asked Abrahamson what she planned after her fellowship, she told him she would like to start an institute which would bring creative thinking to public policy.[32] She even had selected a name, the Jefferson Institute, because she considered him the most imaginative president. Salk told her he admired Jefferson for the same reason and sent her Dos Passos's *The Head and Heart of Thomas Jefferson*. In 1984, with his encouragement, Abrahamson became the president and executive director of the Jefferson Institute, with Salk as the first board chairman. At the same time, he hired her as a consultant at five thousand dollars per month to study the feasibility of a Center for the Study of Human Creativity, similar to the Jefferson Institute.[33] He asked her to establish a base in La Jolla, which she did in 1985, traveling back and forth to see her husband in Los Angeles. That same year she received a fellowship, the so-called genius grant, from the MacArthur Foundation, of which Salk was still a board member.

Spending more time in La Jolla, Abrahamson often accompanied Salk on his daily walk on the beach. That's when they talked; she called it "ritualistic." He loved to go barefoot in the sand and watch the sunset. He called her early in the morning and late at night. "He was all about work," she recalled. "I've just realized such and such," he often said. "I don't want to forget to tell you."[34] Abrahamson knew how sad Salk had been when his laboratory closed; he told her a chapter in his life had ended. She wanted to help him start another by interpreting his night notes, collecting material for an autobiography, planning the Center for Creativity, and later establishing the Jonas Salk Foundation. "Of all the people who came to associate with him," Barbara Robinson noted, "she was the most sincere."[35] Abrahamson provided an intellectual spark, yet, gentle and patient, she focused on him in a way his wife never seemed to. "Everybody knew they were lovers," said one journalist.[36] Others thought not; Joan and Françoise had become friends. Abrahamson herself denied the assertion. With three sons to raise, she would eventually wean Salk from her, but before then she would help him open a significant chapter in his life.

Among several others with whom Salk sought help elucidating the thoughts expressed in his night notes was Heather Wood Ion. An anthropologist, educated at Oxford University, Ion was teaching a course on medicine and the humanities at the University of California, Los Angeles, when they met in the late 1980s. Barbara Beretich, one of Gilot's art dealers, asked Ion, who was visiting, to help her deliver some rugs to Françoise. When Beretich asked to see Salk, Gilot said he was in bed with a strained back. Still, he liked Beretich and came out of his bedroom in his pajamas and dressing gown, surprised to find she had brought a guest. That first conversation with Ion lasted for five hours, despite his back pain. "I've been waiting for you my whole life," she recalled Salk telling her. "No one has been able to understand the breadth of my thinking."[37] Three months later, she moved to San Diego.

Salk once told Ion that he wanted to "create an epidemic of health," and she offered to help craft public policy papers.[38] In addition, he asked her to respond to his night notes—up to 250 pages per month. She took on the role of interpreter, organizing his thoughts into themes and assessing how each evolved. "I am glad to have taken your darshan (vision) in the vortex (whirling mass)," she wrote, "and to have made my own promises to you which you already know as yours. Love, Heather."[39] She occasionally reconfigured his words in verse. "I cannot tell you how immersing in totality these writings and the involvement with them is," she wrote after reading the next installment. "You are giving me amniotic food for the birth of the evolvers, page by poem by page."[40] These letters annoyed Robinson "If there was ever a sycophant," she observed, "she was the epitome."[41]

Joan Abrahamson, too, considered Ion a flatterer and a user from whom Salk could not detach himself. Kathleen Murray, however, thought that he enjoyed their conversations. Ion did go on to spread his word, later founding the Epidemic of Health Corporation. She gave numerous lectures, including a TEDx Talk, "Creating an Epidemic of Health," and workshops such as "Being Good Ancestors." At one conference, a photographer caught her deep in conversation with Barbara Marx Hubbard, two torchbearers side by side.

Salk's most unambiguously physical relationship involved psychologist Lisa Longworth.[42] In 1985, Salk's stepdaughter Aurelia Simon introduced him to Lisa, an undergraduate in fine arts at the University of California, San Diego. Aurelia often invited Lisa and her boyfriend home for dinner, where talk focused on creativity. One night, Lisa revealed she had been treated for a brain tumor, and that experience had opened her up to a larger vision of life. Salk helped her view creativity as a means to heal; Gilot encouraged her to express her spiritual experiences through art. Grateful for their attention, she told the two she considered them her spiritual mother and father. Longworth sensed, however, that something more was brewing between herself and Salk. "I had a crush on him," she confessed. "I was checking out the relationship between him and Françoise, and I could tell it wasn't sexually or physically intimate just by the energy. It felt platonic."[43] She found his penetrating glance, and his celebrity, seductive. For his part, Salk seemed attracted to the tall, slender woman, whose looks caused heads to turn. Still Longworth didn't anticipate what happened next.

She had just broken up with her boyfriend when Salk called to say he and Françoise supported her decision and invited her to their home for dinner. Longworth assumed both would be there. When Salk opened the door, he kissed her—not a peck on the cheek but a sensual kiss. Stunned, Longworth pulled back and looked at this man she had regarded as a mentor. "I realized how much I loved him," she recounted.[44] He took her hand and led her inside. That evening a five-year romance began, and her friendship with Aurelia ended.

Salk called several times each week. The calls began with meditation, with Longworth leading. Once relaxed, Salk would start to talk, primarily about his observations from his night notes, sometimes about the day's events. She found his insights to be profound as well as nourishing, inspiring her to become a psychological healer. What developed between them, Lisa said, was "a very deep, very passionate relationship on many different levels." Salk was clearly drawn to her youth; at the time their relationship began, Longworth was twenty-five. Just the sound of her voice made him feel seventeen again, he told her. "I was like an elixir to him," she recalled. At one point, he said, "If I weren't married, I'd marry you right now."[45] On her thirtieth birthday, he gave her a diamond and emerald ring.

Salk encouraged Longworth to date men her own age, and she knew he had other lovers. (After his death, she attended a formal dinner for him and was seated at a table of women. In the course of the evening, they discovered each had had an affair with Salk.) Eventually Longworth went on to obtain a PhD in psychology and establish a private practice she advertised as "integrating psychology, creativity, and spirituality."[46] Her website states that Jonas Salk mentored her in daily dialogues on creativity and intuition for five years.

When Longworth's affair with Salk began to fade, Carol Anne Bundy filled the void. In 1990, Salk had hired her at the suggestion of his lawyer, former dean of Stanford Law School Bayless Manning, who had been her mentor. Salk and Bundy met to discuss a position at his new foundation, and after they talked for twenty minutes, he asked the bright, physically appealing twenty-seven-year-old lawyer, "When can you move to La Jolla?"[47] Bundy and Peter Salk administered the Jonas Salk Foundation, housed in a small bungalow. "Basically what Jonas couldn't do at the Salk Institute," she said, "I was doing at the foundation."[48] Salk asked Bundy to help write his next book, *The Millennium of the Mind*. When she met Francis Crick and described her job, he replied, "I get it. Jonas needs someone to interpret his polysyllabic sentences."[49]

They never finished the book. "The dialogue took over," she explained, with long walks and late-night conversations. "Ours was a complete and devoted relationship," Bundy mused, "more than just physical, intellectual, philosophical or spiritual." She knew their union seemed strange given their respective ages, but that had been part of the attraction. "We were explorers," she said, "not of the planet but of the mind and of the heart."[50]

Her attentiveness embarrassed Salk's colleagues. At meetings with scientists or Institute officials, Bundy would bring him a glass of water or with a gesture indicate, as Abrahamson put it, "He's mine." Abrahamson blamed herself; Bundy had appeared at a point when she could not devote as much time to Salk as she had in the past. "He wanted someone like me," Abrahamson speculated, "who could help him with some things and that he liked to have around."[51] When, at Salk's request, she had interviewed Bundy for a position at the foundation, Abrahamson thought she had another agenda. She had heard rumors that Carol Anne had a propensity for trysts with high-profile men and thought Jonas might be her next target. After the interview, she had told Salk that Bundy didn't have the proper skills. He hired her anyway.

Kathleen Murray found Bundy's entanglement with Salk uncomfortable and awkward. "People would come to me and ask what was going on, because she began acting and speaking as if she were his partner, almost as if she were his wife." Bundy planned Salk's activities without informing Murray of them, complicating her administrative duties. "You will find discipleship at its highest in her," Murray said.[52] Salk's enchantment in this case seemed to have affected his usual perspicuity. He invited Bundy to his home for a Passover Seder; he took her to Paris with him and Françoise.

One day Bundy appeared in maternity clothes, and the rumors flew. Abrahamson asked Salk if he was the father. "It's not my baby," he replied. "I've never had sex with her."[53] She nonetheless worried a paternity suite might follow until Bundy confirmed the father to be a French scientist who had visited the Institute. Nevertheless, Abrahamson warned Salk, "When she's walking around here pregnant, everyone's going to think it's yours."[54]

When Eva Seilitz Horney heard about Bundy, the news disturbed her deeply. She had corresponded with Salk for decades and visited the Institute almost every year, and neither he nor anyone else had mentioned Bundy until Horney came for his eightieth birthday party. One of his colleagues told her about the affair and how it had become a touchy subject among staff. "I felt he lost some of his glow," Horney admitted, "and I was very upset when I came to know more about his personal life. He was having this kind of double life, which seemed to me rather low level."[55] She considered her own relationship with him to be pure and clean. When she confronted Salk, he said he was afraid she'd be jealous. Even more disturbing, when he introduced Bundy to Horney, Bundy said Jonas had told her all about his relationship with his Swedish friend. And Bundy had her son, who looked just like Salk, with her. When Horney asked if he was the father, Salk denied paternity, yet she was never quite sure.

The day after Salk's birthday, still unnerved, Horney stopped by his home before leaving for Sweden. Gilot had returned to New York, and he sat on the sofa surrounded by the memory books people had given him. "He looked at me," she recalled, "and then he looked at all these books and all the compliments and said, 'Well at least I must have done something good in this life.'" She thanked him for all he had done for her and left. Their flame had burned out. "He was probably missing that full relationship on all levels," she later reasoned, "and perhaps he felt he got it with her. I just don't know."[56]

Salk had told Lisa Longworth that he and Gilot had an understanding: what he did with other women was his own business; she did not want to know about it or hear about it. But she couldn't ignore Carol Anne Bundy. Salk, after all, had the audacity to take her to Paris with them. When a friend told Gilot that she had seen her husband with his mistress, she was furious. He tried to portray Bundy as his collaborator, but Gilot threatened a divorce. Salk asked Abrahamson what he should do, even though he knew the answer. He and Bundy had overstepped the bounds of propriety, and he did not want to risk losing his wife.

Allegations of Salk's romantic interludes surprised several of his male friends. He had never hinted about them to Ted Mohns, with whom he dined monthly. Then again, their conversations tended to be about the larger world. Yet even in a community as small as La Jolla, Mohns had heard no such rumors. When Jack MacAllister learned about his supposed affairs, he responded, "I like him even more now." Salk didn't fit MacAllister's image of a philanderer, not like his associate Louis Kahn, who had open affairs throughout his life. "Jonas was very shy with women," he observed. "And with his high profile, he'd have to be pretty dang clever."[57]

❖

WHY DID JONAS Salk engage in extramarital affairs? Was he simply a womanizer, as Richard Carter, author of *Breakthrough: The Saga of Jonas Salk*, privately asserted?[58] A later colleague agreed: "Jonas had quite an eye for women."[59] Some have argued that he was an innocent victim whose fame made him prey to some women who exaggerated their relationship, such as the one who sent numerous notes addressed to "Schatzi"[60] (sweetheart), signed "your blue-eyed serpent," describing their longtime affair.[61] Murray considered the unwanted attentions of women a burden Salk had to bear. "Fame gives one an enormous sense of responsibility," she thought, "but one can slip, and you have these complex situations."[62] Arnold Mandell recalled entanglements that arose as Salk tried to help women solve financial, family, or career problems. Nevertheless, he did not regard his friend as a naive mark.[63]

Several affairs appeared to be natural extensions of a genuine spiritual bond. Salk told Longworth that women had more evolutionary equipment. "He believed the seeds of his ideas would move forward with these women, and the women they touched."[64] Not all his interactions proceeded from the intellectual to the erotic, however. In his decade-long relationship with Horney, she said he never did anything "come-onish."[65]

Perhaps these romantic interests arose from something missing in his marriage. Friends and colleagues thought it an unusual arrangement from the start. "I am not the usual wife," Gilot maintained. "I am someone with a career of my own."[66] She told a journalist in a rare interview, "A relationship is less demanding and active at this time of life."[67] Abrahamson discerned a vibrant intellectual relationship between Salk and Gilot, sprinkled with playfulness and affection. Not within his earshot, other friends described Gilot as arrogant, cool, self-centered, and calculating. "Françoise is probably the strongest character I've encountered in a woman," Mohns said. "I would characterize her as the oncoming prow of a ship."[68] He never saw her express tenderness toward her husband, either verbally or physically, and Salk never mentioned his wife. Yet to portray theirs as a marriage with no love seems an injustice.

In a television interview after Salk's death, Gilot said she couldn't paint for some time. "It's like you lose an arm," she said.[69]

Longworth thought Salk and Gilot had a deep, soulful love affair. "But it was not physical," she said, at least not later in life. "I know there wasn't and hadn't been for many, many years any sexual connection between the two. She was extremely bright, and I think on a mental level they had this enormous synergy and connection. That was their intercourse."[70] Salk had intimated to Longworth that he and Françoise had an understanding that allowed for extramarital pursuits. Rumors circulated about Gilot's lovers. Salk acted cavalier at times, such as when he seemed to flaunt Carol Anne Bundy in Paris. He may have been showing Françoise that other women found him sexually irresistible. It's possible that feelings of neglect drove Salk's indiscretions; he did tell several women about a deficit in his marriage and his unfulfilled emotional longings.

Some thought he was making up for the perceived lack of respect from his peers. "I think another way he got nourishment was from his intimate, loving, erotic connections," Longworth postulated. "That's the sense I had from comments he made to me even while we were making love."[71] Mandell agreed that women provided comfort for Salk: "Men who have compulsive affairs are mostly fixing their egos. And God knows he was injured. He never saw himself as a success."[72] He told Mandell he felt exploited by the press and ignored by the scientific community.

In trying to comprehend the underlying reasons for Salk's infidelities, the clearest insight came from his youngest son, Jonathan, although he did not acknowledge the women in his father's life. He thought his father had a great and unmet need to connect with others on an intimate level. He didn't know how, except thorough his work, especially his philosophical work. "But nested within that was always a desire to connect."[73] Ion considered Salk himself partly to blame for his isolation; he had constructed an emotional shell to deal with his domineering mother, to survive his rebuff by scientists, to save himself from public scrutiny. In one unguarded moment, he told Ion, "I have encapsulated relationships which are very specific about one aspect of my thinking or one aspect of what I care about. I don't have any relationship which encompasses it all."[74] Still, each woman in her own way brought him some measure of happiness.

It matters little to history if Jonas Salk had one affair or two or ten. In no way do they detract from his enormous contributions and achievements. Nevertheless, they do point out that, although he was considered a saint by much of the public, he was human. As he told Barbara Beretich, "I discovered early on that everybody puts on his pants one leg at a time."[75] In the end, Salk yearned for what most people want—to connect fully with someone in an intimate way, to be loved completely. Having failed in that quest, he had turned to his disciples, sycophants, and lovers. He curtailed his forays abruptly, however, when he heard the clarion call of AIDS.

AIDS:
Salk's Next Mountain

ON OCTOBER 14, 1984, Salk closed the door to his laboratory; his life as a scientist had ended. That same week, officials shut down San Francisco's bathhouses. Although more than eleven thousand cases of AIDS had been recorded in the United States, the public dismissed the disease as one of gay men.[1] A handful of physicians worried that the deadly new virus, if unchecked, could engulf the world; most expressed only passing interest. By now, Salk had found the role of elder statesman frustrating and that of philosopher peripheral in his personal commitment to combating disease. He was a man of action. When a journalist asked him what he considered his failures, Salk replied: "Failure is not a term that I would use. My whole life has been made up of challenges.... How do you know that you can climb a mountain unless there is a mountain there for you to climb?"[2]

⁂

IN THE FALL of 1980, a thirty-year-old man sought medical care for fever and swollen lymph glands. His doctor suspected mononucleosis, but tests returned negative. When his temperature rose to 104°, he was transferred to UCLA Medical Center, sweating profusely and wincing with pain. A thick layer of fungus covered the inside of his mouth and throat; deep ulcers surrounded his anus, and fungating lesions had mutilated his fingertips. With antifungal and antiviral therapy, he improved. Within weeks, however, he returned with a hacking cough, struggling to breathe. A chest radiograph showed something filling his lung airspaces; brushings revealed *Pneumocystis carinii*—a highly infectious microbe. Despite antibiotics, his oxygen level plummeted. Two days later, he died.[3]

No one at the Center for Disease Control in Atlanta suspected a new epidemic when UCLA professor Michael Gottlieb notified them of the five young men he had treated for *Pneumocystis* pneumonia (PCP), a rare infection that usually preys on those whose immune systems have been suppressed by cancer chemotherapy or organ transplant. These five previously healthy men shared two traits: all had faulty immune systems, and all were homosexual. Gottlieb couldn't dismiss these cases as coincidental and postulated the cause to be some sexually transmitted or environmental agent particular to their lifestyle. He barely had time to ponder this when doctors in New York reported eleven gay men with PCP. Eight had died already.

Within a month, the CDC received notification of another strange outbreak, Kaposi's sarcoma (KS).[4] This rare, slow-growing skin cancer generally occurs in older men of Mediterranean descent. Now twenty-six young men had developed reddish-purple nodules on the face and chest, initially mistaken for bruises. Biopsies revealed KS, which resembled that seen in elderly men. Yet in homosexuals KS behaved like a different disease, spreading to major areas of skin, mouth, lung, and brain, sparing no organ. Disfigurement could be substantial. KS soon became a stigma of this new illness, marking afflicted gay men as lepers.

Still another infirmity plagued homosexuals. Herpes simplex, the virus that causes cold sores and genital herpes, morphed into a demon, causing painful anal vesicles which coalesced into large ulcers, spreading onto the buttocks and into the rectum. The CDC received reports of other rampant "opportunistic" infections, so called because a healthy immune system normally controlled them. By year's end, they counted 293 cases nationwide; almost half had died.[5] Fearing an epidemic, the CDC formed a task force to study this illness they now called acquired immunodeficiency syndrome—AIDS for short. No one could begin to comprehend the entire spectrum of the disease, but when they assembled the pieces, the composite appeared horrific.[6]

Because of its innocuous onset, physicians didn't recognize the disease at first. Patients complained of fever, rash, sore throat, muscle aches, and enlarged lymph nodes, much like mononucleosis. Most cases resolved in a week or two, only to wax and wane, sometimes over years. When the immune system failed, organisms that rarely caused significant illness in healthy people struck. Victims suffered from profuse, bloody diarrhea as a host of bacteria and parasites penetrated the intestines. With the entire gastrointestinal tract from tongue to anus damaged, patients wasted away. Hemorrhage and blindness resulted when cytomegalovirus infected the eyes, meningitis when microbes invaded the spinal fluid. Then in a cruel turn, the unidentified evil that caused AIDS assaulted the brain. Forgetfulness and lack of concentration progressed to dementia, loss of balance, and incontinence. Patients became agitated, delusional, paranoiac, robbing them and their loved ones of much-needed intimacy during their last months.

Immunologists found that AIDS patients had a specific derangement of the immune system: it retained the ability to make antibodies— humoral immunity—but the other function of the immune system, cell-mediated immunity, faltered, worsening with time. Lymphocytes, cells that play a major part in defending the body against microbial invasion, became depressed in number. Typically, healthy individuals have a balance of helper T-cell lymphocytes, which activate the immune response against invasion, and suppressor T-cell lymphocytes, which switch off helper cells when the threat has passed. AIDS patients had a reversal of the normal proportion of the two, so that the suppressor T-cells disabled the helper cells. The underlying cause stymied scientists.

Although the CDC predicted an epidemic, most physicians still considered this a homosexual disease, confined to New York City, San Francisco, and Los Angeles, a puzzle for the CDC to solve. President Reagan ignored those suffering from AIDS, and the press barely covered its devastation. What a contrast to the outbreak of Legionnaire's disease in the late 1970s, when there was an outpouring of national sympathy for the stricken veterans. AIDS didn't concern the general public; many considered it God's retribution for gay promiscuity.

Then in 1982 a heterosexual man from Denver developed AIDS. For years, the fifty-nine-year-old hemophiliac had received factor VIII, the blood clotting factor he lacked. This set off an alarm: since factor VIII was extracted from donated blood plasma, that meant the causative agent might have contaminated the nation's blood supply.[7] Because of the long incubation period, AIDS patients could appear healthy enough to donate blood, only to manifest the disease years after some unknowing individual had been transfused with it.[8] The National Institutes of Health (NIH) called a conference to determine blood-bank policy but reached no consensus. By this time, AIDS was spreading rapidly, with one or two new cases diagnosed daily in twenty-seven states and ten foreign countries.

The CDC expected that before long the disease would spread to women. And it did. They received reports of forty-three women who had contracted AIDS from husbands and partners.[9] Worse yet, pediatricians found that mothers could transmit AIDS to their newborns before or during birth. Health care workers contracted the disease, too. AIDS must be caused by a microbe, CDC epidemiologists thought, passed to others through sexual contact, shared needles, or blood.

In May of 1983, Luc Montagnier of the Pasteur Institute announced that he had discovered a virus responsible for AIDS. So did Robert Gallo of the National Cancer Institute (NCI).[10] Both virologists suspected a new class of infectious agent, the retrovirus, because of its propensity to destroy T-cell lymphocytes. Gallo had made history a few years earlier when he identified two retroviruses that caused leukemia—human T-cell leukemia viruses (HTLV-I and HTLV-II)—the first proof that a virus can induce human cancer. He thought one of these viruses caused AIDS.

Montagnier took a different tack: He searched for the virus in the early stage of infection before all the T-lymphocytes had been destroyed. He cultured lymph tissue from a gay man suffering from node enlargement and weight loss, suspected of having AIDS, who divulged more than fifty sexual partners during travels to North Africa, India, and New York City. Montagnier detected a retrovirus that appeared quite different from Gallo's leukemia viruses. He called it lymphadenopathy associated virus (LAV).[11] American scientists were skeptical. Nevertheless, Montagnier measured antibodies against LAV in 40 percent of AIDS patients tested and filed a patent for an AIDS blood test with the US patent office. At the same time, Gallo announced he had recovered HTLV from blood lymphocytes of two AIDS patients.[12] *Science* published reports from both virologists in the same issue. Because the editor placed Gallo's paper first, it appeared Montagnier was just confirming his remarkable discovery. Gallo insisted that LAV was a variant of HTLV; Montagnier disputed his contention. So Gallo asked for one of Montagnier's specimens to prove it, and they agreed tentatively to a collaboration.

On April 23, 1984, Margaret Heckler, the secretary of the Department of Health and Human Services, called a press conference to announce that Robert Gallo had found the AIDS virus. A blood test for AIDS would be available within six months, she proclaimed, a preventive vaccine within two years. Gallo had violated his agreement with Montagnier to compare their viruses first and then make a joint announcement. Furthermore, Gallo was wrong. His AIDS virus did not turn out to be HTLV-I or II but a variant, which he called HTLV-III. When the Pasteur Institute and NCI cloned DNA from Montagnier's LAV and Gallo's HTLV-III, they found them to be identical. The two agreed to call it the human immunodeficiency virus (HIV). At that point Montagnier began to suspect that Gallo had used the LAV sample he had given him in 1983 to develop his AIDS blood test.

With these discoveries, the structure and action of the virus became clear.[13] Most organisms contain DNA at their core, from which messenger RNA is transcribed. RNA coordinates production of proteins needed for cellular functions. Like all viruses, HIV cannot replicate itself but must utilize DNA from other cells, acting like a parasite. Retroviruses are unique in that they contain RNA and an enzyme, reverse transcriptase, which allows them to make DNA from their own RNA. The spherical-shaped AIDS virus has a core, consisting of its RNA and this enzyme, encased in an envelope, composed of a glycoprotein (protein with a sugar attached). The envelope attaches the virus to cells that have a particular receptor—CD4—on their surface, such as T-helper lymphocytes. Once fused, the virus thrusts its core, containing reverse transcriptase and RNA, into the host cell. Using the enzyme, it converts its RNA into DNA, which integrates with the cell's own DNA, thus commandeering the cell for its own purposes.

Having infected these lymphocytes, HIV often remains dormant for years, invisible to the immune system, until stimulated by some other infectious or environmental agent to multiply, destroying the cell that has housed and sustained it. Newly made viruses enter the bloodstream and infect more lymphocytes. Thus when it spreads, HIV destroys the very cells the human immune system uses to try to contain it. Scientists soon perceived that when the CD4 count fell and the ratio of T-helper to T-suppressor cells became reversed, it meant the immune system was losing the battle against HIV. Once a person's cellular immunity had been destroyed, his body became fertile ground for microbes that pose no problem to healthy people. And that was how most AIDS victims died.

The gay community saw its world crumbling as friends and lovers suffered gruesome deaths. They spent most weekends attending funerals, seeing beautiful, talented, vibrant men reduced to ashes. Bereavement overlay a deepening fear as death touched everyone around them. The toll AIDS extracted was heartbreaking for them and their families, but still somehow not for the American public. It took the death of a movie star, Rock Hudson, of AIDS in October 1985 to make the country at last take notice. With that, the finger-pointing escalated. Gay men were ostracized for bringing this scourge upon morally upright citizens. So were those infected through other means. Ryan White, an Indiana teenager with hemophilia-associated AIDS, was barred from his middle school. By the end of 1985, almost twenty-three thousand Americans had contracted AIDS; more than eleven thousand had died.[14] That was when Jonas Salk knew he had to get involved.

⁂

NONE OF SALK'S friends or family remember him talking about AIDS; his sudden interest surprised them. He attributed it to Joan Abrahamson. On one of their beach walks, she asked him why some were saying that there would be no AIDS vaccine in their lifetime. Salk replied that he didn't know why. "It may not be that difficult." She asked what he would do, and he told her that, as with polio, he would isolate the virus, kill it, potentiate it with adjuvant, inject it into volunteers, and see if he could stimulate an immune response. But, he added, he had no intention of getting back into all that "meanness." The last thing he wanted to do was awaken that again. "I've had it. I've closed my lab. I'm done." When Abrahamson suggested, "Maybe if you got involved, other scientists would, too, because they would rather kill themselves than see you get credit again," he laughed.[15]

It just so happened Robert Gallo was coming to the Institute the next week to seek Salk's advice. "I realized that no one [in the public health service] was responsible for an HIV vaccine," Gallo explained. "It was going to be us. Holy cow. I didn't know anything about vaccines. I thought I'd ask Jonas what to do." They met at the Institute on April 15, 1986. Salk told Gallo that, just as with polio, the day he had identified the HIV virus and succeeded in growing it in tissue culture, he had solved the problem. Gallo knew they could not depend on classical vaccinology, however; an AIDS vaccine required expertise working with retroviruses and proficiency with sophisticated immunologic techniques, and Salk had neither. "Comparing polio to HIV," he told Salk, "is like comparing a baby lamb to a lion."[16] Months later, with no vaccine in sight, Salk ventured into the lion's den.

In June of 1986, Salk and Abrahamson attended the Second International Conference on AIDS in Paris. This annual event brought together scientists, clinicians, community advocates, and the press. As the number of AIDS victims increased, so did the audience. That year, attendees came to witness the debate between Gallo and Montagnier. Gallo had not yet experienced the press's aggressiveness. "I was literally hounded," he recalled. Leaving the podium, a horde of reporters chased him, shouting out questions, snapping pictures. Suddenly Salk appeared at his side, grabbed his arm, and said, "Follow me. I know what to do."[17] He pushed Gallo into the men's room and stood guard. When it became clear Salk would stand there all night if necessary, the reporters left. Besides, they had picked up the scent of Lawrence Lasky.

Lasky, a Genentech scientist, and his colleague Phillip Berman had developed a vaccine to prevent herpes simplex. When Genentech obtained a contract to produce an AIDS blood test, the two had ready access to HIV and set out to make a vaccine. Rather than use a whole virus, they chose a portion of the virus, the glycoprotein envelope. And applying the same genetic-engineering techniques they had used to make the herpes vaccine, they synthesized an HIV envelope protein to use as the vaccine. They vaccinated rabbits and guinea pigs with the envelope protein and found it stimulated production of antibodies that neutralized HIV. When Lasky first revealed their results, a coworker declared, "Larry, they're going to carry you in a sedan chair down Castro Street after this."[18]

Most scientists who considered developing an HIV vaccine planned to use a genetically engineered HIV envelope protein to stimulate antibody formation as Lasky and Berman had done, using a variety of techniques. At the Paris conference, Murray Gardner, chair of the Department of Physiology at the University of California, Davis, reported a different approach. He had isolated a retrovirus, which he thought might be the AIDS virus, from rhesus monkeys ailing from a wasting disease similar to AIDS. He proceeded to make a vaccine from the whole virus, much like Salk's polio vaccine, not from the envelope only. When he inoculated monkeys, they produced neutralizing antibodies. His presentation in Paris piqued Salk's interest. Gardner, a large, unpretentious man, most comfortable in a flannel shirt, jeans, and cowboy boots, soon found himself sipping wine on the balcony of Salk's Paris apartment. He couldn't believe the famous man was serving him hors d'oeuvres, talking as if they were old friends.[19]

Before long, Salk unveiled his strategy for controlling AIDS, one that had a new twist: he intended to vaccinate those already infected with HIV who had not yet developed AIDS. He thought a therapeutic vaccine might provoke the patient's own immune system to attack the virus. In diseases with a short incubation period, like polio and influenza, a vaccine only worked if given prior to exposure. Salk postulated that the prolonged period between HIV infection and progression to AIDS resulted from the immune system's ability to keep the virus in check. If they could boost that response with a vaccine, made from whole, killed virus, they might reduce the viral burden and prevent full-blown AIDS.

Many scientists thought his approach foolhardy, not based on modern immunologic concepts and not using current genetic-engineering techniques. "He missed fifty years of cellular and molecular biology," Lasky observed.[20] As a case in point, when Salk inactivated the virus, the envelope—the cellular component most scientists were utilizing to induce antibody formation—fell off. Salk said he preferred that. As opposed to Lasky and others who focused on neutralizing antibodies, namely, humoral immunity, Salk considered cellular immunity to be far more important in fighting HIV.[21] He thought the exposed virus core could stimulate cell-mediated immunity better than the envelope. Neutralizing antibodies did kill virus in the bloodstream, as with polio, but HIV spent most of its time inside the cells it had taken over. Those were the cells they needed to kill. At the time, Gardner was one of the few who agreed with him.

A review on vaccine strategies in *Science*, a popular journal, predicted Salk's approach would be a disaster. Some thought the immune system had been overly stimulated already; others worried it might accelerate disease progression. "They dismissed it," Salk told Gardner. "I'm willing to start with the premise that they are right, killed virus isn't going to work.... I would like to do the experiments to prove that they are right, and if in the course, we find that they are wrong, then hallelujah."

"Déjà vu," Gardner replied.[22]

While a number of lab groups were trying to determine what part of the protein envelope they should use to make a vaccine, Salk charged ahead. "I can now begin to see how to proceed expeditiously," he dictated into his night notes—now labeled his "AIDS journal"—at 2:30 one morning, calling his approach "a major turning point." A few hours later he wondered, "Can I now plan these in a way that is more certain of success than heretofore and without the pitfalls that were encountered previously?" He knew obtaining FDA approval for human studies would present a high hurdle. "I must move with caution and sensitivity," he dictated the next day at 5:10 a.m., "yet with the courage of my convictions."[23]

UC Davis presented its own obstacles when it came to human studies. AIDS had already generated a tremendous amount of bias and stigma. "Everybody was panicky; everybody was scared," Gardner recalled.[24] Associate Dean Faith Fitzgerald agreed. "There was concern that the ravening hordes would come up from San Francisco and contaminate the community." Only four AIDS patients could be admitted to the hospital at one time; many medical staff refused to care for them. "It was a grim situation," she reported, "with Kaposi and *Pneumocystis* patients dying all around us. The syphilitics were treated better. It was Armageddon."[25] Fitzgerald and infectious disease specialist Neil Flynn pressed the hospital director to designate eight beds for AIDS patients at the back of the hospital, staffed by volunteer nurses.

Work at UC Davis was progressing too slowly for Salk, when, in the spring of 1986, Kevin Kimberlin, a thirty-three-year-old entrepreneur, contacted him about starting a company to produce an AIDS vaccine. Fresh from obtaining an MBA at Harvard, Kimberlin had moved to New York City, where the tragedy of AIDS shocked him. "I was a child of the sixties," he said, "of the culture where you really did believe John Lennon when he said we could change the world."[26] He started reading about AIDS and talking to leaders in health care. "AIDS had been neglected in the face of the daunting horror of HIV," he concluded. One day, while browsing through periodicals in a medical library, he came upon a notice in a microbiology journal about the celebration of the fortieth anniversary of the polio field trial, with an accompanying photograph of Jonas Salk. "It was very strange, because he just seemed to come alive in that picture and talk to me."[27] Compelled to contact Salk, Kimberlin began calling the Institute, leaving numerous messages but getting no reply.

Weeks later, Kimberlin traveled to the West Coast to talk to AIDS specialists. He had returned to his hotel room, discouraged by the defeatist attitude, when the phone rang. "I was in the shower, a full head of soap," he recalled. "I reached out and picked up the phone to hear 'Jonas Salk, returning your phone call.'" After waiting for weeks, "I didn't dare say, 'Let me call you at a more convenient time.' So I just stood there stark naked, giving Dr. Salk my impassioned plea that this was the time for a new vaccine."[28] Leery of biotechnology salesmen, Salk demurred. Still, Kimberlin persisted until he agreed to meet.

Sitting in Salk's La Jolla living room, they talked about vaccines in general. When Kimberlin tried to direct the discussion to AIDS, Salk remained reticent, not yet revealing his UC Davis work. Kimberlin knew it would take time to build trust. To converse with Salk, he had to understand basic immunology. So he started a crash course—on his honeymoon. His wife snapped a photo of him sitting on an isolated Caribbean beach with an immunology textbook on his lap.

Subsequently, Kimberlin and Salk took many walks on the La Jolla beach or met at Gilot's Fifth Avenue apartment. A warm relationship developed between them. Kimberlin found Salk more endearing than he imagined. "I'm just a foot soldier in the battle against AIDS," Salk used to tell him. "I'm just a volunteer."[29] He had never been associated with a corporate endeavor; the sources of capital for the polio vaccine had been the March of Dimes. Kimberlin told Salk the fastest way to produce and test an AIDS vaccine would be to gather together a dedicated group of scientists and fund them properly. He thought he could raise a hundred million dollars and help Salk attract the right kind of talent. "Let's build a company," Kimberlin said with boyish enthusiasm.[30]

Salk became intrigued after he looked at a draft of the business plan, which read in part: "There is a necessity and the opportunity to accelerate a program for developing, testing, and making available products to arrest the progress of the AIDS pandemic.... A unique and cost-effective strategy has been proposed based on concepts conceived and designed by Jonas Salk to bring product development, approval and clinical testing in less than two years."[31] The plan called for establishing a research and manufacturing facility to produce a therapeutic vaccine for those testing HIV positive. Salk began to understand that the world of science had changed; industry had become a major source of funding for research. He agreed to serve as a consultant and advisory board chairman for their new company, Immune Response Corporation (IRC), but insisted his payment be in the form of an honorarium. According to Kimberlin, "This whole association with the corporate world was not in his comfort zone."[32]

"Everyone loses and no one wins if the problem of AIDS goes unchecked, if it goes uncontrolled, if it goes unsolved," Salk wrote in his AIDS journal. "Immune Response Corp is a new entity for this purpose, unencumbered by the past." He called the proposal "liberating."[33] As they began specific planning, their mutual excitement grew. Kimberlin didn't tell Salk he was paying the bills for their fledgling company with his personal credit card. Before the year had ended, however, he had raised millions of dollars, and IRC became incorporated. They were going to change the world.

At the same time, Salk was playing another crucial role in the HIV saga—as a Solomon the Wise for Robert Gallo and Luc Montagnier, who were quarreling over who deserved credit for discovering the AIDS virus.[34] The argument had erupted in 1985 when the Pasteur Institute sued the US government, charging that Gallo's lab had misappropriated Montagnier's virus in developing his AIDS blood test. A legal battle had been raging for two years. Neither contender had public appeal. Abrupt and brash, forty-five-year-old Gallo welcomed debate and could be heard shouting as he challenged colleagues. Some called him charismatic; others haughty, egotistical. Montagnier, five years his senior, did not like to argue. Formal in demeanor and taciturn, he remained aloof. "I was hit hard by the controversy," Salk told a journalist. He felt it had so contaminated the field that if it wasn't settled, it might do damage to those seeking to help with the AIDS crisis. "I had no authority. I wasn't asked by anybody. It just occurred to me that there may be some way of mediating this so everybody gets something."[35]

Gallo trusted Salk, as did the French scientific community, but the task proved arduous. Over a two-year period, Salk made numerous transcontinental flights, meeting in Paris cafes, Washington cocktail lounges, and San Diego restaurants, talking to each scientist alone, then together, moving slowly, point by point. Salk listed the commonalities between the two accounts and the chronology, trying to construct a single storyline. Without blame, reprimand, or secret deals, he got them to sign a seven-page document detailing an agreed-upon chronology, including their individual contributions.[36] On April 1, 1987, President Reagan and Prime Minister Jacques Chirac, in a formal ceremony, announced that Montagnier and Gallo shared credit for discovering the AIDS virus and jointly owned the blood test patent.

While Salk was negotiating a peace settlement, Kimberlin was setting up the Immune Response Corporation. He moved quickly, as he estimated the first AIDS vaccine would monopolize a $100 million market. He hired Jim Glavin, a top Wall Street analyst and CEO of Genetic Systems, to run the company and Dennis Carlo as the chief scientific officer/chief operating officer. Smart and experienced, Carlo had worked on vaccine development for years at Merck and Eli Lily and was, as one colleague called him, "a superb salesman of science."[37]

Many thought the friendship between Carlo, a burly, fast-talking entrepreneur, and Salk, an elegantly dressed, soft-spoken scientific philosopher, surprising—"a portrait of opposites,"[38] the "odd couple."[39] Perhaps in Carlo Salk detected a bit of Basil O'Connor with a gold chain instead of a white carnation. And Carlo found the energy of the seventy-three-year-old Salk amazing. He recalled a typical day together: During a trans-Atlantic flight, Salk didn't sleep or watch a movie; he designed new experiments. Upon landing, they attended an hours-long meeting; during dinner Salk suggested a new way to interpret their data, "all with the mind of a forty-year-old." At midnight, he called Carlo about a graph he was looking at from a different angle, then asked, "I didn't wake you up, did I?" The next day he showed Carlo thoughts he had written in his journal, marked 2:00 a.m. "He was always going, always moving," Carlo observed. "He was consumed by AIDS." Carlo began to appreciate something else about Salk: "When Jonas thought he was right, he would never give up. Never. He would just keep on preaching his concept, no matter what anyone said."[40] A hard-charging executive scientist, Carlo seemed the perfect match for Salk. "Nothing was going to get in their way," an IRC coworker said. "We were going to get this trial done and get this to work."[41]

Like Salk, Carlo believed the whole-killed-virus vaccine made the most sense. "We thought the key to the treasure was cell-mediated immunity." Since the virus was hiding inside cells, they planned to make a vaccine that would induce T-cells to recognize and destroy infected cells. "If we're right," Salk warned Carlo, "they'll never forgive us," referring to members of the scientific community.[42]

Soon IRC had four million dollars in the bank. Although their business plan included immune therapies for several diseases, their first undertaking was an AIDS vaccine, starting with experiments on chimps. Since they had no lab at the time, they contracted with NIH researcher Joseph Gibbs. Carlo found a small commercial lab in Orange County, which, with Salk's guidance, prepared the inactivated vaccine. After inoculating the chimpanzees, Gibbs could measure antibodies against HIV as well as changes in cell-mediated immunity. It would take a year, however, to determine if the vaccine could protect the animals when exposed to live HIV. In 1987, *Nature* published Salk's first AIDS article, "Prospects for the Control of AIDS," which outlined his theory for using a whole-killed-virus vaccine to treat those already infected.[43] "A Tough Old Soldier Joins the Fight against AIDS" reported *Business Week*.[44] "New, Unorthodox Strategy on AIDS Proposed by Salk," read a headline in the *New York Times*.[45]

Washington, DC, hosted the Third International Conference on AIDS in June 1987. French scientist Dan Zagury gave the most publicized presentation on the first human vaccine trial. Zagury had made an AIDS vaccine, inoculated himself, and then with no animal studies to test for efficacy or safety proceeded to vaccinate healthy children in Zaire. The trial generated more ethical debates than advances in the field. He had not obtained informed consent and had ignored international consensus that children should not be used in AIDS vaccine trials. He had no way to determine if the vaccine would protect them from infection and refused to let NIH investigators review his records.[46]

Salk and Carlo returned from the conference anxious to start their own human trial. They knew their vaccine was safe and could generate an immune response. It seemed unnecessary to wait another year or more to finish the animal trial, but that was an FDA requirement. So they proceeded to maneuver around the FDA. With the support from the gay population and California governor George Deukmejian, Salk appealed to the state legislature to pass a law allowing the California Department of Health Services to authorize regulatory approval for testing and sales of new AIDS drugs as long as investigators conducted the trials in state.[47] And they assented. Carlo submitted paperwork to the Food and Drug Branch of the California Department of Health Services seeking permission for toxicity testing of the Salk AIDS immunotherapeutic, as IRC called it to distinguish this therapeutic vaccine from a preventive one.[48] That end run perturbed the FDA and would prove problematic later when IRC sought approval to extend their studies outside California.

Salk continued collaborating with Murray Gardner and AIDS specialist Neil Flynn at UC Davis. Flynn had recruited fifty HIV-positive men desperate to try anything to survive. Salk insisted upon keeping the work confidential to avert a media frenzy as well as the expected disparagement from the scientific community. He may have managed that in the early 1950s at the Watson Home, but openness in research had changed substantially, and UC Davis was a public university. Still, he insisted on secrecy. Gardner assured him he would say nothing.

"Somewhere down the line I was giving a talk," Gardner recounted, "and, by golly, I let the cat out of the bag." A *Sacramento Bee* reporter was present, and Gardner extracted a promise from her to keep their plans confidential. "By God," Gardner lamented, "it came out in the headlines: 'Salk Vaccine to Be Tested in Patients in Sacramento.' I was just devastated. I couldn't sleep. I called Jonas and begged for his forgiveness." Salk told him this had happened to him a number of times. "You live and you learn," he consoled Gardner.[49] He started to pull away from UC Davis after that, and Gardner blamed himself. But his faux pas was not the main reason; Salk found the UC Davis medical school administration unwelcoming. They considered him manipulative, using the school for his own aggrandizement; they didn't want a one-man show.

In the summer of 1987, Randy Shilts's best-selling book, *And the Band Played On*, shocked the public with its graphic description of AIDS and the devastating effect on the gay community. Florida's Desoto County School Board refused to allow HIV-positive brothers Ricky, Robert, and Randy Ray to attend school in the county. When a federal judge ordered the board to reinstate the three hemophiliacs, who contracted HIV through contaminated factor VIII, outraged residents refused to let their children go to school. Someone set fire to the Ray home, destroying it. That summer, the FDA approved the first human testing of an AIDS vaccine, but it was not Salk's.

Salk and IRC needed to find a compatible clinical team for their human trials. Walking on the beach one day, Salk happened across Brian Henderson, chief of oncology at the University of Southern California (USC) in Los Angeles. When Salk mentioned his problem, Henderson told him that he had the perfect collaborator. Clinician-scientist Alexandra Levine was studying AIDS-associated lymphomas as well as the early stages of HIV infection before patients developed any symptoms. At the time, she had taken a leave, grieving the recent deaths of both her parents from cancer. "That was the worst time of my life," Levine recalled. "I didn't seem to have a reason to live."[50] A week after her mother's death, Henderson called to say Jonas Salk would like to speak with her. In deference to her period of ritual mourning, Salk offered to fly to Los Angeles and meet after she finished morning prayers at the synagogue.

When Salk entered the USC conference room, the first thing he did was give Levine a hug and tell her how appreciative he was of her being there. Levine could not equate this Jonas Salk with the figure some called egotistical, a limelight seeker. Over time, she got to know a different man, a kind and considerate man who was uncomfortable with public recognition. "He ended up bringing me back to life."[51]

Together Levine and Salk wrote their first human trial. In study 1A/B, patients with known HIV infection at an early stage would be inoculated with the Salk AIDS immunotherapeutic. Three months later, patients would receive a booster shot. Immune function and viral load would be measured before and after vaccination. After they submitted their protocol, Salk, Carlo, Henderson, and Levine spent an entire day with officials from the Food and Drug Branch of the California Department of Health Services in intense negotiations trying to persuade them to approve the study. "They put us through our paces," Carlo recalled. At the day's end, they approved the trial. Salk and Carlo flew back to San Diego in high spirits. "I'm going to take a little vacation," Salk told Carlo.

"You deserve one," he said. "Where are you going?"

"I'm going to the hospital," Salk replied. "I have to have some minor surgery." Carlo asked if he had a prostate problem. Salk laughed. "No." he said. "I'm going to have a triple bypass."[52] Carlo was even more shocked when Salk's secretary met him at the airport and drove him straight to Sharp Hospital, where he had open-heart surgery the next day. When Levine found out, she delayed initiating the trial until Salk could return to USC. She would not start without him.

⁂

ON A NOVEMBER day in 1987, the first injection of the Salk AIDS immunotherapeutic took place at the USC medical center. A photo of the occasion shows a muscular thirty-year-old white male lying in bed, Levine sitting next to him. On the far side stand Salk, Carlo, and several others. No one from the press witnessed or even knew about the event. As they proceeded to vaccinate other subjects, Salk insisted on meeting them, thanking them for participating. Levine noticed their excitement when they met Salk; several cried when he touched them. "The patients in our study adored him," she recalled, "and he, in turn, knew each of them, knew their stories, and genuinely cared for them and for their families.... They were numbers in our study, but they were people to Jonas."[53]

In June of 1988, Salk presented an early analysis of their trial at the Fourth International AIDS Conference in Stockholm. When he arrived, a cadre of reporters followed him—"like the Pied Piper," Gardner observed—taking pictures, trying to elicit comments.[54] Some of the younger scientists were surprised to see Salk was still around. When he started to speak about a whole, inactivated immunogen, harking back to his polio vaccine, several in the audience got up and left. Senior virologist Joseph Melnick called Salk "the Rip Van Winkle of virology," returning after a long sleep. "And when he came back, he thought science was exactly where he left it."[55]

Unperturbed, Salk proceeded to present preliminary data on their study: Of nineteen patients inoculated with their immunotherapeutic, sixteen had no progression to AIDS.[56] CD4 T-helper lymphocyte count increased, indicating their immune systems were regaining strength. And they experienced no toxicity. In the questions that followed, Levine found several to be deprecating, as if the scientists were implying, "Here's an old-fashioned scientist doing this killed vaccine like this was polio. We have the technology of molecular biology. We will solve this."[57] Salk made no promises to the AIDS community, but his presence in the field brought them hope.

Meanwhile, Neil Flynn had anticipated opening a trial with Salk at UC Davis. When he learned in Stockholm that Salk had already started a study with Levine, he was upset. "UCD Drops Plan to Test Salk's AIDS Vaccine," reported the *Sacramento Bee*.[58] University officials said they had withdrawn from the trial because data compiled on the Salk vaccine was insufficient to justify inoculating their volunteers. An interview with an AIDS patient conducted three days later revealed the depth of disappointment felt by the ninety-five people waiting to enter the trial. "We don't know why Dr. Salk did not turn over the vaccine to us," Flynn told the reporter. "You'll have to ask him."[59]

Salk usually ignored what was said about him in the press, but the words of the distraught individual prompted him to write Dean Hibbard Williams to set the record straight. He had planned to test HIV-positive volunteers at UC Davis once he had prepared a vaccine, but Flynn had told him he had to secure FDA permission first, and he did not yet have FDA approval. Furthermore, Salk explained, "Dr. Flynn announced prematurely, without consulting me, the initiation at UC Davis of studies of the 'Salk vaccine.'" He chose to interview patients and keep them on hold. "I do not usually comment to the press," he added, "and hope that UC Davis will not put me in a position where I will be forced to do so."[60] With that, the squall ended.

Meanwhile, IRC and USC opened a larger study, 1C, involving fifty-four HIV-infected people who had not yet shown symptoms or signs of AIDS.[61] Half received vaccine, half no treatment. At twenty-eight weeks, they found more than a third of those vaccinated had no measurable virus in their blood. After six months, they inoculated the untreated group and found improved immunity in those subjects as well.

It looked as if they were making headway, when Salk developed severe back pain and lost sensation in his lower left leg, requiring a laminectomy to remove fragments of a shattered disc. He recovered in time to travel to Montreal for the Fifth International Conference on AIDS, held in June of 1989. There he presented his and Gibbs's animal study.[62] They had inoculated one uninfected and two HIV-infected chimpanzees with their immunotherapeutic. A year later, Gibbs had injected live HIV into all three. The two previously infected chimps mounted a cellular response and no longer had any evident infection. "Salk says tests of vaccine show halt of AIDS infection in chimps," reported the *New York Times*. A prominent AIDS researcher from Duke, Dani Bolognesi, told the Montreal audience that Salk's results represented "the beginning of piercing the armor."[63] And Salk was quoted as saying, "It's becoming clear that a diagnosis of HIV positivity need not be regarded as a death sentence."[64]

What the IRC needed to do now was confirm its findings from the USC trials. That meant conducting a randomized, blinded study, comparing vaccine to placebo in a large number of HIV-infected individuals. Because they planned on using sites outside California, they needed FDA approval. The relationship between the FDA and IRC was far from congenial. After all, IRC had maneuvered around them and obtained approval from the California Department of Health Services. Negotiations soon became charged. IRC wanted to use "intermediary" endpoints—clearing of HIV from the blood and enhanced immune function—to prove vaccine efficacy. The FDA required a comparison of death rates between the two groups as the trial's endpoint. Since they were enrolling subjects early in the course of the disease, this meant that the trial could take up to seven years to complete. They argued this point for some time. CEO James Glavin thought, in retrospect, that IRC's approach to the FDA worked against them. He described Salk as "passive resistant" in meetings. "He'd give them this Aristotelian response, sort of dismiss them in a fatherly way." Nor did the FDA like Salk's ready access to the press or the way he used it. Glavin also thought Dennis Carlo acted too aggressively, in essence telling the FDA, "Just get out of our way, and we'll fix this thing for you." At some point, Glavin recalled, the FDA simply "dug in their heels regardless of what we showed them."[65]

The pressure was on, however. In 1989, the CDC tallied eighty-eight thousand deaths from AIDS. One of them was Frederic de Hoffmann. Five years earlier, de Hoffmann had undergone a coronary bypass operation at Harvard, where he had sought out the nation's best cardiac surgeon.[66] While still recovering in the hospital, he developed a high fever and pronounced personality change, later determined to be an acute but rare manifestation of HIV infection. Blood transfused during his operation was traced to a donor who had died of AIDS. After he recovered, de Hoffmann returned to the Salk Institute, but he never seemed the same. As his thinking became more deranged, staff tried to avoid him. "It was terrible to watch," recalled the chief financial officer, Delbert Glanz. "Here was one of the smartest men I've ever known, and to see him go downhill mentally was shattering."[67] The man who had controlled the Institute for fifteen years could no longer control himself. In October of 1989, de Hoffmann died at age sixty-five from complications of AIDS. How ironic that the scientist de Hoffmann had tried to expel from the Institute was developing a therapeutic vaccine which, if effective, might have saved him.

At the Sixth International Conference on AIDS, held in San Francisco in 1990, Alexandra Levine updated results from the USC studies, conducted in collaboration with IRC.[68] To date they had vaccinated eighty-two HIV-positive individuals with the Salk immunotherapeutic and observed no toxicity. They measured enhanced cellular immunity in 60 percent, and those patients cleared the virus from their systems more readily. The FDA, she announced, had approved a large-scale, randomized trial to begin in several months. In his talk, "Perspectives on an AIDS Vaccine," Salk told the audience, "I must say that the confrontation with HIV is a very humbling experience. The ingenuity of this virus has really outwitted us thus far... [but] we will not be outwitted for long."[69] Daniel Hoth, an AIDS director at the NIH, admired Salk's energy—he recalled him "running up to the microphone, making points, questioning speakers, highly engaged." At the same time, Hoth described the IRC group as "slick and fast with its presentations," and Salk as "a master" at bedazzling the press and public.[70]

◈

By THE END of 1990, almost twice as many Americans had died from AIDS-related diseases as had perished in the Vietnam War. Thus, British scientist James Stott's announcement in May of 1991 generated great interest. Stott had injected live simian immunodeficiency virus (SIV), the monkey equivalent of HIV, into macaques and found those previously inoculated with a vaccine made from genetically engineered envelope proteins became infected; those inoculated with a whole, killed vaccine did not. These results gave credence to Salk's approach. For years, he had been stressing that the key to attacking the AIDS virus lay not in antibody production but in cell-mediated immunity, whereby lymphocytes identified and annihilated cells infected by HIV. And the whole, killed vaccine was better at stimulating cellular immunity. "It's as if I continue to be invisible," he told a reporter. "A number of times I've gotten up and spoken about cell-mediated immunity at these meetings, and there's been dead silence."[71]

At the Seventh International Conference on AIDS in Florence, Italy, the NIH AIDS division posted results from all the animal trials to date. Genetically engineered envelope vaccines protected 13 percent of monkeys from infection; the whole, killed vaccine, 69 percent. Salk's approach had trumped the one favored by most scientists, at least in monkeys. When talk of large trials began and a researcher asked if they should consider a whole, inactivated vaccine, Carlo stated: "It's almost unethical not to."[72] IRC's stock rose.

As 1993 began, AIDS made the front pages again. Ballet dancer Rudolf Nureyev and tennis star Arthur Ashe both died from AIDS-related illnesses. That year saw the first Hollywood film on AIDS,

Philadelphia, starring Tom Hanks as a lawyer suffering from the disease. *Angels in America*, Tony Kushner's play about AIDS, won the Tony Award for best play and the Pulitzer Prize for drama. And three antiviral drugs began to show promise in delaying the onset of AIDS in HIV-infected individuals.

In early June, fifteen thousand gathered at the Ninth International Conference on AIDS, held in Berlin. Activists delivered the opening speeches, filled with fiery rhetoric, "urging scientists to collaborate on finding a cure," reported *Global AIDSnews*, "rather than competing with each other in order to win a Nobel prize."[73] The AIDS community worried that if the conference ended on a pessimistic note, scientists, physicians, and the government would assume a defeatist stance. They needed to hear positive news, and for that many looked to Salk.

Levine had been selected to present the results of their latest trial of their therapeutic vaccine at the plenary session. As she and Salk entered the auditorium, a crush of reporters obstructed the aisle, making a ruckus as they followed the two to their seats, shouting out, "Does it work? Does it work?" Levine was puzzled by the attention, unaware that a press release, crafted by Carlo, had preempted her presentation. At issue was the randomized trial of their HIV immunotherapeutic, now known as the "Salk vaccine." Conducted in nine US medical centers, it involved 103 asymptomatic HIV-infected subjects. Half received three doses of vaccine, half placebo. Carlo had disclosed to the press that they had just unblinded the results and that the treated group had substantial improvement in cellular immunity and reduction of viral load.[74] Thus it was with high expectations that the audience awaited Levine's talk. But she did not start by announcing, "The vaccine works," as many had anticipated. Instead she concluded that the time frame had been too short to determine whether or not the vaccine could halt the progression to AIDS.[75]

Salk tried to absorb the brunt of what followed. Scientists said the techniques used by Levine and Salk had not yet been validated; they considered the differences between the two groups minor. "I'm less than enthusiastic," said David Ho, a New York AIDS researcher. "We simply don't know what these markers mean," remarked Dani Bolognesi. The small changes didn't make him confident of the vaccine's benefit. British virologist Robin Weiss called the presentation "a dog-and-pony show."[76]

"Jonas was practically dragged into a press conference," Kimberlin recounted. "He was trying to settle everybody down, but it was a paparazzi kind of thing."[77] The *Los Angeles Times* called it "a media jamboree that only Salk, with his love-hate relationship with the limelight, could attract." The paper went on to report: "As cameras rolled and reporters scribbled during a news conference that was linked by satellite to the United States, the 78-year-old scientist simply smiled and shrugged off the attacks." When confronted about their inconclusive results, Salk replied, "It's the first whiff of spring, you might say."[78]

Then came the outcry from AIDS activists. They had been awaiting a miracle, and when none emerged, their animosity was palpable. "Hopes Are Dashed on AIDS Therapy," announced the *New York Times*.[79] IRC stock dropped. Well-known AIDS epidemiologist Don Francis put the situation into perspective, however, when he told the press, "Now we should try to ignore the hype and the past and look at the data." Others retracted their skepticism once they read the published report. Bolognesi, who earlier had expressed no confidence in the results, now called them "enticing."[80]

The time had come for a large national field trial to test whether Salk's vaccine could delay or prevent progression to AIDS in those infected with HIV. As 1993 came to a close, the cumulative number of cases topped four hundred thousand; more than half had died. "Dennis," Salk told Carlo, "we've got to do this before I die."[81]

Unbowed

Thirty-four-year-old NIH researcher Ron Moss had just moved to California to direct the clinical trials for the Immune Response Corporation when Salk invited him and his family over on Thanksgiving Day. He was surprised to find Salk alone. "Come on in," Salk said. "Let me get some toys for your kids and see if I have anything for them to eat."

As they sat talking, Moss asked his five-year-old son, Ben, "Do you have any questions for the famous Dr. Salk?" Looking up at the ceiling, his son replied, "Yes. Dr. Salk, why do you have so many cobwebs on your ceiling?"

"Don't you wish you knew what goes on in their little heads," the amused Salk said to Moss. Then he smiled and asked Ben, "Would you like something else to eat?"[1]

⦙⦙⦙

Jonas Salk was a solitary man. Françoise's new book, *Matisse and Picasso: A Friendship in Art*, had come out, keeping her busy with its publicity. After interviewing her, a *Los Angeles Times* writer commented: "While the public's fascination with Gilot stems largely from her intimate relationships with two great men—a source of great annoyance for her—she would prefer to be thought of not as their significant other, but as their equal." By this point Gilot lived in California only a couple of months each winter and summer. "If not for my husband," she told the writer, "I would not spend five minutes in La Jolla."[2] She did return for Jonas's eightieth birthday party but left the next day.

Salk enjoyed spending time with his five grandsons whenever he could, but Jonathan had a busy psychiatry practice in Los Angeles, and Darrell worked for a biotechnology firm in Seattle. Although Peter lived in La Jolla, he and his family spent most summers in Ohio. When in town, they invited Jonas for occasional dinners. Peter's wife, artist Ellen Schreibman, noted that Salk didn't like small talk. "It's all concerns about the world," she told a journalist.[3] Friends thought he spent more time with his housekeeper and gardener, Jose, than with his family.

Both of Salk's brothers had died. Herman, a beloved Palm Springs veterinarian, had a heart attack, then a series of strokes, and passed away on February 23, 1992. Lee, a popular New York child psychologist, author, and television personality, succumbed to esophageal cancer two months later. In August of 1990, Lee had undergone an esophagectomy, followed by numerous complications, including eight weeks in intensive care, seven weeks on a respirator, kidney failure requiring dialysis, infections, and heart problems. Lee's young wife, Mary Jane, married to him less than two years, felt bewildered. Jonas came for the surgery and stayed, checking Lee's medical chart and making suggestions to his physicians. He maintained an aura of calm while his brother faced one problem after another—inability to eat, cancer recurrence, chemotherapy, uncontrollable pain—providing nursing for Lee and support for Mary Jane. "He gave up his own life to help us," she said.[4] The brothers bonded again, laughing, mainly about their mother, and crying. On May 2, 1992, Lee had just received a chemotherapy infusion when he had a cardiac arrest and died.

Seeking companionship, Salk resumed his monthly dinners with Ted Mohns, the occasional lunch with Antonio Damasio, nightly calls to Joan Abrahamson, and visits from Carol Anne Bundy and Heather Wood Ion. Nevertheless, he spent most of his time thinking about AIDS, working mainly with Ron Moss, the young medical director of IRC who had been hired to help initiate the large clinical trial of the Salk vaccine. Sub rosa, he was to serve as the go-between for Salk and IRC, keeping Salk updated on the vaccine's progress and relating back his ideas on its testing. Although Salk had served on IRC's scientific advisory board for years, Moss was told that he was not to attend its meetings. He understood why. In order to get its vaccine approved by the FDA, IRC needed to work with key AIDS opinion leaders, several of whom had expressed annoyance about Salk's entry into the field. A number of them told Carlo they would not work with IRC if Salk was involved. So Moss met with him at the Institute or in his home.

Moss soon discovered that, although fifty years his senior, Salk had a phenomenal understanding of biology—and that his relegation to the sidelines disheartened him. He wanted to be actively involved with the AIDS vaccine. As their discussions moved from data analysis to Judaism to life's lessons, Moss became quite fond of Salk, calling every moment with him "magical." Salk enjoyed their chats, too. "It seemed to me he lived a lonely life for such an eminent man," Moss said.[5]

Abrahamson disagreed. She thought Salk was a good loner. He needed solitude; it had not been imposed upon him.[6] Still optimistic at eighty, Salk was wrestling nonetheless with a number of unresolved challenges: The Public Health Service had not yet adopted a standardized approach to influenza, and he feared another devastating pandemic. Although Sabin's vaccine caused most cases of paralyzing polio in the United States, it had become entrenched. Salk had not cured cancer or multiple sclerosis. Now IRC had reached an impasse with the FDA. The Salk Institute had never realized his vision of melding science and humanism. And few understood his metabiological concerns about man's future.

In actuality, not all of these issues remained unresolved forever and should be considered part of his legacy. Just out of medical training, Salk and Thomas Francis, Jr., had made the first effective influenza vaccine. Beyond that, Salk had found that by adding mineral oil adjuvant, he could enhance the antibody response, requiring a smaller amount of virus per vaccine dose. That meant multiple viral strains could be incorporated into one shot, giving broader protection. Although concerns that mineral oil might cause cancer had hampered acceptance of his idea, the scientific community eventually recognized the benefits of adjuvants. In 2008, adjuvant-containing vaccines against avian flu would be approved for use in the European Union.[7] NIH scientist Anthony Fauci would write in 2010, "Adjuvants may be critically important in future vaccination programs."[8] And even though Salk had been unsuccessful in his efforts to effect widespread influenza vaccination, in 2010 the US Advisory Committee on Immunization Practices recommended influenza vaccination for everyone older than six months. Salk would have been astounded to see drugstores and groceries offering on-site vaccination while patrons shopped.

The prevention of poliomyelitis represents Salk's greatest achievement—and in some ways the source of his greatest dismay. Since 1979, when fifteen unvaccinated Amish contracted polio from contacts in Ontario, Canada, the United States had had no further cases from the natural virus. Still, eight to ten people developed paralysis each year from the live vaccine (OPV) developed by Sabin. Modern molecular techniques determined the cause to be the poliovirus used in OPV, yet it remained the US vaccine of choice. Several countries already had switched to inactivated polio vaccine (IPV), including France, Canada, the Netherlands, Iceland, and the Scandinavian countries; all remained polio-free. Salk, who likened the live/killed polio vaccine debate to "a holy war," had fought for more than twenty years to get OPV delicensed and IPV reinstated. Trying every tactic possible, he had been blocked in large part by the politics of science. "I keep looking for a court of last resort," he once said in an interview, "a supreme court, where I can go to see to it that ethics prevail."[9]

Eventually Salk realized that to convince American physicians and public health officials about the superiority of IPV he had to design a better vaccine, one that overrode all their criticisms. With pharmaceutical magnate Charles Mérieux and Dutch scientist Toon van Wezel, he developed an enhanced inactivated vaccine, eIPV, which could be mixed in one shot with other childhood vaccines. Still, the major US decision-makers resisted change. "Before, the limiting factor was technology," Salk told a reporter. "Now it is human nature. The world needs more creative, more wise compassion."[10]

Sabin's voice had weakened as his health deteriorated. Even after his open-heart surgery and with the residual weakness from a mysterious

paralysis that followed neck surgery, the octogenarian continued to oppose Salk. Their decades-long dispute ended when Sabin suffered a stroke
and became comatose. Debbe Sabin informed the medical team treating
her father: "Years ago, he told me if he ever had a stroke and became veg-
etative, to take a gun and shoot him. So please put him on morphine and
let him die."[11] Albert Sabin died on March 4, 1993, and was buried in
Arlington National Cemetery. He died believing that he alone would be
credited with ridding the world of polio. Two years after Sabin's death, the
Institute of Medicine and the Centers for Disease Control and Prevention
held a meeting to consider a change in vaccine policy. "It's about time,"
Salk told Abrahamson.[12] In 1999, the US government would replace the
Sabin vaccine with the newer version of Salk's vaccine.

No one would contest that the Salk Institute remains one of the
world's premier research institutes. "It's only half my dream, the biology
half of my dream," Salk told CEO Charles Massey in 1995. "The humanity half of my dream has not been fulfilled. So I'm only half happy."[13]
Some had thought the whole concept foolhardy from the beginning. "It
was a romantic vision of science," concluded researcher Larry Lasky:
"put people in a beautiful place, and they will come up with beautiful
ideas. But what drives a scientist is funding and publishing his next
paper."[14] Damasio thought Salk was simply ahead of his time, a visionary
trying to marry two disparate partners. Although initially called "The
Thirty Million Dollar Temple of Thought" by the press, it has, since its
inception, attracted a cadre of National Academy of Science members
and Nobel Prize laureates.[15] And Louis Kahn's masterpiece represents
one of the country's finest architectural achievements.

Salk had imagined the Institute, perched on a cliff above the ocean,
would serve as his refuge, yet the conflicts he faced in its founding would
have defeated a lesser man. Some Institute scientists respected neither
his work, nor his ideas, nor him. Frederic de Hoffmann had tried to banish
him altogether. Salk told Massey he felt like a pariah in his own house. Yet
when he walked up the steps onto the plaza and gazed out to sea, especially
as the sun set, he felt a sense of awe, as if he were seeing it for the first time.

While engaged in battle over the polio vaccine and building the
Institute, Salk had set out to harness the immune system. That meant
initiating research in cancer and multiple sclerosis that ranged from

laboratory to clinical studies. Although cancer biologists did not recognize any contribution of import, neuroscientists at the time held him in high regard for his work on EAE and MBP. His human trial looked promising until Harry Weaver died and Salk ran out of funds. Still in a field dominated by basic scientists, Salk had goaded researchers to move toward clinical application and in doing so raised public awareness of the disease.

Prevention of polio and influenza and treatment of multiple sclerosis were concrete endeavors; Salk's foray into metabiology was not. His books and lectures expressed his concern for mankind's future, emphasizing the need to be good ancestors. In his night notes, he wrote that he viewed himself as "a scientist-humanist, a scientist devoted to trying to understand what human life is all about."[16] He attempted to spread his message, and many of his torchbearers have done so to some extent. Yet, as Carol Anne Bundy put it, "He suffered the angst of a visionary."[17]

And now, toward the end of his life, there was his AIDS vaccine. Salk's self-worth had always centered on his physician-scientist role, and it was slipping away. When the desperate need for an AIDS vaccine became apparent, Salk found a raison d'être. Kevin Kimberlin entered his life at a pivotal point. He, Dennis Carlo, Murray Gardner, and Alexandra Levine revered Salk, empowered him, and became his friends. In doing so, they revitalized him.

The time had come to prove whether or not the Salk AIDS vaccine could halt this devastating disease. By 1993, negotiations between IRC and the FDA had gone on for nearly a decade. Although the FDA did not believe in a whole-virus therapeutic vaccine, it could no longer rebuff IRC, as the company had demonstrated the vaccine's safety and its efficacy in stimulating immunity, reducing the viral load. The FDA finally allowed the company to proceed with a randomized trial of 2,500 HIV-positive individuals at seventy-seven medical centers. To avoid conflict of interest, an outside group was selected to conduct the trial. San Francisco AIDS specialist James Kahn and Harvard statistician Stephen Lagakos agreed to serve as national co-leaders. They added one stipulation, which, although ethical, proved fatal to the trial's ultimate analysis: while on the trial, patients could take antivirals, newly approved drugs which block HIV's life cycle. By 1995, more than a half million Americans had contracted AIDS. The definitive trial of Salk's vaccine was set to begin.

When the final chapter of AIDS is written, its story will feature hundreds of virologists, epidemiologists, immunologists, pathologists, and clinicians who spent their careers trying to decipher, treat, and prevent AIDS. Pharmaceutical and biotechnology companies rose and fell, rushing to be the first to capture the world market on a vaccine. Few will associate Salk's name with AIDS. If mentioned at all, he will be portrayed as a minor character in this great saga. Some dismissed his efforts as those of an old man attempting to recapture his former glory. "That's bullshit," Robert Gallo argued. "Anyone who says that didn't know the man."[18] Others called him innovating, inspiring, a pioneer, and his entry into the AIDS arena a noble gesture. When Gallo and Montagnier seemed at an impasse, one that threatened to obstruct progress in the field, Salk took it upon himself to help mediate the dispute. When researchers scoffed at Salk's idea of using a whole, killed virus vaccine to stimulate cellular immunity, he dared them to prove him wrong, and in so doing challenged them to reconsider their stance. When few were considering therapeutic interventions, waiting until they had deciphered how HIV destroyed the immune system, Salk charged forward, knowing thousands would die for every year of procrastination. And by attracting the media, Salk helped make the public understand AIDS wasn't just about gay men, but an illness with which they all had to deal.

Perhaps Salk's greatest, yet unstated, disappointment was not scientific or administrative but rather his inability to form an all-encompassing, intimate relationship with another human being. His family, friends, wives, and lovers never provided that missing piece. "My dad had a deep loneliness," attested Jonathan, "a need for connection and companionship that was never really fully satisfied in his life."[19] Although he was genuinely warm and social, his drive to solve the world's problems isolated him. In later years, when he focused somewhat more on relationships, he often approached them from a philosophical instead of emotional standpoint. Once, when asked about Françoise, he told a journalist, "She's one of the most highly evolved people I know."[20] In a sense, Salk had more concern for mankind than for himself; he always had. "How can I use my self or allow my self to be used in a way that might be able to influence the human future for the better?" he wrote on June 19, 1995, probably his last night note. "I must give some thought to this since this is, in effect, the mission in my life."[21]

For Jews, good deeds define a person, and from childhood Salk had set out to fulfill his duty of *tikkun olam*. He had been a religious child, praying daily, but that practice had fallen by the wayside, at least so as far as anyone knew. Though rarely seen at synagogue, he told Ron Moss that Judaism had influenced his life; he had inherited his tenacity from his Jewish ancestors who had persevered from biblical times. He observed Yom Kippur, the holiest day for Jews, a day of atonement for sins, a day of fasting and prayer. He didn't share his beliefs with his family, however. Jonathan sensed his father had his own philosophy or religion, which had to do with the principles of nature. On the other hand, in discussions with Eva Seilitz Horney, Salk talked about God. "That was quite an unknown side of him," she said. "He had a humble conviction of God's power working through him."[22]

This man who always looked to the future never talked about it in terms of his own death. He did reveal his belief in a spiritual afterlife, *olam ha-ba*, in the eulogies he gave at his brothers' funerals. "We love you Herman, and our time will come when we will join with you in your heavenly paradise," he had recited at the memorial service.[23] In his tribute to Lee, he said, "We too, will join you in your heavenly paradise to go on forever more."[24] He told Heather Wood Ion he did not fear death; dying was a natural process.[25] Near the end of his life, he witnessed a tragedy that touched him deeply and tested that faith. James Dillon Aronson, Joan Abrahamson's son and Salk's godson, suddenly died on June 4, 1995.[26] Not yet two, James was found at autopsy to have a viral cardiomyopathy; without warning a virus had attacked his heart muscles. Salk tried to comfort his longtime companion, tried to help her understand why an innocent child had died.

Still, Salk was not anticipating his end; he felt he had more to do. In mid-June, 1995, flying home from a New York AIDS meeting, he stood for almost the entire trip, talking to Kevin Kimberlin, urging him, "You've got to keep on."[27] In one of his last night notes, he wrote: "I must find a way to achieve the peace and serenity that I will need to make the most of a rich life experience...that now needs to become a life of greater fulfillment than disappointment. Can I turn all this around in one day? Can I do so in one week, one month, or one year? Can I do so...step by step and day by day? I shall try."[28]

AT THREE O'CLOCK on Saturday afternoon, June 17, 1995, Dr. Patrick Whelan, a second-year medical resident at Scripps Hospital, got called to urgent care.[29] He was surprised to learn that Dr. Jonas Salk had just come in complaining of chest pain. When Whelan entered the exam room, he found Salk lying on a gurney, looking fatigued, uncomfortable, and anxious.

"I understand you've been having some pain," he said.

"Not really pain," Salk replied, "but I've been feeling like I can't quite catch my breath."[30] He explained that he had had a cardiac catheterization a few months before and had been doing well until the last few days. He had attended a reception where he consumed sushi and other Japanese dishes with high salt content. Since then he had had difficulty breathing and awoke from sleep short of breath. He apologized for being overly cautious, but with his wife away he was home by himself. Whelan realized that Salk, who likely had heart failure and might be having a heart attack, had driven himself five miles to Scripps Hospital. He ran an EKG, sent off blood tests, and admitted Salk to the intensive care unit. A subsequent cardiac catheterization showed a partially blocked right coronary artery.

On rounds the next morning, Whelan found Salk sitting in bed, reading the newspaper, his breathing improved with diuretics, his anxiety gone. He appreciated his room's sweeping view—the golf course, lined by Torrey pines, in the foreground; a show of hand gliders launching from the cliffs; and the ocean beyond. It puzzled Whelan that such a prominent man had no visitors, but Salk said he had no family members in the area at the time. So Whelan had the man he had admired for years to himself. They spent several hours each day talking. Whelan couldn't believe how unaffected and forthcoming Salk was. At one point, Whelan mentioned a quote he had just read from Speaker of the House Newt Gingrich. When asked at a press conference if the government ever got anything right, Gingrich replied, "Well, they do some things right, like curing polio." Salk laughed. "The government didn't have anything to do with it."[31]

Salk did call Ron Moss, who was preparing for an advisory hearing with the FDA. "I'm in the hospital," he said. "I have some arteries that are closed. I'm getting myself ready for the FDA meeting. Don't worry. It's just a tune-up, Ron."[32] Salk seemed stable, so his cardiologist discharged him on Monday and scheduled an elective stent placement. That evening, Salk drove back to the hospital, saying he felt ill; perhaps he had been premature in leaving.

Before undergoing the angioplasty, Salk called Jonathan and Peter, who was vacationing in England. Later Jonathan wondered if he had called to say goodbye in case he didn't survive the procedure.[33] If he was nervous, he didn't indicate it. Bundy, who was at his side, recalled how amiable he had been to the staff while being wheeled into the procedure suite.[34]

During the angioplasty, the cardiologist inserted a balloon catheter through Salk's groin into the blood vessel that fed the right heart. He blew up the balloon and crushed the atherosclerotic plaque, then inserted a stent. When Whelan visited him after the procedure, Salk took his hand and looked at him with amazement. "You just won't believe the sensation that I had when they opened up that blood vessel," he said. "It was as if a tide of well-being washed over me. It was extraordinary. It was supernatural....It wasn't just that I could breathe easier....My whole outlook on life dramatically improved in an instant."[35]

Salk checked out of the hospital on Wednesday, telling Bundy he had to do a satellite interview. That same day, Françoise felt the sudden urge to fly home, even though she had a number of appointments. "I had the intuition," she recalled. "There was a voice in my head that said, 'Change your ticket. Go away today.'"[36] Jonas tried to dissuade her, but she insisted.

On Thursday, Lisa Longworth called to tell Salk she was leaving for Tahiti. She worried something was wrong, as he had a flat affect. Salk then spent most of the day getting the house in order for his wife's return. His assistant Barbara Robinson came over to help. He had papers scattered everywhere, and he didn't want Françoise to see the house like that. After she arrived, they went out for Chinese food.

Salk sat up all that night, struggling to breathe. Not wanting to bother his cardiologist, his physician sons, or his wife, he waited until morning and called an ambulance. Françoise alerted Jonathan that his father was on his way to the hospital. Salk insisted on talking to his son on the phone, but he could only whisper, "Hey, buddy."[37]

Patrick Whelan was making rounds that Friday, June 23, morning when he heard a page, "Code blue—code blue—intensive care unit."[38] He ran to the room where the lights were flashing. On the bed lay a frail-looking man, surrounded by a host of doctors and nurses, a tube down his throat with one physician trying to ventilate him with a resuscitator bag, another pumping his chest, a lead doctor shouting out orders. Whelan realized they were attempting to resuscitate Jonas Salk. A physician yelled to stand back as he turned on the defibrillator and delivered a shock. With no response, he delivered another. Everyone looked at the monitor, which registered a flat line. Afterward Whelan learned Salk had felt well at discharge, but at home he had become nauseated and overwhelmingly weak, barely able to breathe. The emergency room doctor found him in kidney failure with a dangerously high potassium level. When the ICU team tried to insert a dialysis catheter to lower his potassium, he started to bleed at the puncture site. Then his heart stopped.

Probably Salk had developed acute kidney failure from the injection of contrast dye given during the catheterization and angioplasty. Elderly patients and those with congestive heart failure are more prone to this complication. Had he stayed in the hospital for close monitoring, the high potassium would have been detected. Unchecked, it can generate irregular heart rhythms, leading to a cardiac arrest. The man who had spent his life trying to prevent disease likely died from a preventable condition. For an hour and a half, the cardiac team tried to restart his heart, but to no avail.

⁂

JONAS SALK ACHIEVED a level of public recognition accorded few in the history of medicine. On April 12, 1955, his life changed forever. Considering that day, he told a writer for the *New York Times*, "It's as if I've been a public property ever since....It's brought me enormous gratification, opened many opportunities, but at the same time, placed many burdens on me. It altered my career, my relationships with colleagues; I am a public figure, no longer one of them."[39] His image spread across magazines and newspapers, making it impossible for him to go anywhere unrecognized; people wanted to touch him, embrace him, thank him. Organizations honored him into his later years.

Some in the scientific community accused Salk of seeking the limelight. For the most part, however, he rejected his celebrity. "If only I'd known how many of these dinners I'd have to address," he said at a California bar association event, "I would have developed some sort of vaccine against them."[40] In a moment of despair, he told Lorraine Friedman he wished this had never happened to him.[41] To endure his popularity, Salk developed a shell that allowed him to project a positive public persona while keeping his true sentiments hidden. Occasionally, he did use his fame to leverage other opportunities, though never financial. When he spoke, the public listened; he had access to other famous people. Salk's friend Christine Forester called him "the two Jonases."[42] He may have wearied of the publicity, but she thought on occasion he enjoyed showing off to those who had snubbed him by posing with Eleanor Roosevelt, Indira Gandhi, or Coretta Scott King.

Did fame change him? Saint Augustine argued that even the virtuous are keen for recognition and find it hard to resist the temptations of earthly praise. Commendations by five US presidents had to have affected Salk's view of himself. Yet the all-but-canonized Salk felt he had not been altered by his public acclaim. When a journalist said she couldn't believe success had not turned his head, Salk replied that she reminded him of the farmer who, seeing a giraffe for the first time, said, "Aw, there ain't no such animal."[43] Although he became a bit more bold—some would say hubristic—in his behavior, if anything, life under the microscope enhanced his isolation as he tried to maintain his privacy.

Inherently shy, Salk extended himself to the public in ways no scientist had. He tried to temper premature rumors about a vaccine on the radio, showed how to make a vaccine on television, gave interviews to *Good Housekeeping* and *Parenting*. In large part, he was responding to Basil O'Connor's expectations. He served as the March of Dimes spokesman and willingly became a folk hero to generate support for the organization. In attempts to help the public grasp the obscure concept behind the Salk Institute, he allowed *Life* to do a photo shoot of him and his family on vacation, portraying the common man swimming in the lake or cooking hamburgers. Some of those efforts had backfired. His detractors considered them publicity stunts. Yet Salk sought to close the chasm between ordinary citizens and ivory-tower academicians. He had insisted that every one of the letters he received, numbering in the thousands, be answered; the public deserved to be heard and responded to, he told Friedman.

Even-tempered and composed, Salk seemed to generate controversy no matter what he set out to do. That wasn't his intent, but he defied conventional wisdom—"marched to a different drummer," as he said.[44] Two aspects of his personality both contributed to his success and generated friction. One was that he held strong convictions. Certain about the merit of the things he had done, the things he wanted to do, he rarely expressed self-doubt. Connected to this, he was unrelenting, repeating his view over and over, never seeming piqued or tired. Once he determined a course of action, he would not waver from it. His persistence exasperated those on the receiving end.

Some felt he was an ingenuous man, simply trying to do his work; others, that he was a shrewd tactician who connived to reach his ends, such as his large lab or favored status with the National Foundation. Although Salk once told a journalist, "When a reporter approaches, I generally find myself wishing for a martini," he knew perfectly well how to charm them.[45] He advised a colleague to develop a good relationship with the press. That cooperation, along with Salk's saintly status, likely kept journalists from divulging the less savory side of his private life, about which a number of them whispered.

When attacked, Salk rarely struck back. He had an ability to absorb hits and rebound as if untouched. Gilot observed that, despite the enmity Salk faced at the Institute, he never once expressed anger. He personified equanimity, which he achieved in part by absenting himself. "Whatever was going on around him," Jonathan explained, "he found a way to rise above it and go to another plane." Yet his night notes reveal a man who did feel the wounds and agonized over why they had been inflicted. In the early morning hours, he asked himself, "How did that happen? What was that person thinking? What did I do that enraged him?"[46]

Salk received among the highest awards from heads of state—the Congressional Gold Medal, Presidential Medal of Freedom, French Legion of Honor, Jawaharlal Nehru Award, to name a few. Yet he received almost no recognition from the scientific world, aside from the Lasker Award and admission into the Institute of Medicine at the age of seventy-eight. Some contended he made no true scientific discovery. His was called "kitchen chemistry," and he was likened to a director of product development at a pharmaceutical company. "He's no Watson-and-Crick," said a former chairman of molecular and cell biology at Berkeley.[47] Others disagreed. "The fact that a fundamental advance in human health could not be recognized as a scientific contribution," countered Nobel laureate Renato Dulbecco, "raises the question of the role of science in our society."[48] Even Larry Lasky, the Genentech scientist who disparaged Salk's AIDS work, admitted, "There is no denying he made one of the most important contributions as a single person. It's not like Pfizer did this. A single guy did this. It was enormous."[49]

Surely his accomplishments merited admission into the National Academy of Sciences or earlier election into the Institute of Medicine. Some blamed Albert Sabin for Salk's ostracism. Sabin seized every opportunity to discredit his vaccine competitor. Still, Salk contributed to his own rejection with his unconventional approach to science—his emphasis on intuition and sometimes abstract principles—matched by a convoluted manner of writing and a love of metaphor. In other words, he didn't behave like an academic scientist. Somehow, though, this doesn't seem enough of an explanation for the disparity between Salk's scientific achievements and his recognition. "Don't discount envy," Arnold Mandell said. "Envy is fierce in the world of science."[50]

Salk remained unbowed. When people asked him why he didn't get the Nobel Prize, Robert Gallo recalled Salk's answer: "Everybody thinks I got it. So that's fine."[51] But when Salk started to put together autobiographical material, he wrote, "My intention and purpose has been to do good in the world through the advancement of knowledge; that of others is only the advancement and dissemination of knowledge. That's the difference....That's what they can't forgive me for." He wasn't referring just to those involved in the polio saga but scientists at the Institute as well. "What crime or crimes have I committed against the Salk Institute," he asked himself, "to have deserved the punishment and treatment that I received—the banishment?"[52]

Some considered Salk noble, others egotistical. Those in the latter group cite the *Salk* vaccine and *Salk* Institute as examples, the use of his name suggesting a preening vanity. But he didn't choose either. The media attached his name to the vaccine, and O'Connor forced him to allow the Institute to bear his name. Friends and family noted that Salk usually focused the conversation on his activities, not on theirs, yet arguably he wasn't directing attention to himself personally but to what he was trying to do. To accomplish what he did, one had to have a strong ego, not necessarily an inflated ego. Julius Youngner lambasted him for failing to share credit for the vaccine with his laboratory coworkers, and the UC Davis deans thought he tried to use the school for his own aggrandizement. On the other hand, so many who worked with and under him found him unpretentious; he insisted that everyone call him Jonas.

Nonetheless, nobility of purpose doesn't preclude conceit. In a 1954 *Times* article, when a reporter asked why he devoted his life to research, Salk answered, "Why did Mozart compose music?"[53] His denigrators assumed he was comparing himself to Mozart. Yet by "Mozart" Salk likely meant that people with creative drive devote what time they have to their passion. Even the oft-quoted statement Salk made when Edward R. Murrow asked who owned the vaccine patent—"How can you patent the sun?"—conveys a degree of magnanimity or self-adulation.

Jonas Salk was an enigmatic man. After 1955, he forged a protective shield, making it difficult to reconcile the paradoxes of his life. He was far more complex than the public image of him—America's beloved hero— and yet far more sensitive and caring than the distorted image suggested by some scientists: a stubborn, standoffish, glory-seeking dilettante. Introspective and mild-mannered, he presented a calm demeanor to the world while he carried enormous inner burdens; he loathed confrontation yet was surrounded by controversy; he longed to be accepted but challenged prevailing norms with unremitting tenacity. Above all, Jonas Salk was an idealist. As a boy, he prayed that one day he would perform some noble deed. And he did. That same boy craved acceptance from his peers and a connection with someone that transcended the ordinary; he never realized either. His dreams and ambitions, his passion to solve the problems of the world both enshrined and isolated him, vaulted him to fame and confined him to loneliness. In the end, Salk's drive to aid humanity trumped his inner needs, and the world is better for it.

Acknowledgments

AS A CHILD, I worried every summer that I or my family might be stricken with polio. Every time we went to the movies, I cringed when the newsreel came on, showing children in iron lungs or those struggling to walk with metal braces. My hometown of Kingsport, Tennessee, was selected as a site for the National Foundation's trial of the Salk vaccine. On April 28, 1954, I stood in line with my second-grade class to receive the polio vaccine and a red lollipop. My mother saved my Polio Pioneer button, never suspecting I might write about the man we considered our hero—Jonas Salk.

My love for biography began at Andrew Johnson Elementary School, where I anticipated reading about the next great figure in the Bobbs-Merrill biography series, among the most popular books in our library. I never found one on Jonas Salk, however. My first serious writing endeavor started partway through my medical career when I was fortunate to study with Ehud Havazelet, an outstanding mentor, winner of the Pushcart Prize and the Whiting Writer's Award. After a decade of weekly seminars, I can still hear him whisper in my ear if I become sloppy or try a shortcut. My biography writing was facilitated in large part by an endowed professorship from Drs. Ben and A. Jess Shenson, who bestowed upon me the gift of academic freedom. I am grateful for residencies at the Virginia Center for the Creative Arts, Ragdale Foundation, MacDowell Colony, and the Djerassi Resident Artists Program, each of which provided a retreat from the workaday world and a creative atmosphere in which to write. While at the Djerassi Program, I was surprised to be awarded the Patricia E. Bashaw and Eugene Segre Fellowship in support of my writing.

As opposed to medicine, where I have many colleagues and receive instant gratification from patients, writing is a lonely endeavor. Fortunately, I learned of Biographer's International, founded by James McGrath Morris to promote the art and craft of biography. With its monthly newsletter, "The Biographer's Craft," and a yearly conference, I came to know fellow biographers who shared their wisdom. Nigel Hamilton and Debbie Applegate, along with Jamie, stand out for their tireless efforts to help other writers.

Every biographer knows that there is no one as invaluable as the archivist, for whom the appellation "unsung hero" couldn't be more apt. Having spent years reading through the Jonas Salk Papers at the University of California, San Diego, I gained respect and regard for Lynda Claassen, director of Special Collections and Archives. I appreciate beyond measure the professional help and constant encouragement she and her staff provided. At the March of Dimes Foundation, archivist David Rose—part historian, part sleuth—helped me utilize the enormous amount of archival information, provided me with marvelous videos and photos, and helped me understand the important relationship between Jonas Salk and Basil O'Connor. His ready access with answers to every inquiry, peppered with wit, made working with him a joy.

As I began my research on Salk, I was thankful to those who provided background and insights through their published works: David Oshinsky with his Pulitzer Prize–winning history, *Polio: An American Story*; Richard Carter, who recounted conversations with Salk in *Breakthrough: The Saga of Jonas Salk*; Jane Smith, who introduced me to the polio vaccine saga in *Patenting the Sun*; Suzanne Bourgeois's *Genesis of the Salk Institute: The Epic of Its Founders*; and Jon Cohen's remarkable account of the early attempts to make an AIDS vaccine, *Shots in the Dark: The Wayward Search for an AIDS Vaccine*. David Roll's *The Hopkins Touch* served as a beacon in my last months of writing. How blessed we both are to share the same editor, Timothy Bent.

My thanks go to all those who were gracious enough to spend time talking about their experiences with Salk and his endeavors. They are listed individually in the bibliography. I am particularly grateful to Peter and Jonathan Salk. They spent hours talking with me and never seemed to tire of my incessant emails and questions. In their honesty and equanimity, I could see the best parts of their father shine through. I appreciate how difficult it must be for children to read the life story of a parent, finding out pieces of his or her life they never knew, reading about incidents they remembered or would have interpreted differently. To Jonathan and Peter, I give my sincerest thanks.

As a first-time biographer, I felt overjoyed to be represented by the inveterate Robert Lescher, who with great attentiveness shepherded my first biography, *Henry Kaplan and the Story of Hodgkin's Disease*, to publication. The literary world lost a great man when he died on November 28, 2012. Feeling a bit afloat, I contacted friend and colleague Abraham Verghese. Always ready to help, he put me in touch with his agent, Mary Evans, who recommended Rachel Vogel. With amazing enthusiasm and skill, Rachel placed Salk's biography with Oxford University Press in what I consider record time. She has gone way beyond what I anticipated from a literary agent. I will be forever grateful for her dedication, wisdom, and guidance.

When I first talked with Timothy Bent at Oxford University Press, I had to keep pinching myself to be sure I wasn't dreaming. How privileged, how delighted I feel to be working with such an experienced, talented editor. His astute insights and thoughtful edits enhanced my biography substantially. Assistant editor Keely Latcham provided sound advice, readily answering my question of the day. I count myself incredibly fortunate to have senior production editor Joellyn Ausanka bring my biography down the final stretch with such expertise. I admire the work she did with *The Hopkins Touch* and *Polio: An American Story*. "Brilliant" best describes Ben Sadock, the copy editor for Salk's biography. He is a true Renaissance man, and I am indebted to him for his detailed editing.

I could never have written the Salk biography without the love and support of my family and friends. My late father, George, and my mother, Lucille DeCroes Wilson, instilled in me curiosity about the lives of others. My sons, Ben and Adam, stepsons Graham, Chris, and Scott, and daughters-in-law Shahla, Anne, Liz, and Maggie have been infinitely patient with "the book." My thanks to surgeon Sherry Wren, who provided thoughtful suggestions, and to Fred Dotzler, a Salk Institute trustee, for his assistance and encouragement. My gratitude and love goes to my wonderful girlfriends Linda Ara, Lucy Berman, and Ellen King, who have sustained me through the journey with their friendship, gift packages, and good humor. I am grateful to Ellen for her eleventh-hour rescue.

Ten years ago, Jonas Salk moved into our home, and he has not yet left. Not once has my incredible husband, Rod Young, threatened to evict him. My selfless companion, home editor, and dear heart, Rod has supported my efforts with enormous respect, sage advice, and above all patience. Dedication of this book to him represents a tiny fraction of what he has given me.

Notes

ABBREVIATIONS

ABS   *Albert Bruce Sabin*

ASA   *Albert B. Sabin Archives, Henry R. Winkler Center for the History of the Health Professions, University of Cincinnati Libraries, Cincinnati, OH*

BOC   *Basil O'Connor*

JES   *Jonas Edward Salk*

JSP   *Jonas Salk Papers, Mandeville Special Collections Library, University of California, San Diego*

MOD   *March of Dimes Archives*

PROLOGUE

1   On the history of the 1916 polio epidemic: Gould, *A Summer Plague: Polio and Its Survivors*; Paul, "Epidemiology of Poliomyelitis," 9–57; Seavey, Smith, and Wagner, *A Paralyzing Fear: The Triumph over Polio in America*; articles from unknown New York newspapers, 1916, Jonas Salk Papers (henceforth JSP): "Call in the Doctor if Baby has Cold," "Twenty P.C. Mortality in Epidemic," "How to Guard Your Children in An Epidemic," "Twenty-One Deaths," "Sixty-Eight New Cases of Paralysis, Two Hundred in Hospital," "Mothers Hurrying Out of City With Children," "Rushing More Cribs for Babies in the Hospital," "No Child to Quit State Without Health Certificate," "Mothers Will Do Anything to Keep Their Sick Babies at Home."

2 "46 More Infantile Paralysis Cases; Girl of Fourteen Dies," unknown New York newspaper, 1916, JSP.
3 "Paralysis Kills 42 Brooklyn Children in a Week," unknown New York newspaper, 1916, JSP.
4 Debre, "Symptomatology and Diagnosis of Poliomyelitis," 109–36.
5 On the history of the 1918 influenza: Aimone, "The 1918 Influenza Epidemic in New York City: A Review of the Public Health Response," 71–79; Beveridge, *Influenza: The Last Great Plague*; Crosby, *America's Forgotten Pandemic*; Iezzoni, *Influenza 1918*; Kolata, *Flu: The Story of the Great Influenza Pandemic of 1918 and the Search for the Virus That Caused It*; Woolley, "The Epidemic of Influenza at Camp Devens, Mass."
6 Williams, *Virus Hunters*, 196.
7 Iezzoni, *Influenza 1918*, 136.
8 www.flu.gov/pandemic/history/1918/.
9 *Arizona Republican*, November 9, 1918.

CHAPTER 1

1 Jonathan Salk interview.
2 Jonas E. Salk (henceforth JES) interview, November 14, 1990, March of Dimes archives (henceforth MOD), A/V Collection.
3 On the history of the Russian Jews: Greenberg, *The Jews in Russia: The Struggle for Emancipation*; Sachar, *The Course of Modern Jewish History*.
4 On Dora Press and Daniel Salk families and marriage: Department of Commerce, Bureau of the Census, Fifteenth Census of the United States, 1930; Salk to Eltermann, September 17, 1956, JSP; Jonas Salk to Jacob Salk, June 28, 1954, JSP; Harriet Press Brown, Robert Dribbon, Francoise Gilot, Eileen Kessner, Mortimer Kramer, Jonathan Salk, Peter Salk, Sylvia Salk, and Anne Meltzer Selikov interviews.
5 Keller, *Diaspora: The Post-Biblical History of the Jews*, 431.
6 Antin, *From Plotzk to Boston*, 11–12.
7 I. Howe, *World of Our Fathers*; Rischin, *The Promised City*.
8 I. Howe, *World of Our Fathers*, 131.
9 Harriet Press Brown interview.
10 Harriet Press Brown interview.
11 JES childhood: Carter, *Breakthrough: The Saga of Jonas Salk*; McPherson, *Jonas Salk: Conquering Polio*; Jonathan Salk, Peter Salk, and Anne Meltzer Selikov interviews.
12 JES interview, November 14, 1990, MOD, A/V Collection.
13 Anne Meltzer Selikov interview.
14 Kurtzman Laser to JES, February 8, 1959, JSP.
15 McPherson, *Jonas Salk*, 13.
16 Jonas Salk interview, Academy of Achievement: A Museum of Living History, available online at http://achievement.org/autodoc/page/sal0int-1.
17 Sylvia Salk interview.
18 L. Salk, *My Father, My Son*, 10.
19 L. Salk, *My Father, My Son*, 10.

20 Françoise Gilot interview.
21 JES interview, November 14, 1990, MOD, A/V Collection.
22 JES interview, November 14, 1990, MOD, A/V Collection.
23 Jonathan Salk interview.
24 Jonathan Salk interview.
25 JES interview, November 14, 1990, MOD, A/V Collection.
26 Carter, *Breakthrough*, 30.
27 Peter Salk interview.
28 I. Howe, *World of Our Fathers*, 254.
29 Jonas Salk interview, Academy of Achievement: A Museum of Living History, available online at http://achievement.org/autodoc/page/sal0int-1.
30 Carter, *Breakthrough*, 30.

CHAPTER 2

1 Lebow, *The Bright Boys: A History of Townsend Harris High School*; Rudy, *The College of the City of New York: A History, 1847–1947;Crimson and Gold* (Townsend Harris High School Yearbook), 1931, available at Seth Poppel's Celebrity Yearbooks; Harold Goldstein, Murray Nathan interviews.
2 *Crimson and Gold*, 1931, 41.
3 Jonas Salk interview, Academy of Achievement: A Museum of Living History, available online at http://achievement.org/autodoc/page/sal0int-1.
4 *Crimson and Gold*, 1931, 41.
5 Murray Nathan interview.
6 Fabricant to Salk, January 13, 1958, JSP.
7 Available online at http://emersoncentral.com/selfreliance.htm.
8 Ayres, *The Wit and Wisdom of Abraham Lincoln: An A–Z Compendium of Quotes from the Most Eloquent of American Presidents*, 44.
9 Stanley Gitenstein interview.
10 Murray Nathan interview.
11 *Crimson and Gold*, 1931, 29.
12 *Crimson and Gold*, 1931, 40.
13 *Crimson and Gold*, 1931, 20.
14 *Crimson and Gold*, 1931, 79.
15 *Crimson and Gold*, 1931, 37.
16 *Crimson and Gold*, 1931, 9.
17 Rudy, *College of the City of New York*.
18 I. Howe, *World of Our Fathers*, 282.
19 I. Howe, *World of Our Fathers*, 283.
20 Harold Goldstein interview.
21 Transcript, CCNY Archives.
22 Oshinsky, *Polio: An American Story*, 98.
23 Carter, *Breakthrough: The Saga of Jonas Salk*, 31.
24 Jonas Salk interview, Academy of Achievement: A Museum of Living History, available online at http://achievement.org/autodoc/page/sal0int-1.

25 JES Interview, 11/14/1990, MOD.

26 Jonas Salk interview, Academy of Achievement: A Museum of Living History, available online at http://achievement.org/autodoc/page/sal0int-1.

27 Curson, *Jonas Salk*, 21.

28 Heaton and Dumont, *The First One Hundred Twenty-Five Years of the New York University School of Medicine.*

29 New York University School of Medicine Archives; Frances Bailen-Rose, Isidor Bernstein, Murray Glusman, Walter Kees, Herman Zuckerman interviews.

30 John Stetler interview.

31 Walter Kees interview.

32 Isidor Bernstein interview.

33 Mrs. Karl Paley interview.

34 Isidor Bernstein, Herman Zuckerman, Rudy Drosd, Walter Kees, and Frances Bailen-Rose interviews.

35 JES Interview, 11/14/1990, MOD.

36 Blake to Salk, March 4, 1942, JSP (includes a summary of a paper by Salk entitled "The Alkali Denaturation of Crystalline Hen's Egg Albumin," read at a meeting of the NYU Medical Society, January, 1937).

37 Carter, *Breakthrough*, 33.

38 Salk, "Methods for Separation of Micro-organisms from Large Quantities of Broth Culture."

39 JES Interview, 11/14/1990, MOD.

40 JES Interview, 11/14/1990, MOD.

41 Carter, *Breakthrough*, 35.

42 Carter, *Breakthrough*, 35–36.

43 Bendiner, "Adulation, Animosity, and Achievement;" JES Interview, 11/14/1990, MOD.

44 *The Medical Violet 1939*, New York University School of Medicine Archives, 93.

CHAPTER 3

1 McPherson, *Jonas Salk: Conquering Polio*, 23.

2 Jonathan Salk interview.

3 Sylvia Salk interview.

4 Jessica Franken interview.

5 Jessica Franken, David Korr, Jonathan Salk, Peter Salk, and Sylvia Salk interviews; "Donna Lindsay Salk, 85; Prominent Civic Activist," *San Diego Union-Tribune*, May 31, 2002; Carter, *Breakthrough: The Saga of Jonas Salk*; McPherson, *Jonas Salk*.

6 Jonathan Salk interview.

7 Carter, *Breakthrough*, 37.

8 Oshinsky, *Polio: An American Story*, 100.

9 Bailen-Rose interview.

10 Jonathan Salk interview.

11 Oshinsky, *Polio*, 99.

12 Jonathan Salk interview.
13 John DeHoff and Arthur Seligmann interviews; JES Interview, 11/14/1990, MOD; *Mt. Sinai Hospital Manuel of Procedures for the House Staff*, 1940, JSP; Mount Sinai Hospital website, http://www.mountsinai.org.
14 Carter, *Breakthrough*, 37.
15 Arthur Seligmann interview.
16 Arthur Seligmann interview.
17 Carter, *Breakthrough*, 38.
18 Arthur Seligmann interview.
19 Arthur Seligmann interview.
20 John DeHoff interview.
21 history.amedd.army.mil.
22 Carter, *Breakthrough*, 39.
23 Carter, *Breakthrough*, 42; Rivers to JES, February 3, 1941, JSP.
24 Francis to JES, September 29, 1941, JSP.
25 Francis to JES, October 21, 1941, JSP.
26 JES to Francis, October 21, 1941, JSP.
27 JES to Francis, December 12, 1941, JSP.
28 JES to Francis, December 12, 1941, JSP.
29 Francis to JES, December 18, 1941, JSP.
30 Kopetzky to JES, March 13, 1942, JSP.
31 Francis to Selective Service Board, February 13, 1942, JSP.
32 Notice from the University of Michigan to JES, March 5, 1942, JSP.
33 Blake to JES, March 4, 1942, JSP.
34 Clerk to JES, March 17, 1942, JSP.

CHAPTER 4

1 On the history of influenza: Beveridge, *Influenza: The Last Great Plague*; Crosby, *America's Forgotten Pandemic*; Iezzoni, *Influenza 1918*; Kolata, *Flu: The Story of the Great Influenza Pandemic of 1918 and the Search for the Virus That Caused It*; Williams, *Virus Hunters*.
2 Flexner and Flexner, *William Henry Welch and the Heroic Age of American Medicine*; Vaughan, *A doctor's Memories*; Woolley, "The epidemic of influenza at Camp Devens, Mass."
3 Flexner and Flexner, *William Henry Welch*, 376.
4 Flexner and Flexner, *William Henry Welch*, 376.
5 Flexner and Flexner, *William Henry Welch*, 376.
6 Iezzoni, *Plague*, 68.
7 Iezzoni, *Plague*, 51.
8 Beveridge, *Influenza*; Smith, Andrewes, and Laidlaw, "A Virus Obtained from Influenza Patients"; Williams, *Virus Hunters*.
9 On the life of Francis: Griffin, "Epidemiologist to the Military"; Paul, "Thomas Francis, Jr., 1900–1969"; Williams, *Virus Hunters*; June Mack and Paul Stumpf interviews.

10 June Mack interview.
11 Paul, "Thomas Francis, Jr.," 86.
12 Paul, "Thomas Francis, Jr.," 86.
13 Salk, "The Restless Spirit of Thomas Francis, Jr. Still Lives."
14 Francis, "Transmission of Influenza by a Filterable Virus."
15 Francis and Magill, "Immunological Studies with the Virus of Influenza."
16 Francis, "A New Type of Virus from Epidemic Influenza."
17 Plotkin and Mortimer, *Vaccines.*
18 Hirst, "The Quantitative Determination of Influenza Virus and Antibodies by Means of Red Cell Agglutination."
19 Francis, "Influenza: Methods of Study and Control."

CHAPTER 5

1 On Ann Arbor circa 1942: "The War Hits Home," Ann Arbor District Library, available online at http://moaa.aadl.org/book/export/html/3045.
2 Carter, *Breakthrough: The Saga of Jonas Salk,* 45.
3 June and Walter Mack, and Paul Stumpf interviews; Carter, *Breakthrough.*
4 Notice from the University of Michigan to JES, March 5, 1942, JSP.
5 June and Walter Mack interviews.
6 Walter Mack interview.
7 Paul Stumpf interview.
8 June Mack interview.
9 June Mack interview.
10 Carter, *Breakthrough,* 45.
11 Francis and Salk, "A Simplified Procedure for the Concentration and Purification of Influenza Virus."
12 Ibbotson, *Eloise: Poorhouse, Farm, Asylum and Hospital, 1839–1984,* 128.
13 Christopher Zbrozek, "Opening Its Doors Again," *Michigan Daily,* September 28, 2005.
14 Francis et al., "Protective Effect of Vaccination Against Induced Influenza A"; Salk et al., "Protective Effect of Vaccination against Induced Influenza B."
15 Salk, Wilbur, and Francis, "Identification of Influenza Virus Type A in Current Outbreak of Respiratory Disease"; Lusk to JES, June 8, 1943, JSP; JES to Frisch, July 10, 1943, JSP.
16 JES to Bartemeier, May 19, 1943, JSP.
17 Members of the Commission on Influenza et al., "A Clinical Evaluation of Vaccination against Influenza."
18 Science Service, August 25, 1944, JSP.
19 Salk, Menke, and Francis, "A Clinical, Epidemiological and Immunological Evaluation of Vaccination against Epidemic Influenza."
20 J. Salk and D. Salk, "Control of Influenza and Poliomyelitis with Killed Virus Vaccines."
21 Bayne-Jones to JES, January 4, 1945, JSP.
22 Notice from the University of Michigan to JES, January 23, 1943, JSP.
23 Agreement with Parke, Davis and Co., January, 1945, JSP.

24 Stimpert to JES, November 21, 1946, JSP.
25 Salk and Francis, "Immunization against Influenza," 451.
26 JES to Bayne-Jones, June 14, 1945, JSP; JES to Cosigel, July 13, 1945, JSP; Rakosy to JES, June 12, 1945, JSP.
27 Bayne-Jones to JES, June 18, 1945.
28 Notice from University of Michigan to JES, July 31, 1945, JSP.
29 Sabin to JES, May 4, 1944, JSP.
30 JES to Veldee, September 5, 1946, JSP.
31 Invitation to present paper in Copenhagen, March 19, 1945, JSP.
32 Horsfall to JES, February 25, 1946, JSP.
33 Carter, *Breakthrough*, 51.
34 "Michigan State Prisons in Ionia County," Ionia County MIGenWeb, http://ionia .migenweb.net/history/prisons.htm.
35 Curphey, "Fatal Allergic Reaction Due to Influenza Vaccine."
36 Salk, "Reactions to Influenza Virus Vaccines."
37 JES to Scott, April 18, 1947, JSP.
38 Carter, *Breakthrough*, 48.
39 JES to Moore, July 6, 1945, JSP.
40 JES to Mrs. Joel Moor, November 21, 1946, JSP.
41 JES to Slevin, March 29, 1943, JSP.
42 JES to Moore, November 21, 1946, JSP.
43 Science Service, May 17, 1946, JSP.
44 *Parents Magazine* to JES, August 30, 1946, JSP.
45 Carter, *Breakthrough*, 51.
46 Carter, *Breakthrough*, 51.
47 Carter, *Breakthrough*, 51.
48 McPherson, *Jonas Salk: Conquering Polio*, 30.
49 Paul Stumpf interview.
50 JES to Wayne, May 2, 1947, JSP.
51 Carter, *Breakthrough*, 51.
52 Pearson to Salk, May 28, 1947, JSP.
53 Carter, *Breakthrough*, 51.
54 Carter, *Breakthrough*, 51.
55 Lauffer to JES, May 27, 1947, JSP.
56 Paull, *A Century of Medical Excellence*, 163.
57 Lennette to JES, June 11, 1947, JSP.
58 JES to Lauffer, June 27, 1947, JSP.
59 Carter, *Breakthrough*, 53.
60 Carter, *Breakthrough*, 46.

CHAPTER 6

1 Smith, *Patenting the Sun*, 116.
2 JES to Dammin, July 30 and August 7, 1947, JSP.

3   JES to Shwartzman, February 26, 1948, JSP.
4   Paull, *A Century of Medical Excellence*, 163.
5   Peter Salk interview.
6   JES to Barlow, November 10, 1947, JSP.
7   JES to Francis, December 4, 1947, JSP.
8   Lorraine Friedman interview.
9   Carter, *Breakthrough: The Saga of Jonas Salk*, 55.
10 Carter, *Breakthrough*, 56.
11 JES to Daer, December 9, 1950, JSP.
12 JES to McEllroy, December 19, 1947, JSP.
13 JES to McEllroy, December 9, 1947, JSP.
14 JES to McEllroy, November 4, 1947, JSP.
15 Alexander to Lauffer, August 25, 1947, JSP.
16 JES to McEllroy, January 27, 1948, JSP.
17 JES to McEllroy, February 27, 1948, JSP.
18 Carter, *Breakthrough*, 66.
19 JES to McEllroy, September 24, 1948, JSP.
20 Paull, *Century of Medical Excellence*, 200.
21 JES to Schlesinger, July 2, 1948, JSP.
22 Paull, *Century of Medical Excellence*, 177–78.
23 JES to Richmond, March 19, 1948, JSP.
24 JES to Doutt, December 8, 1948, JSP.
25 JES to Francis, December 4, 1953, JSP.
26 Salk and Suriano, "Importance of Antigenic Composition of Influenza Virus Vaccine in Protecting against the Natural Disease."
27 JES to Kierstein, February 15, 1952, JSP.
28 JES to Weinblatt, June 11, 1950, JSP.
29 Hansen to JES, March 12, 1951, JSP.
30 JES to Rapalski, June 5, 1950, JSP.
31 Bauer to JES, November 29, 1950, JSP.
32 JES to Rapalski, December 24, 1952, JSP.
33 JES to Nigg, October 8, 1948, JSP.
34 JES to Francis, October 14, 1949, JSP.
35 JES to Francis, April 10, 1950, JSP.
36 JES to Francis, April 10, 1950, JSP.
37 Salk, "An Interpretation of the Significance of Influenza Virus Variation for the Development of an Effective Vaccine," 761.
38 JES to Stimpert, December 21, 1951, JSP.
39 VanRooyen to JES, October 8, 1952, JSP.
40 JES to Bell, December 12, 1952, JSP.
41 JES to Bell, December 12, 1952, JSP.
42 JES to Stimpert, February 11, 1952, JSP.
43 *The Evening Bulletin*, April 2, 1953.
44 *Newsweek*, April 20, 1953, 100.

45 "They've Been Learning a Lot About Influenza," draft for *Collier's*, September 29, 1953, JSP.

46 DeCoursey to Surgeon General, June 3, 1953, JSP.

47 Minutes of the Meeting of the AFIP to Discuss General DeCoursey's Memorandum, July 1, 1953, JSP.

48 Silliphant to Dixon, March12, 1954, JSP.

49 "Follow-up on Individuals Injected Nine Years Ago with the Influenza Vaccine and Adjuvants," undated draft, JSP.

50 Cox to Workman, July 9, 1953, JSP.

51 Carter, *Breakthrough*, 30.

52 Interview of Dr. Jonas Salk by Gabriel Stickle in La Jolla, California, September 8, 1984, MOD.

CHAPTER 7

1 Interview of Dr. Jonas Salk by Gabriel Stickle in La Jolla, California, September 8, 1984, MOD.

2 Jonas Salk interview, Academy of Achievement: A Museum of Living History, available online at http://achievement.org/autodoc/page/sal0int-1.

3 On the history of polio: Oshinsky, *Polio: An American Story*; Paul, *A History of Poliomyelitis*; Wilson, *Margin of Safety*; Seavey, Smith, and Wagner, *A Paralyzing Fear: The Triumph Over Polio in America*.

4 Paul, *History of Poliomyelitis*, 28.

5 Paul, *History of Poliomyelitis*, 7.

6 Caverly, "Preliminary Report of an Epidemic of Paralytic Disease, Occurring in Vermont, in the Summer of 1894," 15.

7 Caverly, "Preliminary Report of an Epidemic of Paralytic Disease, Occurring in Vermont, in the Summer of 1894," 17.

8 Caverly, "Notes of an Epidemic of Acute Anterior Poliomyelitis," 23.

9 Caverly, "Epidemic Poliomyelitis: A Review of the Epidemics of 1914 and 1915," 117.

10 Caverly, "Anterior Poliomyelitis in Vermont in the Year 1910," 54.

11 Caverly, "Epidemic Poliomyelitis," 142.

12 On Roosevelt's illness: Gallagher, *FDR's Splendid Deception*; Gould, *A Summer Plague*; Paul, *History of Poliomyelitis*.

13 Gallagher, *FDR's Splendid Deception*.

14 On the life of O'Connor: Henry Beckett, "Master Humanitarian," *New York Post*, August 2, 1944; biographical data, MOD; Fishbein to BOC, January 10, 1957, MOD; *American Magazine*, September 1955; "One Man's War Against Disease," *Medical World News*, January 31, 1964; Carter, *Breakthrough: The Saga of Jonas Salk*; Charles Massey oral history, October 3, 1983, MOD; Oshinsky, *Polio*.

15 Gould, *A Summer Plague*; Oshinsky, *Polio*; Smith, *Patenting the Sun*.

16 *New York Times*, March 10, 1972, 40.

17 Henry Beckett, "Master Humanitarian," *New York Post*, August 2, 1944.

18 Henry Beckett, "Master Humanitarian," *New York Post*, August 2, 1944.
19 Carter, *Breakthrough*, 12.
20 Carter, *Breakthrough*, 12.
21 *Polio Chronicle*, vol. 2, no. 5, December 1932.
22 Gould, *A Summer Plague*, 60.
23 *Medical World News*, January 31, 1964.
24 History of NFIP: Carter, *Breakthrough*; Cohn, *Four Billion Dimes*; Gould, *A Summer Plague*; Oshinsky, *Polio*; Paul, *History of Poliomyelitis*.
25 Paul, *History of Poliomyelitis*, 310.
26 Rosenfeld, "The March of Dimes as People," MOD.
27 Gomery, "Two Documents: 'Your Priceless Gift' and 'The 1946 Film Daily Yearbook.'"
28 Cohn, *Four Billion Dimes*, 68.
29 Van Riper to Crabtree, January 29, 1948, MOD; "In Daily Battle," A/V collection, MOD.
30 Melvin Glasser Eulogy of O'Connor, March 13, 1972, JSP.
31 Paul, *History of Poliomyelitis*, 311.
32 *Medical World News*, January 31, 1964.
33 Wilson, *Margin of Safety*, 59.
34 Gomery, "Two Documents."
35 Ducas, "Unto the Least of These," 6.
36 Wilson, *Margin of Safety*, 40.
37 On the life of Harry Weaver: Benison, *Tom Rivers: Reflections on a Life in Medicine and Science*; Paul, *History of Poliomyelitis*.
38 Weaver, "Poliomyelitis Research: Four Eras of Progress," address, January 26, 1953, 10–11, MOD.
39 Klein, *Trial by Fury: The Polio Vaccine Controversy*, 22.
40 Paul, *History of Poliomyelitis*, 315.
41 Benison, *Tom Rivers*, 424.
42 Carter, *Breakthrough*, 69.
43 Benison, *Tom Rivers*, 405.
44 Benison, *Tom Rivers*, 417.
45 Paul, *History of Poliomyelitis*, 413.
46 Weaver to Salk, December 15, 1947, JSP.
47 Round-Table Conference on the Immunogenic Types of the Virus of Poliomyelitis, January 7–8, 1948, JSP.
48 On the life of Sabin: "Albert Sabin," *People*, July 2, 1984; Benison, *Tom Rivers*; Debbe Sabin interview; "Dr. Albert Sabin, Developer of Oral Polio Vaccine, Dies," *Los Angeles Times*, March 4, 1993; Katz, "From Culture to Vaccine: Salk and Sabin;" Paul, *History of Poliomyelitis*; Sabin interviews by Benjamin Felson and Saul Benison, August 12, 1978, Albert B. Sabin Archives (henceforth ASA).
49 Benison, *Tom Rivers*, 235.
50 Benison, *Tom Rivers*, 235.
51 ABS to JES, May 23, 1944, ASA.
52 Benison, *Tom Rivers*, 443.
53 Benison, *Tom Rivers*, 409.

54　PBS, *American Experience* website, pbs.org/wgbh/americanexperience/features/biography/polio-bio-morgan/.
55　JES to Weaver, January 19, 1948, JSP.
56　Fitzgerald to O'Connor, January 5, 1949, JSP.

CHAPTER 8

1　On the typing project: Benison, *Tom Rivers: Reflections on a Life in Medicine and Science*; Weaver to JES, August 24, 1948, JSP; Carter, *Breakthrough: The Saga of Jonas Salk*; Curson, *Jonas Salk*; Paul, *A History of Poliomyelitis*.
2　JES to McEllroy, October 9, 1950, JSP.
3　On the lab staff: Bendiner, "Salk: Adulation, Animosity, and Achievement"; Carter, *Breakthrough*; Lorraine Friedman interview; JES to the Editor of *Science*, June 10, 1949, JSP.
4　Names of strains and telegrams, JSP.
5　JES to Gebhardt, September 28, 1949, JSP.
6　JES to Gebhardt, November 8, 1950, JSP.
7　JES to Lepine, April 15, 1949, JSP.
8　Weaver to JES, March 28, 1949, JSP.
9　Benison, *Tom Rivers*, 417.
10　JES to Kessel, February 15, 1950, JSP.
11　Salk, Lewis, Youngner, and Bennett, "The Use of Adjuvants to Facilitate Studies on the Immunologic Classification of Poliomyelitis Viruses."
12　Weaver to JES, June 21, 1951, JSP.
13　Benison, *Tom Rivers*, 492.
14　Carter, *Breakthrough*, 81.
15　Carter, *Breakthrough*, 81.
16　JES to Weaver, November 10, 1950, JSP.
17　Weaver to JES, May 1, 1950, JSP.
18　Melnick to JES, September 12, 1950, JSP.
19　Lepine to JES, January 7, 1952, JSP.
20　Enders to JES, January 28, 1952; JES to Enders, February 4, 1952, JSP.
21　Enders to JES, June 22, 1952, JSP.
22　ABS to JES, March 29, 1949, JSP.
23　JES to ABS, March 14, 1952, JSP.
24　ABS to JES, May 26, 1950, ASA.
25　Benison interview of Sabin, August 12, 1978, ASA.
26　JES to Enders, September 14, 1949, JSP.
27　Enders to JES, December 9, 1950, JSP.
28　Youngner, Ward, and Salk, "Studies on Poliomyelitis Viruses in Cultures of Monkey Testicular Tissue: I. Propagation of Viruses in Roller Tubes."
29　Carter, *Breakthrough*, 106.
30　Enders to JES, January 28, 1952, JSP.
31　Bodian to JES, February 6, 1952, JSP.

32 Ethel Bailey interview.

33 Paul, *A History of Poliomyelitis*, 235.

34 Weaver to Board of Trustees of NFIP, January 26, 1953, JSP.

35 JES to Bodian, June 4, 1952, JSP.

36 Bodian to JES, August 1, 1951, JSP.

37 Kane, "The Second International Poliomyelitis Conference."

38 Paul, *A History of Poliomyelitis*, 235.

39 Website for the *Queen Mary*: http://queenmary.com.

40 On the transatlantic crossing: Carter, *Breakthrough*; Oshinsky, *Polio: An American Story*; Smith, *Patenting the Sun*; Salk interview by Gabriel Stickle, September 8, 1984, MOD; Melvin Glasser Eulogy, March 13, 1972, MOD.

41 Salk oral history, September 8, 1984, MOD.

42 Smith, *Patenting the Sun*, 170.

43 JES to BOC, December 8, 1966, JSP.

44 Carter, *Breakthrough*, 121.

45 Lorraine Friedman interview.

46 JES to Evans, May 2, 1952, JSP.

47 Peter and Sylvia Salk interviews.

48 Sylvia Salk interview.

49 JES to Francis, April 13, 1954, JSP.

50 Carter, *Breakthrough*, 68–69.

CHAPTER 9

1 NFIP Annual Statistical Review, JSP.

2 Elaine Vitone, "Among My Souvenirs," *Pitt Med*, August 7, 2005, 33–34.

3 Carter, *Breakthrough: The Saga of Jonas Salk*, 107.

4 JES to Weaver, June 16, 1950, JSP.

5 Committee on Immunization, May 17, 1951, JSP.

6 Committee on Immunization, July 6, 1951, JSP.

7 Hammon, Coriell, and Stokes, "Evaluation of Red Cross Gamma Globulin as a Prophylactic Agent for Poliomyelitis: 1. Plan of Controlled Field Tests and Results of 1951 Pilot Study in Utah."

8 Hammon et al., "Evaluation of Red Cross Gamma Globulin as a Prophylactic Agent for Poliomyelitis: 3. Preliminary Report of Results Based on Clinical Diagnoses."

9 Oral history, Gabriel Stickle, August 17, 1983, MOD.

10 "35,000 To Get Polio Shots in Elmira Area," *Chicago Daily Tribune*, July 9, 1953.

11 Troan, *Passport to Adventure*, 199.

12 Benison, *Tom Rivers: Reflections on a Life in Medicine and Science*; Klein, *Trial By Fury: The Polio Vaccine Controversy*; Paul, *A History of Poliomyelitis*.

13 Klein, *Trial By Fury*, 52.

14 Paul, *History of Poliomyelitis*, 260.

15 H. A. Howe, "Antibody Response of Chimpanzees and Human Beings to Formalin-Inactivated Trivalent Poliomyelitis Vaccine."

16 On Koprowski: Margalit Fox, "Hilary Koprowski, Who Developed First Live-Virus Polio Vaccine, Dies at 96," *New York Times*, April 20, 2013.
17 Oshinsky, *Polio: An American Story*, 133–38.
18 Oshinsky, *Polio*, 136.
19 Oral history, Alexander Langmuir, September 5, 1984, MOD.
20 Donald Wegemer interview.
21 Ethel Bailey interview.
22 Anita Srikameswaran, "Polio Pioneers," *Pittsburgh Post-Gazette*, July 2, 2002.
23 Donald Wegemer interview.
24 Schlesinger, Morgan, and Olitsky, "Transmission to Rodents of Lansing Type Poliomyelitis Virus in the Middle East."
25 *Sunny Hill World*, March 1953, JSP.
26 Salk, Youngner, and Ward, "Use of Color Change of Phenol Red as the Indicator in Titrating Poliomyelitis Virus or Its Antibody in a Tissue-Culture System."
27 Oshinsky, *Polio*, 175–76.
28 Troan, *Passport to Adventure*, 185–89.
29 Troan, *Passport to Adventure*, 180.
30 "Pitt to Test Polio Serum on Humans," *Pittsburgh Press*, May 13, 1952.
31 Troan, *Passport to Adventure*, 191.
32 Bernard Fisher interview.
33 JES to Robinette, January 31, 1951, JSP.
34 JES to Tyler, 1953, JSP.
35 Proceedings of the Committee on Immunization, December 4, 1951, JSP.

CHAPTER 10

1 "Polio Nears Epidemic Stage: Eight in One Family Stricken," *Chicago Daily Tribune*, September 12, 1952.
2 "Fifth Polio Case on North Carolina Campus Strikes Freshman Guard on Football Squad," *New York Times*, October 4, 1952.
3 Silver and Wilson, *Polio Voices: An Oral History from the American Polio Epidemics and Worldwide Eradication Efforts*, 28.
4 Silver and Wilson, *Polio Voices*, 54–55.
5 Carter, *Breakthrough: The Saga of Jonas Salk*, 137.
6 Consent form, JSP.
7 *Sunny Hill World*, March 1953, JSP.
8 *Sunny Hill World*, March 1953, JSP.
9 Anita Srikameswaran, "Polio Pioneers," *Pittsburgh Post-Gazette*, July 2, 2002.
10 Anita Srikameswaran, "Polio Pioneers."
11 Anita Srikameswaran, "Polio Pioneers."
12 Anita Srikameswaran, "Polio Pioneers."
13 Carter, *Breakthrough*, 139.
14 Carter, *Breakthrough*, 139.
15 Salk, "Studies in Human Subjects on Active Immunization against Poliomyelitis."

16 Troan, *Passport to Adventure*, 197.
17 Sylvia Salk interview.
18 Walker to JES, April 11, 1952, JSP.
19 Walker to JES, July 14, 1953, JSP.
20 JES to Walker, April 8, 1953, JSP.
21 Committee on Immunization Minutes Summary, January 23, 1953, JSP.
22 Committee on Immunization Minutes Summary, January 23, 1953, JSP.
23 Carter, *Breakthrough*, 142.
24 Benison, *Tom Rivers: Reflections on a Life in Medicine and Science*, 245.
25 Committee on Immunization Minutes Summary, January 23, 1953, JSP.
26 Committee on Immunization Minutes Summary, January 23, 1953, JSP.
27 Committee on Immunization Minutes Summary, January 23, 1953, JSP.
28 Benison, *Tom Rivers*, 495.
29 Committee on Immunization Minutes Summary, January 23, 1953, JSP.
30 Committee on Immunization Minutes Summary, January 23, 1953, JSP.
31 Carter, *Breakthrough*, 144.
32 Committee on Immunization Minutes Summary, January 23, 1953, JSP.
33 Committee on Immunization Minutes Summary, January 23, 1953, JSP.
34 Committee on Immunization Minutes Summary, January 23, 1953, JSP.
35 Committee on Immunization Minutes Summary, January 23, 1953, JSP.
36 Committee on Immunization Minutes Summary, January 23, 1953, JSP.
37 Committee on Immunization Minutes Summary, January 23, 1953, JSP.
38 Carter, *Breakthrough*, 146.
39 Troan, *Passport*, 197–98.
40 Bendiner, "Salk: Adulation, Animosity, and Achievement," 208.
41 NFIP Annual Statistical Review, JSP.
42 Carter, *Breakthrough*, 150.
43 "The Scientist Speaks for Himself," March 26, 1953, JSP.
44 "The Scientist Speaks for Himself," March 26, 1953, JSP.
45 "The Scientist Speaks for Himself," March 26, 1953, JSP.
46 Salk, "Studies in Human Subjects," 1096.
47 Robert P. Laurence, "Jonas Salk: Optimism Still Motivates Him," *San Diego Union*, Sunday, April 10, 1983.
48 Carter, *Breakthrough*, 158.

CHAPTER 11

1 Carter, *Breakthrough: The Saga of Jonas Salk*, 171.
2 Carter, *Breakthrough*, 173.
3 Carter, *Breakthrough*, 179.
4 Carter, *Breakthrough*, 170–71.
5 Carter, *Breakthrough*, 176.
6 Benison, *Tom Rivers: Reflections on a Life in Medicine and Science*, 503–4; Carter, *Breakthrough*, 175–76.

7   Charles Massey interview.

8   Weaver to JES, September 1, 1953, JSP.

9   Carter, *Breakthrough*, 189.

10 BOC to JES, September 14, 1953, JSP.

11 Benison, *Tom Rivers*; Klein, *Trial by Fury: The Polio Vaccine Controversy*.

12 Carter, *Breakthrough*, 179.

13 "Mass Field Test Slated for Pitt Polio Vaccine," *Pittsburgh Press*, July 14, 1953, JSP.

14 Benison, *Tom Rivers*, 511.

15 Carter, *Breakthrough*, 228–29.

16 JES to BOC, October 16, 1953, JSP.

17 "Many Thousands to Get Polio Vaccine Next Year," Science Service, October 9, 1953, JSP.

18 Paul, *A History of Poliomyelitis*, 424.

19 Paul, *History of Poliomyelitis*, 425.

20 Paul, *History of Poliomyelitis*, 424.

21 Carter, *Breakthrough*, 196.

22 Cohn, *Four Billion Dimes*, 109.

23 BOC to JES, October 28, 1953, JSP.

24 Charles Massey interview.

25 John Troan, "Polio Vaccine Called Only 'Booster Shot,'" unknown newspaper, June 5, 1953, JSP.

26 ABS to JES, February 9, 1953, JSP.

27 ABS to McGuinness, December 15, 1953, JSP.

28 Donald Wegemer interview.

29 "D-Day against Polio," *Time*, November 23, 1953.

30 JES to *American Journal of Public Health*, December 10, 1953, JSP.

31 Kempe to McGuinness, November 27, 1953, JSP.

32 Sabin to McGuinness, December 15, 1953, JSP.

33 Francis to McGuinness, December 22, 1953, JSP.

34 JES to McGuinness, January 7, 1954, JSP.

35 JES to McGuinness, January 18, 1954, JSP.

36 JES to Bell, September 16, 1953, JSP.

37 Carter, *Breakthrough*, 207.

38 JES to BOC, December 1, 1953, JSP.

39 Benison, *Tom Rivers*, 511.

40 Carter, *Breakthrough*, 216.

41 Donald Wegemer interview.

42 Engel to JES, December 23, 1953, JSP.

43 Anita Srikameswaran, "Salk Team's 'Mr. Inside' Honored for Work on Polio Vaccine," *Pittsburgh Post-Gazette*, August 9, 2001, available online at http://old.post-gazette.com/healthscience/20010809poliohealth4p4.asp.

44 "Slow Hurry Led to Polio Vaccine," *New York Times*, October 11, 1953, JSP.

45 Seavey, Smith, and Wagner, *A Paralyzing Fear*, 199.

46 *National Foundation News*, vol. 13, 1954, JSP.

47   "Climax of the Strange Medical Drama," *New York Times Sunday Magazine*, January 10, 1954.

48   Harmon to JES, February 5, 1954, JSP.

49   John Troan, "He's the Man Who May Lick Both Polio and Flu," *World Telegram*, 1953.

50   Carter, *Breakthrough*, 166.

51   JES to Lieberson, June 28, 1954, JSP.

52   JES to Rivers, November 16, 1953, JSP.

53   Seavey, Smith, and Wagner, *Paralyzing Fear*, 185.

54   "Polio Fighter Salk: Is This the Year?," *Time*, March 1954.

55   Smith, *Patenting the Sun*, 255.

56   "Several States Balk at Tests of Polio Vaccine," *Chicago Daily News*, January 15, 1954.

57   Paul, *History of Poliomyelitis*, 422.

58   Troan, *Passage to Adventure*, 216.

59   Miller to JES, March 23, 1954, JSP.

60   Carter, *Breakthrough*, 224.

61   Cohn, *Four Billion Dimes*, 116.

62   Carter, *Breakthrough*, 231–32.

63   Soffel to JES, April 6, 1954, JSP.

64   Seavey, Smith, and Wagner, *Paralyzing Fear*, 187.

65   Carter, *Breakthrough*, 232.

66   Oshinsky, *Polio: An American Story*, 197.

67   Carter, *Breakthrough*, 233.

68   Carter, *Breakthrough*, 234.

69   Minutes from the Vaccine Advisory Committee meeting, April 25, 1954, JSP.

70   Carter, *Breakthrough*, 236.

71   Seavey, Smith, and Wagner, *Paralyzing Fear*, 204.

72   Jonas Salk interview, Academy of Achievement: A Museum of Living History, available online at http://achievement.org/autodoc/page/sal0int-1.

73   Peter Salk interview.

74   Ayres, *The Wit and Wisdom of Abraham Lincoln: An A-Z Compendium of Quotes from the Most Eloquent of American Presidents*, 44.

CHAPTER 12

1   Field trial: Carter, *Breakthrough: The Saga of Jonas Salk*; Francis et al., *Evaluation of the 1954 Field Trial for Poliomyelitis Vaccine: Final Report*; Oshinsky, *Polio: An American Story*; Seavey, Smith, and Wagner, *A Paralyzing Fear: The Triumph Over Polio in America*; Sills, *The Volunteers*; Smith, *Patenting the Sun*.

2   *National Foundation News*, December, 1953.

3   *American Weekly*, February 28, 1954.

4   Carter, *Breakthrough*, 228.

5   Oshinsky, *Polio*, 190.

6   *True Strange Medical Facts*, September, 1954.

7   "Polio Fighter Salk: Is This the Year?" *Time*, March 29, 1954.

8   "Polio: Free Shots for Nine Million," *Newsweek*, November 1, 1954.

9   "269,000 Needles," *Time*, May 10, 1954.

10 "1955—Polio's Last Year?," *Michigan Alumnus*, January 15, 1955, 165.

11 Paul, "Thomas Francis, Jr., 1900–1969."

12 "1955—Polio's Last Year?," *Michigan Alumnus*, January 15, 1955, 165.

13 Paul, "Thomas Francis, Jr."

14 Van Riper to Brown, November 15, 1954, JSP.

15 JES to von Magnus, November 8, 1954, JSP.

16 JES to Meltzer, May 18, 1954, JSP.

17 JES to Larson, 1954, JSP.

18 JES to Dietrich, May 4, 1954, JSP.

19 Bauer to JES, February 25, 1955, JSP.

20 JES to Bauer, March 22, 1955, JSP.

21 On the Rome conference: Carter, *Breakthrough*; Correspondent, "International Conferences: Poliomyelitis"; Smith, *Patenting the Sun*; International Poliomyelitis Congress, "Third International Poliomyelitis Conference," September 6–10, 1954, JSP.

22 Unknown date or author, JSP.

23 Salk, "Studies with Noninfectious Poliomyelitis Virus Vaccines," paper for the Third International Poliomyelitis Conference in Rome, September 8, 1954, JSP.

24 Benison, *Tom Rivers: Reflections on a Life in Medicine and Science*, 543.

25 Van Riper to JES, July 6, 1954, JSP; Weller, *Growing Pathogens in Tissue Cultures*, 86.

26 "Salk Vaccine: The Business Gamble," *Fortune*, September 1955, JSP.

27 Weller, *Growing Pathogens in Tissue Cultures*, 87.

28 Carter, *Breakthrough*, 249.

29 Klein, *Trial by Fury: The Polio Vaccine Controversy*, 106.

30 JES to Workman, December 27, 1954, JSP.

31 JES to BOC, February 7, 1955, JSP.

32 JES to BOC, November 8, 1954, JSP.

33 Cohn, *Four Million Dimes*, 109.

34 Carter, *Breakthrough*, 262–63.

35 Carter, *Breakthrough*, 262–63.

36 Seavey, Smith, and Wagner, *Paralyzing Fear*, 206.

37 JES to Kovener, November 30, 1954, JSP.

38 Braverman to JES, February 17, 1955, draft response attached, JSP.

39 Coe to BOC, December 13, 1954, JSP; JES to BOC, December 28, 1954, JSP.

40 JES to Ducas, October 13, 1954, JSP.

41 Smith, *Patenting the Sun*, 303.

42 Carter, *Breakthrough*, 264.

43 NFIP to Friedman, March 23, 1955, JSP.

44 Paul, "Thomas Francis, Jr."

45 Carter, *Breakthrough*, 243.

46 Seavey, Smith, and Wagner, *Paralyzing Fear*, 189.

47 Williams, *Virus Hunters*, 312.

48 Paul, *History of Poliomyelitis*, 432.

49 Benison, *Tom Rivers*, 548.

CHAPTER 13

1 "Annual Report 1955, The National Foundation for Infantile Paralysis," JSP; Ann Arbor Michigan footage, April 12, 1955, MOD A/V collection; Benison, *Tom Rivers: Reflections on a Life in Medicine and Science*; Carter, *Breakthrough: The Saga of Jonas Salk*.; Gould, *A Summer Plague: Polio and its Survivors*; Klein, *Trial by Fury: The Polio Vaccine Controversy*; Kluger, *Splendid Solution: Jonas Salk and the Conquest of Polio*; Oshinsky, *Polio: An American Story*; Paul, *A History of Poliomyelitis*; Salk talk at the National Organization's Conference of the NFIP, September 11,1955, JSP; Seavey, Smith, and Wagner, *A Paralyzing Fear: The Triumph Over Polio in America*; Smith, *Patenting the Sun*; Williams, *Virus Hunters*.

2 Carter, *Breakthrough*, 258.

3 Ann Arbor Michigan footage, April 12, 1955, MOD A/V collection; "Annual Report 1955, The National Foundation for Infantile Paralysis," JSP; "History of the Rackham Building," http://www.rackham.umich.edu/about/what-is-rackham/history-of-the-rackham-building.

4 Peter Salk interview.

5 Smith, *Patenting the Sun*, 318; John Troan, "The Impact of Dr. Francis's Announcement," *Pittsburgh Press*, April 12, 1955.

6 Williams, *Virus Hunters*, 314.

7 Ann Arbor Michigan footage, April 12, 1955, MOD A/V collection; "Annual Report 1955, The National Foundation for Infantile Paralysis," JSP; secretary of Gregg to JES, March 28, 1955, JSP.

8 Ann Arbor Michigan footage, April 12, 1955, MOD A/V collection; Francis et al., *Evaluation of the 1954 Field Trial for Poliomyelitis Vaccine: Final Report*.

9 Francis et al., *Evaluation of the 1954 Field Trial for Poliomyelitis Vaccine: Final Report*, 1.

10 Remarks at Ann Arbor, April 12, 1955, JSP.

11 Smith, *Patenting the Sun*, 323.

12 Salk, "Vaccination against Paralytic Poliomyelitis Performance and Prospects," 576.

13 Salk, "Vaccination Against Paralytic Poliomyelitis Performance and Prospects," 578.

14 Carter, *Breakthrough*, 281.

15 Remarks at Ann Arbor, April 12, 1955, JSP.

16 "Polio Is Conquered," *Pittsburgh Press*, April 12, 1955.

17 Smith, *Patenting the Sun*, 318.

18 "Triumph Over Polio," *South China Morning Post*, April 13, 1955.

19 Carter, *Breakthrough*, 271.

20 Paul, *History of Poliomyelitis*, 433.

21 "City May Get Its Supply in Forty-Eight Hours," *Pittsburgh Press*, April 12, 1955.

22 *See It Now*, CBS, April 12, 1955, MOD, A/V collection.

23 *National Jewish Monthly*, May 1955.

24 *See It Now*, CBS, April 12, 1955, MOD, A/V collection.

25 Carter, *Breakthrough*, 283.

26 Jonas Salk interview, Academy of Achievement: A Museum of Living History, available online at http://achievement.org/autodoc/page/sal0int-1.

27 Carter, *Breakthrough*, 285.

28 Carter, *Breakthrough*, 267.

29 Seavey, Smith, and Wagner, *Paralyzing Fear*, 207.

30 Peter Salk interview.

31 Peter Salk interview.

32 Carter, *Breakthrough*, 287.

33 Carter, *Breakthrough*, 286.

34 "Salk's Polio Vaccine is a Medical Milestone," CBC Digital Archives, http://www
    .cbc.ca/player/Digital+Archives/Health/Public+Health/Polio/ID/1824791244/.

35 Johnson to JES, April 21, 1955, JSP.

36 Fett to JES, n.d., JSP.

37 Carter, *Breakthrough*, 288.

38 Seavey, Smith, and Wagner, *Paralyzing Fear*, 216–17.

39 Seavey, Smith, and Wagner, *Paralyzing Fear*, 207–8.

40 *Pittsburgh Press Roto*, June 5, 1955, JSP.

41 Moore to Mrs. Salk, April 27, 1955, JSP.

42 "It's Anti-Climax for Dr. Salk," *Pittsburgh Press*, April 12, 1955.

43 BOC telegram to JES, April 22, 1955, JSP.

44 Notes, awards, offers, JSP.

45 Gertrude Salk, April 14, 1955, with clipping from the *New York Times*, April 14,
    1955, JSP.

46 Seavey, Smith, and Wagner, *Paralyzing Fear*, 208–9.

47 Specter to JES, April 18, 1955, JSP.

48 A grateful mother to JES, April 14, 1955, JSP.

49 Elliott to JES, May 4, 1955, JSP.

50 Cherre to JES, n.d., JSP.

51 Casper to JES, April 24, 1955, JSP.

52 Pietta to JES, April 23, 1955, JSP.

53 Vance to JES, April 23, 1955, JSP.

54 Michael to JES, May 2, 1955, JSP.

55 Bostron to JES, n.d., JSP.

56 Doeblen to JES, April 19, 1955, JSP.

57 Paul to JES, May 3, 1955, JSP.

58 Walker to JES, April 15, 1955, JSP.

59 Manning to JES, n.d., JSP.

60 Notes, awards, offers, JSP.

61 Fialkoff to JES, April 19, 1955, JSP.

62 Marc Selvaggio, "The Making of Jonas Salk," *Pittsburgh Magazine*, June 1984, 50.

63 Notes, awards, offers, JSP.

64 Notes, awards, offers, JSP.

65 "The Jonas Salk Congressional Gold Medal," *E-Sylum*, http://www.coinbooks.org/
    esylum_v17n36a20.html.

66 Carter, *Breakthrough*, 294–95.

67 Salk acceptance speech, Presidential Citation, April 22, 1955, JSP.

68   Carter, *Breakthrough*, 296.
69   "Where's the Vaccine?," *Time*, May 2, 1955.
70   Peter Salk interview.
71   *New York Times Magazine*, July 17, 1955.
72   "Thieves Visit Salk Auto," *New York Times*, April 24, 1955.
73   Jonas Salk interview, Academy of Achievement: A Museum of Living History, available online at http://achievement.org/autodoc/page/sal0int-1.
74   Carter, *Breakthrough*, 281.
75   Carter, *Breakthrough*, 281.
76   Rivers to JES, November 21, 1955, JSP.
77   Benison, *Tom Rivers*, 550.
78   Paul, *History of Poliomyelitis*, 433.
79   Carter, *Breakthrough*, 273.
80   Paul, *History of Poliomyelitis*, 432–33.
81   "Fanfare Ushers Verdict on Tests," *New York Times*, April 13, 1955.
82   Greer Williams, "Polio Post-mortem. What Really Happened?," *Medical Economics*, August, 1955.
83   Greer Williams, "Polio Post-mortem. What Really Happened?," *Medical Economics*, August, 1955.
84   "Annual Report 1955, The National Foundation for Infantile Paralysis," JSP.
85   Carter, *Breakthrough*, 269.
86   Editorial, "Narrow is the Way," 1096.
87   Carter, *Breakthrough*, 3.
88   Carter, *Breakthrough*, 122.
89   Jonas Salk interview, Academy of Achievement: A Museum of Living History, available online at http://achievement.org/autodoc/page/sal0int-1.

CHAPTER 14

1   *Newsweek*, April 25, 1955; Beasley to all physicians, April 20, 1955, JSP; US Department of Health, Education, and Welfare press release, April 22, 1955.
2   *Hong Kong Standard*, April 15, 1955; Wilson, *Margin of Safety*.
3   *Hong Kong Standard*, April 14, 1955; "Triumph Over Polio," *South China Morning Post*, April 13, 1955; *South China Morning Post*, April 14, 1955.
4   *Hong Kong Standard*, April 17, 1955.
5   Von Magnus to Friedman, June 4, 1955, JSP.
6   Beasley to all physicians, April 20, 1955, JSP; "The Polio Scramble," *Newsweek*, May 2, 1955.
7   "Where's the Vaccine?," *Time*, May 2, 1955.
8   Carter, *Breakthrough: The Saga of Jonas Salk*, 306.
9   Slack to NFIP, n.d., JSP.
10   Carter, *Breakthrough*, 304.
11   "The Polio Scramble," *Newsweek*, May 2, 1955.
12   "The Polio Scramble," *Newsweek*, May 2, 1955.

13 "Where Are We Now on Polio?," *Saturday Evening Post*, September 10, 1955.

14 US Department of Health, Education, and Welfare press release, April 22, 1955, JSP.

15 On the Cutter incident: Carter, *Breakthrough*; Neal Nathanson interview; Nathanson and Langmuir, "The Cutter Incident: Poliomyelitis Following Formaldehyde-Inactivated Poliovirus Vaccination in the United States during the Spring of 1955. I. Background"; Offit, *The Cutter Incident*; Oshinsky, *Polio: An American Story*; Troan to JES, draft of article for *Family Magazine*, August 29, 1955; Wilson, *Margin of Safety*.

16 "Leonard Andrew Scheele (1948–1956)," http://www.surgeongeneral.gov/about/previous/bioscheele.html.

17 Seavey, Smith, and Wagner, *A Paralyzing Fear: The Triumph Over Polio in America*, 198.

18 Wilson, *Margin of Safety*, 106.

19 Carter, *Breakthrough*, 315.

20 Saul Benison interview of Sabin, August 12, 1978, ASA.

21 Seavey, Smith, and Wagner, *Paralyzing Fear*, 210.

22 Carter, *Breakthrough*, 323.

23 US Department of Health, Education, and Welfare, press release from Surgeon General Leonard A. Scheele, May 8, 1955, JSP.

24 Carter, *Breakthrough*, 326.

25 Neal Nathanson interview.

26 "Great Polio Vaccine Snafu," *Democratic Digest*, July 1955.

27 Editorial, *Detroit Times*, May 15, 1955.

28 Williams, *Virus Hunters*, 326.

29 "Where Are We Now on Polio?," *Saturday Evening Post*, September 10, 1955.

30 *Time*, May 23, 1955.

31 Carter, *Breakthrough*, 327.

32 *Time*, May 30, 1955.

33 Williams, *Virus Hunters*, 330.

34 "Salk Vaccine: The Business Gamble," *Fortune*, September, 1955.

35 Offit, *Cutter Incident*, 81–82.

36 Cutter to "Dear Friends," n.d., JSP.

37 Williams, *Virus Hunters*, 218.

38 JES to Elliot, copy of editorial from the *Vancouver Province*, July 6, 1955, JSP.

39 Donald Wegemer interview.

40 Salk et al., "Formaldehyde Treatment and Safety Testing of Experimental Poliomyelitis Vaccines."

41 Ward to JES, July 5, 1955, JSP.

42 JES to Ward, August 18, 1955, JSP.

43 "Salk Shots for My Child," *American Magazine*, April 1955.

44 Salk's discovery of sediment: Memo to Technical Committee on Polio Vaccine, "Interim Report on Possible Influence of Precipitates on Inactivation of Virus," Fall 1955, JSP; JES to Shannon, October 5, 1955, JSP.

45 JES to WHO, November 11, 1955, JSP.

46 Salk, "Poliomyelitis Vaccine in the Fall of 1955."
47 Wilson, *Margin of Safety*, 113.
48 Carter, *Breakthrough*, 335.
49 Williams, *Virus Hunters*, 336.
50 Williams, *Virus Hunters*, 337.
51 Troan to JES, draft of an article for *Family Magazine*, August 29, 1955, JSP.
52 Williams, *Virus Hunters*, 338.
53 Paul to JES, June 27, 1955, JSP.
54 *Time*, July 4, 1955.
55 Carter, *Breakthrough*, 337.
56 ABS to BOC, June 25, 1955, ASA.
57 BOC to ABS (draft), July 12, 1955, MOD.
58 BOC to ABS, July 13, 1955, ASA.
59 ABS to BOC, August 1, 1955, JSP.
60 Analysis of Cutter incident: Bodian et al., "Interim Report, Public Health Service Technical Committee on Poliomyelitis Vaccine"; Nathanson and Langmuir, "The Cutter Incident: Poliomyelitis Following Formaldehyde-Inactivated Poliovirus Vaccination in the United States during the Spring of 1955. II. Relationship of Poliomyelitis to Cutter Vaccine"; Offit, *Cutter Incident*; Salk and Gori, "A Review of Theoretical, Experimental, and Practical Considerations in the Use of Formaldehyde for the Inactivation of Poliovirus"; Shorter, *The Health Century*, 68–69; Troan to JES, draft of article for *Family Magazine*, August 29, 1955, JSP; US Department of Health, Education, and Welfare, PHS Progress Report on the Poliomyelitis Vaccination Program, January 24, 1956, JSP; US Department of Health, Education, and Welfare press release, August 25, 1955, JSP.
61 Enders to Francis, November 18, 1955, JSP; Neva to JES, December 27, 1955, JSP; Philbrook and Ingalls, "Poliomyelitis Vaccination in Southeast Massachusetts in 1955."
62 Shorter, *Health Century*, 70.
63 JES to Hobby, February 24, 1956, JSP.
64 JES to Scheele, June 30, 1956, JSP.
65 "Salk Vaccine: The Business Gamble," *Fortune*, September, 1955.
66 Offit, *Cutter Incident*, 132–53.
67 "The Blue Sheet," January 8, 1958, 1, 3–14.
68 Belli to JES, January 20, 1958, JSP.
69 "Cutter Verdict—Families Awarded Total of $147,300," *San Francisco Chronicle*, January 18, 1958.
70 "Cutter Verdict," *Time*, September 5, 1955.
71 "Cutter Verdict—Families Awarded Total of $147,300," *San Francisco Chronicle*, January 18, 1958.
72 *Barron's*, September 12, 1955.
73 Statistical review issued by the NF-March of Dimes, MOD.
74 Editorial from local paper sent by Langmuir to JES, July 13, 1955, JSP.
75 JES to Diamond, October 20, 1955, JSP.
76 Van Riper to JES, September 27, 1955, JSP.

77 JES to Van Riper, October 1, 1955, JSP.
78 Van Riper to JES, October 4, 1955, JSP.
79 JES to Von Magnus, August 29, 1955, JSP.
80 JES to Von Magnus, September 22, 1955, JSP.
81 Shannon to JES, December 30, 1955, JSP.
82 Wucher to JES, June 3, 1955, JSP; Kipling, *Rewards and Fairies.*
83 JES to Wucher, n.d., JSP.

CHAPTER 15

1 Jonas Salk interview, Academy of Achievement: A Museum of Living History, available online at http://achievement.org/autodoc/page/sal0int-1.
2 Jane Krieger, "What Price Fame—To Dr. Salk," *Times Sunday,* July 17, 1955.
3 All letters from JSP; those quoted are separately referenced only if sender identified.
4 Baumann to JES, January 5, 1956, JSP.
5 Garcia to JES, December 26, 1955, JSP.
6 JES to Ritter, February 8, 1956, JSP.
7 Tauber to JES, January 27, 1957, JSP.
8 JES to Tauber, February 19, 1957, JSP.
9 Harris to JES, n.d., JSP.
10 JES to Alpert, November 5, 1956, JSP.
11 JES to Valchuela, February 4, 1957, JSP.
12 JES to Sanders, January 28, 1957, JSP.
13 JES to Glueck, January 28, February 17, 1956, JSP.
14 Lorraine Friedman interview.
15 National Father's Day Committee to JES, 1957, JSP.
16 JES to Spock, May 21, 1956, JSP.
17 JES to Enders, March 12, 1957, JSP.
18 Jane Krieger, "What Price Fame—To Dr. Salk," *Times Sunday,* July 17, 1955.
19 *Jewish Criterion,* April 15, 1955, JSP.
20 Huschel to JES, December 23, 1955, JSP.
21 JES to Miller, January 30, 1956, JSP.
22 JES to Coughlan, September 24, 1956, JSP.
23 President of Glycolator to Friedman, February 6, 1956, JSP.
24 Hassard to JES, February 6, 1956, JSP.
25 Albany Chamber of Commerce telegram to JES, February 27, 1956, JSP.
26 Fratzke to JES, February, 1956, JSP.
27 Evans and Wilson, *Fame: The Psychology of Stardom,* 63.
28 Peter Salk interview.
29 Seavey, Smith, and Wagner, *A Paralyzing Fear: The Triumph Over Polio in America,* 217–18.
30 Jonathan Salk interview.
31 Hirsch to JES, June 12, 1957, JSP.

32　Peter Salk interview.

33　Itinerary: JSP.

34　"Salk Back from Europe, Antique Buyer Bobo Too," *New York World-Telegram and Sun*, August 6, 1957.

35　*New York Herald Tribune*, August 6, 1957.

36　Darrell Salk in conversation with author.

37　"All Virus Vaccine Eyed by Dr. Salk," January 7, 1957, unknown newspaper, JSP.

38　Jane Krieger, "What Price Fame—To Dr. Salk," *Times Sunday*, July 17, 1955.

39　Donald Wegemer interview.

40　Anita Srikameswaran, "Salk Team's 'Mr. Inside' Honored for Work on Polio Vaccine," *Pittsburgh Post-Gazette*, August 9, 2001, available online at http://old.post-gazette.com/healthscience/20010809poliohealth4p4.asp.

41　Smith, *Patenting the Sun*, 323.

42　Carter, *Breakthrough: The Saga of Jonas Salk*, 214.

43　Anita Srikameswaran, "Salk Team's 'Mr. Inside' Honored for Work on Polio Vaccine," *Pittsburgh Post-Gazette*, August 9, 2001.

44　Oshinsky, *Polio: An American Story*, 174–75.

45　Donald Wegemer interview.

46　Lewis to JES, February 10, 1958, JSP.

47　Campbell Moses interview.

48　Receipt of the Presidential Citation, April 22, 1955, JSP.

49　"Vaccine's Name Irks Salk," *Pittsburgh Press*, April 12, 1959.

50　JES to Epstein, October 2, 1956, JSP.

51　JES to Bazeley, May 1, 1957, JSP.

52　Seavey, Smith, and Wagner, *Paralyzing Fear*, 218.

53　Lorraine Friedman interview.

54　JES to Neva, December 6, 1956, JSP.

55　Norrby, *Nobel Prizes and Life Sciences*, 11.

56　Norrby, *Nobel Prizes and Life Sciences*, 136.

57　Norrby, *Nobel Prizes and Life Sciences*, 139.

58　Norrby, *Nobel Prizes and Life Sciences*, 140.

59　Boffey, "National Academy of Sciences: How the Elite Choose Their Peers," 738.

60　Boffey, "National Academy of Sciences," 741.

61　Hellman, *Great Feuds in Medicine*, 2001, 126.

62　Klein, *Trial by Fury: The Polio Vaccine Controversy*, 115.

63　Paul Stumpf interview.

64　Campbell Moses interview.

65　JES to Lasker, undated draft, JSP.

66　Robert P. Laurence, "Jonas Salk: Optimism Still Motivates Him," *San Diego Union*, Sunday, April 10, 1983.

67　Campbell Moses interview.

68　Oshinsky, *Polio*, 209.

69　Oshinsky, *Polio*, 208.

70　Lorraine Friedman interview.

CHAPTER 16

1   Carter, *Breakthrough: The Saga of Jonas Salk*, 273–74.
2   Goetz to JES, November 27, 1957, JSP.
3   Bicks to JES, July 31, 1957, JSP.
4   JES telegram to Loynd, March 27, 1953, JSP.
5   JES to Bicks, August 13, 1957, JSP.
6   Beesley to JES, May 12, 1958, JSP.
7   JES to Bazeley, May 1, 1957, JSP.
8   Salk and Ward, "Some Characteristics of a Continuously Propagating Cell Derived from Monkey Heart Tissue."
9   "May Have Stumbled on Way to Cancer Victory," newspaper clipping sent by Sivens to JES, January 2, 1958, JSP.
10 "Salk's New Anticancer Claim," newspaper clipping sent by Rumsly to JES, January 22, 1958, JSP.
11 *Post and Times-Star*, August 1, 1958, JSP.
12 Walter to Lawrence, November 3, 1958, JSP.
13 Kuhn to JES, December 10, 1958, JSP.
14 Bzuro to JES, March 11, 1958, JSP.
15 Waters to JES, January 13, 1959, JSP.
16 Maxia to JES, April 4, 1959, JSP.
17 JES to Crum, January 6, 1958, JSP.
18 Press release from JES, December 27, 1957, JSP.
19 History of live virus vaccine: Carter, *Breakthrough*; Oshinsky, *Polio: An American Story*; Paul, *A History of Poliomyelitis*; Wilson, *Margin of Safety*.
20 "Live Polio Vaccine Tried on Prisoners: Chief Salk Critic Conducting Tests," *Pittsburgh Post*, January 18, 1955.
21 Debbe Sabin interview.
22 Peter Salk interview.
23 Samuel Katz interview.
24 Benison interview of Sabin, July 4, 1976, ASA.
25 Paul, *History of Poliomyelitis*, 455.
26 Debbe Sabin interview.
27 Health Commissioner to Terry, March 22, 1961, JSP.
28 Benison interview of Sabin, February 16, 1978, ASA.
29 *Meet the Press*, NBC, May 1, 1961, JSP.
30 Salk to Blasingame, November 22, 1960, JSP.
31 Critique of report on "The Present Status of Poliomyelitis Vaccination in the United States," approved by the House of Delegates, AMA, July 13, 1961, JSP.
32 Youmans to Salk, July 10, 1961, JSP.
33 Rosenthal to Larsen, July 3, 1961, JSP.
34 Larsen to Rosenthal, August 24, 1961, JSP.
35 Bodian, "Poliomyelitis Immunization."
36 Bodian, "Poliomyelitis Immunization," 21–22.

37   Benison interview of Sabin, February 19, 1978, ASA.
38   Salk to Terry, August 3, 1961, JSP.
39   Salk to Larsen, September 26, 1961, JSP.
40   Youmans to Salk, November 4, 1961, JSP.
41   Salk to Youmans, November 22, 1961, JSP.
42   Salk to Bodian, February 26, 1962, MOD.
43   JES to BOC, January 31, 1962, MOD.
44   Benison interview of Sabin, February 19, 1978, ASA.
45   "Death of a Killer," *Chet Huntley Reporting*, August 10, 1962, JSP.
46   O'Connor Press Conference, March 30, 1962, JSP.
47   BOC to McKelway, September 10, 1962, JSP.
48   Ruskin et al., "Poliomyelitis Following Sabin Type III Vaccine: Report of a Case Stressing Importance of Electro-Diagnostic Studies."
49   Gloucester to Culvertson, December 7, 1962, JSP.
50   BOC to Celebrezze, December 20, 1962, JSP.
51   On the attempt to create the Pitt institute: Bourgeois, *Genesis of the Salk Institute: The Epic of Its Founders*; Paull, *A Century of Medical Excellence*.
52   Personal note, May 25, 1957, JSP.
53   Personal note, May 25, 1957, JSP.
54   Paull, *Century of Medical Excellence*, 220.
55   Bernard Fisher interview.
56   JES to BOC, November 20, 1957, MOD.
57   JES to Gregg, November 24, 1958, JSP.
58   Paull, *Century of Medical Excellence*, 203.
59   Paull, *Century of Medical Excellence*, 220.
60   JES to McCluskey, April 22, 1959, JSP.
61   Paull, *Century of Medical Excellence*, 220.

CHAPTER 17

1   Notes to self, June 26, 1959, JSP.
2   Walsh, "Two Cultures," 652.
3   JES to Beaman, November 25, 1960.
4   Wade, "Salk Institute: Elitist Pursuit of Biology with a Conscience," 846.
5   JES to Lord Cohen, August 26, 1959, JSP.
6   JES to BOC, January 9, 1959, JSP.
7   Statement by Basil O'Connor re Institute, March 15, 1960, JSP.
8   JES to BOC, September 23, 1958, JSP.
9   Szilard to JES, May 7, 1959, JSP.
10   San Diego History Center website, http://www.sandiegohistory.org.
11   JES to Murrow, July 20, 1960, JSP.
12   Revelle to Kerr, August 23, 1959, JSP.
13   JES to Murrow, January 14, 1960, JSP.
14   JES to Murrow, January 14, 1960, JSP.

15 JES to Hazel O'Connor, November 25, 1959, JSP.

16 Bourgeois, *Genesis of the Salk Institute: The Epic of Its Founders.*

17 Jonas Salk, "Horizons into the Future: Reflections on the Thirtieth Anniversary of a Creative Collaboration with Louis Kahn," October 17, 1990, MOD.

18 On the life of Kahn: Wiseman, *Louis I. Kahn, Beyond Time and Style: A Life in Architecture*; Nathaniel Kahn, dir., *My Architect: A Son's Journey* (New York: New Yorker Video, 2003), DVD.

19 Mary Houlihan, "*My Architect* Builds Bridge from a Son to His Father," *Chicago Sun-Times*, February 22, 2004.

20 Jack MacAllister interview.

21 O'Connor press release, March 1, 1960, JSP.

22 JES to Revelle, March 17, 1960, JSP.

23 City Manager to Kerr, April 27, 1960, JSP.

24 Fletcher and Mack to BOC, April 5, 1960, JSP.

25 Whitney to JES, May 21, 1960, JSP.

26 Telegram from Revelle to JES, June 9, 1960, JSP.

27 Shapiro, "Jacob Bronowski: A Retrospective"; Wade, "Salk Institute."

28 Bronowski, "Bruno: A Personal View," 223.

29 Thomas, *A Few Selected Exits*, 206.

30 Bruce Mazlish, personal communication.

31 Salk, "The Next Evolutionary Step in the Ascent of Man in the Cosmos," 237.

32 Salk, "The Next Evolutionary Step in the Ascent of Man in the Cosmos," 237.

33 On Crick: "Francis Crick—Biographical," http://nobelprize.org/nobel_prizes/medicine/laureates/1962/crick-bio.html; Watson, *The Double Helix.*

34 Watson, *Double Helix*, 7.

35 On Szilard: Bourgeois, *Genesis of the Salk Institute*; Lanouette and Szilard, *Genius in the Shadows: A Biography of Leo Szilard, the Man Behind the Bomb.*

36 G. N. Cohen, "The Early Influence of the Institut Pasteur on the Emergence of Molecular Biology."

37 JES to BOC, October 18, 1959, MOD.

38 On Dulbecco: "Renato Dulbecco—Biographical," http://www.nobelprize.org/nobel_prizes/medicine/laureates/1975/dulbecco-bio.html.

39 Renato to JES, December 24, 1960, JSP.

40 JES to Renato, December 30, 1960, JSP.

41 On Benzer: http://www.plosbiology.org/search/simple?from=globalSimpleSearch&filterJournals=PLoSBiology&query=William%20A.%20Harris.

42 On Lennox: Curriculum vitae, JSP; Edwin Lennox interview; Wade, "Salk Institute."

43 Edwin Lennox interview.

44 On Cohn: Edwin Lennox interview; Bourgeois, *Genesis of the Salk Institute*; curriculum vitae in JSP.

45 Paul Berg interview.

46 Paul Berg interview.

47 Edwin Lennox interview.

48 Dulbecco to JES, November 8, 1960, JSP.

49 Cohn to JES, October 22, 1960, JSP.

50 JES to Dulbecco, n.d., JSP.

51 JES to Cohn, July 24, 1961, JSP.

52 Snow to JES, October 19, 1961, JSP.

53 On Weaver: John Henahan, "Warren Weaver Oral History," February 27, 1969, JSP; Mina Rees, *Warren Weaver, 1894–1978: A Biographical Memoir*, available online at http://www.nasonline.org/publications/biographical-memoirs/memoir-pdfs/weaver-warren.pdf.

54 John Henahan, "Warren Weaver Oral History," February 27, 1969, JSP.

55 John Henahan, "Warren Weaver Oral History," February 27, 1969, JSP.

56 JES to BOC, Spring 1961, JSP.

57 Weingarten to JES, May 4, 1961, JSP.

58 Director's Annual Report, February 1971, JSP.

59 Charles Massey interview.

60 David Rose interview.

61 Charles Massey interview.

62 Cohn to JES, July 13, 1961, JSP.

63 Cohn, Benzer, and Lennox to JES, December 22, 1961, JSP.

64 Monod to JES, December 13, 1961, JSP.

65 JES to Cohn, January 8, 1962, JSP.

66 Formal agreement between the NF and the Salk Institute for Biological Studies, February 26, 1962, JSP.

67 By-laws of the Institute for Biological Studies, March 6, 1962, JSP.

68 JES to Bronowski, February 19, 1962, JSP.

69 JES telegram to Cohn, Benzer, and Lennox, March 1, 1962, JSP.

70 Bronowski to JES, May 6, 1962, JSP.

71 "The Salk Institute: Probing the Mystery of Man," *Denver Post Sunday Empire Magazine*, July 24, 1966.

CHAPTER 18

1 Stoller, *The Salk Institute*, 3.

2 Esther McCoy, "Dr. Salk Talks About His Institute," *Architectural Forum*, December 1967; Stoller, *Salk Institute*; Wiseman, *Louis I. Kahn, Beyond Time and Style: A Life in Architecture*; Kahn to JES, August 14, 1961, JSP.

3 Esther McCoy, "Dr. Salk Talks About His Institute," *Architectural Forum*, December 1967.

4 Jonas Salk, "Horizons into the Future: Reflections on the Thirtieth Anniversary of a Creative Collaboration with Louis Kahn," October 17, 1990, MOD.

5 On the design of the Salk Institute: Brownlee and De Long, *Louis I. Kahn: In the Realm of Architecture*; Larson, *Louis I. Kahn: Unbuilt Masterworks*; Leslie, "A Different Kind of Beauty: Scientific and Architectural Style in I. M. Pei's Mesa Laboratory and Louis Kahn's Salk Institute;" Esther McCoy, "Dr. Salk Talks About His Institute," *Architectural Forum*, December 1967; McCarter, *Louis I. Kahn*; Stoller, *Salk Institute*; Wiseman, *Louis I. Kahn*.

6   Leslie, "A Different Kind of Beauty," 209–10.
7   JES to Kahn, August 8, 1962, JSP.
8   Stoller, *Salk Institute*, 2; *The Tribune*, May 17, 1985, JSP.
9   Jack MacAllister interview.
10 Brownlee and De Long, *Louis I. Kahn*, 331.
11 "Alfred Newton Richards Medical Research Laboratories and David Goddard Laboratories Buildings," Docomomo, http://docomomo-us.org/register/fiche/alfred_newton_richards_medical_research_laboratories_and_david_goddard_laboratories_buildings.
12 Jack MacAllister interview.
13 Wiseman, *Louis I. Kahn*, 134.
14 Wiseman, *Louis I. Kahn*, 134.
15 Stoller, *Salk Institute*, 3.
16 Charles Wilson, Summary of meeting with Kahn staff, December 28, 1961, JSP.
17 Jonas Salk, "Horizons into the future: Reflections on the Thirtieth Anniversary of a Creative collaboration with Louis Kahn," October 17, 1990, MOD.
18 Judith Bronowski, prod., *Jonas Salk: Personally Speaking* (San Diego: KPBS, 1999), VHS.
19 Esther McCoy, "Dr. Salk Talks About His Institute," *Architectural Forum*, December 1967.
20 Owner's representative to Kahn, October 25, 1962, JSP.
21 Donald Wegemer interview.
22 Joel Elkes interview.
23 Harvey to JES, July 19, 1962, JSP.
24 JES to Kahn, August 8, 1962, JSP; Leslie, "Different Kind of Beauty," 209.
25 Harvey memorandum, February 2, 1963, JSP.
26 Wiseman, *Louis I. Kahn*, 134.
27 Salk to Kahn, November 16, 1962, JSP.
28 Jack MacAllister interview.
29 JES to Weaver, December 7, 1962, JSP.
30 JES telegram to Kahn, January 2, 1963, JSP.
31 Weaver, "News, Questions and Reflections," February 11, 1963, JSP.
32 Edwin Lennox interview.
33 Harvey to BOC, June 6, 1963, JSP.
34 Langford to Fever, April 5, 1963, JSP.
35 Jack MacAllister interview.
36 Albert Rosenfeld, "The Great New Dream of Dr. Salk," *LIFE*, February 8, 1963.
37 Edwin Lennox interview.
38 Albert Rosenfeld, "The Great New Dream of Dr. Salk," *LIFE*, February 8, 1963.
39 Dulbecco to JES, February 7, 1963, JSP.
40 Dulbecco to JES, February 7, 1963, JSP.
41 Cohn to fellows, January 3, 1963, JSP.
42 Ralph Dighdon, "A Fortress Where War Is Waged on Disease: Commander Salk and His Eight Generals," *Los Angeles Herald-Examiner*, July 8, 1964.
43 Cohn to JES, November 21, 1963, JSP.

44   Murrow to JES, February 6, 1960, JSP.
45   Weaver to fellows, July 1963, JSP.
46   Report of the Director, September 23, 1963, JSP.
47   Wiseman, *Louis I. Kahn*, 120.
48   Brownlee and De Long, *Louis I. Kahn*, 333.
49   McCarter, *Louis I. Kahn*, 199.
50   Brownlee and De Long, *Louis I. Kahn*, 100.
51   Larson, *Louis I. Kahn*, 54.
52   Edwin Lennox interview.
53   Edwin Lennox interview.
54   Paul Berg interview.
55   Wiseman, *Louis I. Kahn*, 135.
56   Peter Salk interview.
57   Stoller, *Salk Institute*, 11.

CHAPTER 19

1   Livingston to JES, March 31, 1964, JSP.
2   Wade, "Salk Institute: Elitist Pursuit of Biology with a Conscience."
3   Crick to Salk, n.d., JSP.
4   "Has Dr. Salk's Dream Come True?" *Medical World News*, December 13, 1968.
5   Edwin Lennox interview.
6   Joel Elkes interview.
7   Edwin Lennox interview.
8   John Henahan, "Warren Weaver Oral History," February 27, 1969, JSP.
9   Weaver to Piel, March 12, 1964, JSP.
10   JES to Weaver, March 20, 1964, JSP.
11   JES to Elkes, April 23, 1964, JSP.
12   Bartemeier to JES, July 12, 1965, JSP.
13   On Kinzel: http://www.nasonline.org/member-directory/deceased-members/53790
     .html.
14   John Henahan, "Warren Weaver Oral History," February 27, 1969, JSP.
15   Edwin Lennox interview.
16   Paul Berg interview.
17   JES to BOC, June 15, 24, 1966, JSP.
18   Morrow to Lancaster, October 16, 1965, JSP.
19   "Andy Williams Tonight," *San Diego Union*, February 7, 1968.
20   Waitley to Williams, November 8, 1967, JSP.
21   *Valley News*, March 30, 1968.
22   Memo, August 4, 1965, JSP.
23   JES to BOC, February 22, 1967, JSP.
24   JES to BOC, March 6, 1967, JSP.
25   JES to BOC, May 20, 1967, JSP.
26   JES telegram to BOC, October 16, 1967, JSP.

27 Kinzel to institute staff, May 1, 1967, JSP.

28 Orgel to JES, May 3, 1967, JSP.

29 Orgel to JES, May 3, 1967, JSP.

30 "Hassle Ends Art Show at Institute," *San Diego Union*, n.d., JSP.

31 "Artists, Salk Official Row Over Paintings," *Los Angeles Times*, May 2, 1967.

32 Stoll to Kinzel, n.d., JSP.

33 Luce, Forward, Hamilton & Scripps to Orgel, May 8, 1967, JSP.

34 Porter to Baltimore, May 8, 1967, JSP.

35 Woodward-Baltimore and Duckworth to Orgel and Cohn, May 9, 1967, JSP.

36 Fellows to Board of Trustees, May 12, 1967, JSP.

37 Walter Eckhart interview.

38 Paul Berg interview.

39 JES to fellows, May 1967, JSP.

40 Shimkin, "Leonell C. Strong, 1894–1982."

41 Glazier to JES, January 16, 1964, JSP.

42 Betty McCraig, "Strong-Salk Trial," *East County Independent*, October 23, 1969.

43 JES to Parsons, June 10, 1969, JSP.

44 Randolph to JES, November 3, 1969, JSP.

45 "Salk Institute Loses Suit to Scientist," *Evening Tribune*, San Diego, December 13, 1967.

46 Betty McCraig, "Strong-Salk Trial," *East County Independent*, October 23, 1969.

47 Board of Trustees meeting, February 5, 1965, JSP; fellows to the Director, August 28, 1967, JSP.

48 Salk remarks at Kinzel memorial, October 27, 1987, JSP.

49 JES to Weaver, July 27, 1967, JSP.

50 On Slater: Kathleen Sullivan, "Joseph E. Slater: Aided WWII Rebuilding," *San Francisco Chronicle*, November 30, 2002, available online at http://www.sfgate.com/bayarea/article/Joseph-E-Slater-aided-WWII-rebuilding-2749434.php.

51 JES to fellows, May 1967, JSP.

CHAPTER 20

1 Milestones, *Time*, May 31, 1968.

2 Bob Lardine, "Dr. Salk Provides Some Answers," *New York Sunday News*, December 14, 1969.

3 JES to Walker Cisler, October 12, 1964, JSP.

4 Sylvia Salk interview.

5 Sylvia Salk interview; "Dr. Lee Salk, Child Psychologist and Popular Author, Dies at 65," *New York Times*, May 5, 1992.

6 Peter Salk interview.

7 Peter Salk interview.

8 Jonathan Salk interview.

9 Peter Salk interview.

10 Jonathan Salk interview.

11 "Mrs. Jonas Salk Happily Anticipates La Jolla Home," *Evening Tribune*, April 13, 1963.

12 Françoise Gilot; June and Walter Mack; Darrell, Jonathan, Peter and Sylvia Salk interviews.

13 Lorraine Friedman interview.

14 Peter Salk interview.

15 Jonathan Salk interview.

16 Sylvia Salk interview.

17 Joan Abrahamson interview.

18 "Mrs. Jonas Salk Happily Anticipates La Jolla Home," *Evening Tribune*, April 13, 1963.

19 Jonathan Salk interview.

20 Sylvia Salk interview.

21 Donna to JES, February 4, 1963, MOD.

22 Donna to JES, February 4, 1963, MOD.

23 Donna to JES, April 23, 1963, MOD.

24 Jonathan Salk interview.

25 "Donna Lindsay Salk, 85; Prominent Civic Activist," *San Diego Union Tribune*, May 31, 2002, available online at http://legacy.utsandiego.com/news/obituaries/20020531-9999_1m31salk.html.

26 Joel Elkes interview.

27 Maureen Dulbecco interview.

28 Barbara Marx Hubbard interview.

29 Hubbard, *The Hunger of Eve*, 15.

30 Barbara Marx Hubbard interview.

31 Barbara Marx Hubbard interview.

32 Hubbard, *Hunger of Eve*, 49.

33 Hubbard, *Hunger of Eve*, 49.

34 Barbara to JES, September 15, 1964, JSP.

35 Barbara Marx Hubbard interview.

36 Hubbard, *Hunger of Eve*, 81.

37 Barbara to JES, October 4, 1964, JSP.

38 Barbara to JES, October 27, 1964, JSP.

39 Barbara to JES, November 12, 1964, JSP.

40 Barbara to JES, December 6, 1964, JSP.

41 Fred Westhall interview.

42 Barbara Marx Hubbard interview.

43 Jon Cohen to author.

44 Salk to Goldsmit, December 16, 1957, JSP.

45 Bainbridge, *Across the Secular Abyss: From Faith to Wisdom*, 132.

46 Hubbard to JES, November 3, 1965, JSP.

47 Hubbard to JES, February 14, 1966, JSP.

48 Hubbard to JES, 1966, JSP.

49 Barbara Marx Hubbard interview.

50 Jessica Franken interview.

51 Peter Salk interview.

52 Peter Salk interview.
53 Darrell Salk in conversation with author.
54 Jonathan Salk interview.

CHAPTER 21

1 "Salk Tests Hint at Cure for Sclerosis," *San Diego Union*, December 1, 1970.
2 Donald Wegemer interview.
3 Report to National Foundation, November 1962–June 1963, JSP.
4 Lorraine Friedman interview.
5 Peter Salk interview.
6 Fred Westall interview.
7 Cruse and Lewis, *Historical Atlas of Immunology*; Salk, "Immunological Paradoxes: Theoretical Considerations in the Rejection or Retention of Grafts, Tumors, and Normal Tissue."
8 Salk, "Immunological Paradoxes," 368–69.
9 Salk and Ward, "Some Characteristics of a Continuously Propagating Cell Derived from Monkey Heart Tissue."
10 Summary of NFIP Grant, January 1 to December 31, 1964, JSP.
11 Rivers, Sprunt, and Berry, "Observations on Attempts to Produce Acute Disseminated Encephalomyelitis in Monkeys."
12 Poskanzer and Adams, "Multiple Sclerosis and other Demyelinating Diseases."
13 Timiras, "Remembrance: Elizabeth Roboz Einstein, (1904–1995)."
14 Einstein to JES, October 25, 1965, JSP.
15 Fred Westall interview.
16 Remarks by Dr. Harry M. Weaver, National Multiple Sclerosis Society in Chicago, March 29, 1969, JSP.
17 Nee to JES, May 1, 1968, JSP.
18 Eylar et al., "Experimental Allergic Encephalomyelitis."
19 JES grant application to the National Multiple Sclerosis Society, June 1, 1973, JSP.
20 Alvord et al., "Encephalitogen-Induced Inhibition of Experimental Allergic Encephalomyelitis: Prevention, Suppression and Therapy."
21 Bornstein, "A Tissue Culture Approach to Demyelinative Disorders."
22 Fred Westall interview.
23 Fred Westall interview.
24 Fredrick Seil interview.
25 Fred Westall interview.
26 Steven Brostoff interview.
27 Carlos Johnson memo, December 2, 1970, JSP.

CHAPTER 22

1 *San Diego Union*, February 19, 1968.
2 Ralph Keyes, "Jonas Salk Unfolding," *Human Behavior*, June 1973.

3   Jack MacAllister interview.
4   Salk to Warren Weaver, October 17, 1971, JSP.
5   Christine Forester interview.
6   Fred Westall interview.
7   Sylvia Salk interview.
8   *Independent Press-Telegram*, November 24, 1968.
9   Arnold Mandell interview.
10 Sylvia Salk interview.
11 Night notes, January 31, 1969, JSP.
12 "An Hour with French Painter Francoise Gilot," *Charlie Rose*, PBS, February 13, 1998.
13 "An Hour with French Painter Francoise Gilot," *Charlie Rose*, PBS, February 13, 1998.
14 On Gilot's life: "An Hour with French Painter Francoise Gilot," *Charlie Rose*, PBS, February 13, 1998; Françoise Gilot interview; Gilot, *Françoise Gilot: An Artist's Journey / Un Voyage Pictural*; Gilot and Lake, *Life with Picasso*; The F. Gilot Archives, http://www.francoisegilot.com.
15 "An Hour with French Painter Francoise Gilot," *Charlie Rose*, *PBS*, February 13, 1998.
16 Gilot, *Françoise Gilot*, 34.
17 Gilot, *Françoise Gilot*, 21.
18 Gilot, *Françoise Gilot*, 21.
19 "An Hour with French Painter Francoise Gilot," *Charlie Rose*, *PBS*, February 13, 1998.
20 Gilot and Lake, *Life with Picasso*, 15.
21 Gilot and Lake, *Life with Picasso*, 31.
22 "An Hour with French Painter Francoise Gilot," *Charlie Rose*, *PBS*, February 13, 1998.
23 Gilot and Lake, *Life with Picasso*, 354–55.
24 Gilot, *Françoise Gilot*, 54.
25 The F. Gilot Archives, http://www.francoisegilot.com.
26 Gilot, *Françoise Gilot*, 70.
27 "An Hour with French Painter Francoise Gilot," *Charlie Rose*, *PBS*, February 13, 1998.
28 Françoise Gilot interview.
29 Sylvia Salk interview.
30 Night notes, January 31, 1969, JSP.
31 "An Hour with French Painter Francoise Gilot," *Charlie Rose*, *PBS*, February 13, 1998.
32 Françoise Gilot interview.
33 Françoise Gilot interview; Jonathan Salk interview.
34 Françoise Gilot interview.
35 Christine Forester interview.
36 Darrell Salk conversation with author.
37 *Harrisburg News*, June 30, 1970.
38 "Jonas Salk Stalks Another Killer," *Philadelphia Enquirer*, January 12, 1978.
39 Françoise Gilot interview.
40 Jack MacAllister interview.
41 Ralph Keyes, "Jonas Salk Unfolding," *Human Behavior*, June 1973.
42 Sylvia Salk interview.
43 Maureen Dulbecco interview.

44 Christine Forester interview.
45 Donald Wegemer interview.
46 Walter Mack interview.
47 Lorraine Friedman interview.
48 Fred Westall interview.
49 Sylvia Salk interview.
50 Jack MacAllister interview.
51 Ralph Keyes, "Jonas Salk Unfolding," *Human Behavior*, June 1973.
52 Jonathan Salk interview.
53 Françoise Gilot interview.
54 Françoise Gilot interview.
55 Joan Abrahamson interview.
56 Françoise Gilot interview.
57 Françoise Gilot interview.
58 Ralph Keyes, "Jonas Salk Unfolding," *Human Behavior*, June 1973.
59 "An Hour with French Painter Francoise Gilot," *Charlie Rose*, PBS, February 13, 1998.

CHAPTER 23

1 Freud, *The Future of an Illusion*, 53.
2 "Narcissism and Responsibility in Science and Man," pamphlet prepared by the editor of the Carnegie Mellon University publications, from a taped record of the Salk lecture, May 1969, JSP.
3 "Salk's Smear," *Lynchburg (VA) News*, November 7, 1970.
4 Night notes, June 3, 1995, Eva Seilitz personal file, JSP.
5 Peter Salk interview.
6 Night notes, January 21, 1969, JSP.
7 Jonathan Salk interview.
8 Salk to Rubin, August 8, 1975, JSP.
9 "Buckminster Fuller," *Wikipedia*, http://en.wikipedia.org/wiki/Buckminster_Fuller.
10 Salk to Rubin, August 8, 1975, JSP.
11 Fuller, *I Seem To Be a Verb*.
12 "Buckminster Fuller," *Wikipedia*, http://en.wikipedia.org/wiki/Buckminster_Fuller.
13 Salk, "Biology in the Future," 430.
14 Salk, "Biological Basis of Disease and Behavior."
15 *Chet Huntley Reporting*, NBC, May 7, 1963.
16 "Narcissism and Responsibility in Science and Man," pamphlet prepared by the editor of the Carnegie Mellon University publications, from a taped record of the Salk lecture, May 1969, JSP.
17 Norman Cousins, "A Litany for Modern Man," *Saturday Review*, August 8, 1953.
18 Cousins to JES, June 29, 1969, JSP.
19 JES to Cousins, November 28, 1969, JSP.
20 Transcription of a taped conversation between Kahn and Salk at the Salk Institute, May 20, 1972, JSP.

21 Transcription of a taped conversation between Kahn and Salk at the Salk Institute, May 20, 1972, JSP.

22 Transcription of a taped conversation between Kahn and Salk at the Salk Institute, May 20, 1972, JSP.

23 Frederick Terzo interview.

24 Salk to Doxiadis, July 8, 1969, JSP.

25 Francoise Gilot interview.

26 *Baton Rouge Louisiana Advocate*, June 1970.

27 "Salk's Smear," *Lynchburg (VA) News*, November 7, 1970.

28 Taped transcript of Kahn's visit to the Salk Institute on May 20, 1972, JSP.

29 Lisa Longworth interview.

30 Jonathan Salk interview.

31 Jonathan Salk interview.

32 Heather Wood Ion interview.

33 Jonathan Salk interview.

34 Arnold Mandell interview.

35 Salk, *Man Unfolding*, 1.

36 Salk, *Man Unfolding*, 7.

37 Salk, *Man Unfolding*, 28.

38 Salk, *Man Unfolding*, 38.

39 Salk, *Man Unfolding*, 97.

40 Salk, *Man Unfolding*, 118.

41 *Triton Times*, December 1, 1972, JSP.

42 JES to Bronfman, May 8, 1972, JSP.

43 JES to Rubin, August 8, 1975, JSP.

44 C. H. Waddington, review of *Man Unfolding*, by Jonas Salk, *New York Times*, October 22, 1972.

45 Kenneth Klivington, "Dr. Salk: Yea-Sayer," *Los Angeles Times*, July 15, 1973.

46 Interview with Elizabeth Campbell, the Humanistic Psychology Institute, San Francisco, November, 1974.

47 Ralph Keyes, "Jonas Salk Unfolding," *Human Behavior*, June 1973.

48 Salk, *The Survival of the Wisest*, 1973; Edie Anderson, "Jonas Salk and Son: A New Reality," *North County Express*, December 15–31, 1981.

49 Lannan to JES, December 18, 1973, JSP.

50 Diefenbach to JES re excerpts from his book in the *Phi Delta Kappan*, June, 1975, JSP.

51 Salk, *Survival of the Wisest*, 91.

52 Salk, *Survival of the Wisest*, 118.

53 Kenneth Klivington, "Dr. Salk: Yea-Sayer," *Los Angeles Times*, July 15, 1973.

54 Dialogue discussion paper by Professor Robert Rosen, May 25, 1973, JSP.

55 Artigiani to JES, April 2, 1986, JSP.

56 Perl to JES, October 18, 1980, JSP.

57 Gough to JES, February 6, 1981, JSP.

58 Flower to JES, February 9, 1981, JSP.

59 Gutterman to JES, May 20, 1980, JSP.

60 Tobin to JES, July 18, 1974, JSP.

61 Horton to JES, April 4, 1974, JSP.

62 Graham to JES, September 24, 1973, JSP.

63 Christine Forrester interview.

64 Floyd Bloom interview.

65 Edwin Lennox interview.

66 Antonio Damasio interview.

67 Walter Eckhart interview.

68 Brian Henderson interview.

69 JES to Hardy and Linowitz, March 10, 1971, JSP.

70 Wiseman, *Louis I. Kahn—Beyond Time and Style: A Life in Architecture*, 135.

71 Arnold Mandell interview.

72 Crick to JES, January 19, 1967, JSP.

73 JES to Slater, March 5, 1968, JSP.

74 "Salk Institute Goes Public."

75 Bronowski to staff, February 17, 1970, JSP.

76 Night notes, January 28, 1969.

CHAPTER 24

1 On Slater's plans: *Scientific Research*, January 6, 1969, JSP.

2 Salk Institute Board meeting, November 9, 1967, JSP.

3 Wade, "Salk Institute: Elitist Pursuit of Biology with a Conscience."

4 Roger Guillemin interview.

5 Wade, "Salk Institute," 848.

6 Wade, "Salk Institute," 848.

7 Note to self, n.d., JSP.

8 "Andy Williams Tonight," *San Diego Union*, February 7, 1968.

9 "Dr. Salk Provides Some Answers," *New York Sunday News*, December 14, 1969.

10 "Armand Hammer," *Wikipedia*, http://en.wikipedia.org/wiki/Armand_Hammer.

11 McCloy memo to file, September 15, 1969, JSP.

12 Delbert Glanz interview.

13 Oral history interview, Gabriel Stickle, August 17, 1983, MOD.

14 Delbert Glanz interview.

15 Oral history interview, Gabriel Stickle, August 17, 1983, MOD.

16 Theodore Gildred interview.

17 John Henahan, Warren Weaver Oral History, February 27, 1969, MOD.

18 Board of Trustees meeting, October 8, 1969.

19 Board of Trustees meeting, February 12–13, 1970, JSP.

20 Board of Trustees meeting, February 12–13, 1970, JSP.

21 Board of Trustees meeting, February 12–13, 1970, JSP.

22 Board of Trustees meeting, February 12–13, 1970, JSP.

23 Nee to McCloy, February 5, 1970, JSP.

24 Board of Trustees meeting, February 12–13, 1970, JSP.

25 Board of Trustees meeting, February 12–13, 1970, JSP.

26 Ryan to Salk Institute, May 14, 1970, JSP.
27 O'Connor to McCloy, May 14, 1970, JSP.
28 Salk, Director's Annual Report, February 1971.
29 "Basil O'Connor: One Man's War against Disease," *Medical World News,* January 31, 1964.
30 "Heroes of our time," *Bulletin of the Overseas Press Club of America,* October 22, 1968.
31 Françoise Gilot interview.
32 JES to BOC, March 1, 1967, JSP.
33 JES to BOC, January 8, 1969, JSP.
34 Hazel O'Connor to JES, October 28, 1969, JSP.
35 JES to McCloy, Hardy, Linowitz, Slater, January 26, 1971, JSP.
36 Charles Massey interview.
37 O'Connor to JES, January 11, 1962, JSP.
38 Seavey, Smith, and Wagner, *A Paralyzing Fear: The Triumph Over Polio in America,* 204–5.
39 Albert Rosenfeld interview.
40 Night notes, January 12, 1969, JSP.
41 Jack MacAllister interview.
42 Night notes, January 12, 1969, JSP.
43 Rose to BOC, July 16, 1970, JSP.
44 McCloy telegram to Board, July 22, 1970, JSP.
45 Nee to McCloy, July 28, 1970, JSP.
46 Salk draft letter, August 17, 1970, JSP.
47 JES to Nee, January 26, 1971, JSP.
48 Guillemin interview; Guillemin to Nee, July 31, 1970, JSP.
49 *Evening Tribune,* San Diego, June 15, 1971.
50 Bourgeois, *Genesis of the Salk Institute: The Epic of Its Founders.*
51 *Daily Report,* January 26, 1972, JSP.
52 JES to Glasser, February 21, 1972, JSP.
53 Wade, "Salk Institute," 849.
54 Basil O'Connor obituary, *Houston Chronicle,* March 9, 1972; "Basil O'Connor, Polio Crusader, Dies," *New York Times,* March 14, 1972.
55 O'Connor Eulogy, March 13, 1972, JSP.
56 McCloy to Glasser, May 15, 1972, JSP.

CHAPTER 25

1 Biographical material, JSP; Delbert Glanz interview.
2 Walter Eckhart interview.
3 Fred Westall interview.
4 Ralph Keyes, "Jonas Salk Unfolding," *Human Behavior,* June 1973.
5 Westall Career Review, JSP.
6 Fred Westall interview.
7 Fred Westall interview.

8   Peter Salk interview.
9   Fred Westall interview.
10 JES to Nee, August 10, 1971, JSP.
11 JES to Bernbach, April 27, 1973, JSP.
12 JES to Linowitz, February 25, 1972, JSP.
13 JES to Nee, February 23, 1972, JSP.
14 Fred Westall interview.
15 Diefenbach to JES, June 13, 1973, JSP.
16 Minutes of the Executive Committee Meeting, July 12, 1973, JSP.
17 Edwin Lennox interview.
18 Delbert Glanz interview.
19 Edwin Lennox interview.
20 Floyd Bloom interview.
21 Arnold Mandell interview.
22 Cohn, Guillemin, Holley, Lennox, and Orgel memo to de Hoffmann, July 22, 1973, JSP.
23 Bronowski, Cohn, Guillemin, Lennox, and Orgel to McCloy, October 8, 1973, JSP.
24 JES to Meyer, July 26, 1973, JSP.
25 Holley to the Executive Committee, October 12, 1973, JSP.
26 Board of Trustees meeting, October 24, 1973, JSP.
27 Lorraine Friedman interview.
28 Arnold Mandell interview.
29 Annual fellows meeting, January 30–31, 1974, JSP.
30 Annual fellows meeting, January 30–31, 1974, JSP.
31 Annual fellows meeting, January 30–31, 1974, JSP.
32 CertainTeed Jonas Salk Foundation brochure, December 10, 1973, JSP.
33 De Hoffmann to Board of Trustees, April 18, 1974; Diefenbach to Stewart, June 27, 1974, JSP.
34 JES to Meads, January 3, 1975, JSP.
35 Diefenbach to Stewart, June 27, 1974, JSP.
36 Board of Trustees meeting, January 22–23, 1976, JSP.
37 Fred Westall interview.
38 Ajl to JES, October 30, 1975, JSP.
39 Fred Westall interview.
40 JES to Weaver, April 23, 1976, JSP.
41 Campbell et al., "Myelin Basic Protein Administration in Multiple Sclerosis."
42 Gonsette, Delmotte, and Demonty, "Failure of Basic Protein Therapy for Multiple Sclerosis."
43 Fred Westall interview.
44 "Study of Myelin Basic Protein as a Possible Therapeutic Agent in Multiple Sclerosis," Salk secretary to Romine, March 29, 1977, JSP.
45 Bornstein to JES, January 3, 1979, JSP.
46 Einstein to JES, January 16, 1978, JSP.
47 "Polio Hero Salk May Be Near Multiple Sclerosis Remedy," *Milwaukee Journal*, January 10, 1978.

48 "Jonas Salk Stalks Another Killer," *Philadelphia Enquirer*, January 12, 1978.
49 Neufeld to JES, January 12, 1978, JSP.
50 Ousley to JES, January 12, 1978, JSP.
51 Mastro to JES, January 19, 1978, JSP.
52 Brotman to JES, n.d., JSP.
53 Meyers to JES, n.d., JSP.
54 Foster to JES, n.d., JSP.
55 Nichols to JES, n.d., JSP.
56 Bachmann to JES, January 17, 1978, JSP.
57 Romine et al., "Preliminary Phase Studies of Myelin Basic Protein in Multiple Sclerosis: II. Clinical Observations."
58 Fred Westall interview.
59 B. T., n.d., JSP.
60 Anonymous patient, n.d., JSP.
61 Patients to JES, October 28, 1978, JSP.
62 JES to Romine, Wiederholt, Smith, September 8, 1978, JSP.
63 Romine et al., "Studies on Myelin Basic Protein Administration in Multiple Sclerosis Patients: 2. Preliminary Report of Clinical Observations."
64 Committee on Investigations involving Human Subjects, UCSD, to Romine, February 9, 1979, JSP.
65 NMSS review of MBP feasibility study, May 10, 1980, JSP.
66 JES to Eidinoff, April 17, 1989, JSP.

CHAPTER 26

1   Howard Taubman, "Father of Biophilosophy," *New York Times*, November 11, 1966.
2   Board of Trustees meeting, June 5, 1969, JSP.
3   Annual fellows meeting, February 3–4, 1972, JSP.
4   On de Hoffmann: William K. Stevens, "Frederic de Hoffmann, 65, Dies; Physicist and Salk Institute Chief," *New York Times*, October 7, 1989.
5   William K. Stevens, "Frederic de Hoffmann, 65, Dies; Physicist and Salk Institute Chief," *New York Times*, October 7, 1989.
6   Roger Guillemin interview.
7   Jack MacAllister interview.
8   Jack MacAllister interview.
9   Delbert Glanz interview.
10 Gibbons, "The Salk Institute at a Crossroads," 360.
11 Edwin Lennox interview.
12 Paul Berg interview.
13 Edwin Lennox interview.
14 Fred Westall interview.
15 Delbert Glanz interview.
16 Paul Berg interview.
17 Maureen Dulbecco interview.

18 On the relationship between Salk and de Hoffmann: Floyd Bloom, Maureen Dulbecco, Walter Eckhart, Theodore Gildred, Delbert Glanz, Roger Guillemin, Edwin Lennox, Jack MacAllister, Al Rosenfeld, Fred Westall interviews.

19 Gibbons, "Salk Institute at a Crossroads," 360.

20 Gerald Edelman interview.

21 Joan Abrahamson interview.

22 Al Rosenfeld interview.

23 Joan Abrahamson interview.

24 Edwin Lennox interview.

25 Victor K. McElheny, "Jacob Bronowski is Dead at 66," *New York Times*, August 23, 1974.

26 Salk memo, August 21, 1974, JSP.

27 Bourgeois, *Genesis of the Salk Institute*, 178.

28 Annual fellows meeting, January 24–25, 1975, JSP.

29 Delbert Glanz interview.

30 Board of Trustees meeting, January 29–30, 1975, JSP.

31 Leslie, "A Different Kind of Beauty: Scientific and Architectural Style in I. M. Pei's Mesa Laboratory and Louis Kahn's Salk Institute," 215–16.

32 Gabe Stickle interview of JES, September 8, 1984, MOD.

33 Vittachi to JES, May 17, 1976, JSP.

34 Hubbard, *The Hunger of Eve*.

35 Hubbard to JES, August 24, 1975, JSP.

36 Priestland, BBC, to JES, December 29, 1977, JSP.

37 Stan Swinton, Associated Press New York, October 27, 1977, JSP.

38 Board of Trustees meeting, January 30–31, 1974, JSP.

39 Board of Trustees meeting, January 29–30, 1975, JSP.

40 Lorraine Friedman, Arnold Mandell interviews.

41 Arnold Mandell interview.

CHAPTER 27

1 On the Fort Dix outbreak: Gaydos et al., "Swine Influenza A at Fort Dix, New Jersey (January–February 1976). I. Case Finding and Clinical Study of Cases"; "Swine influenza A at Fort Dix, New Jersey (January–February 1976). II. Transmission and Morbidity in Units with Cases"; "Swine Influenza A Outbreak, Fort Dix, New Jersey, 1976."

2 Osborn, *History, Science, and Politics: Influenza in America, 1918–1976;* Williams, *Virus Hunters.*

3 Salk, "The Restless Spirit of Thomas Francis, Jr., Still Lives," 275.

4 On the 1976 swine influenza: Boffey, "Anatomy of a Decision: How the Nation Declared War on Swine Flu"; Kolata, *Flu: The Story of the Great Influenza Pandemic of 1918 and the Search for the Virus that Caused It;* Neustadt and Fineberg, *The Swine Flu Affair: Decision Making on a Slippery Disease;* Osborn, *History, Science, and Politics.*

5 Boffey, "Anatomy of a Decision," 638.

6 Neustadt and Fineberg, *Swine Flu Affair*, 147–55.
7 Neustadt and Fineberg, *Swine Flu Affair*, 148.
8 Neustadt and Fineberg, *Swine Flu Affair*, 150.
9 Neustadt and Fineberg, *Swine Flu Affair*, 25.
10 Neustadt and Fineberg, *Swine Flu Affair*, 6.
11 Osborn, *History, Science, and Politics*, 49.
12 Neustadt and Fineberg, *Swine Flu Affair*, 29.
13 "Warning: The Virus is Present and Active," *Los Angeles Times*, April 11, 1976.
14 Neustadt and Fineberg, *Swine Flu Affair*, 30.
15 Neustadt and Fineberg, *Swine Flu Affair*, 46.
16 Night notes, January 8, 1969, JSP.
17 *Medical Post*, May 11, 1976.
18 Testimony before Subcommittee on Health and Environment, House of Representatives re HR 14409, June 28, 1976, JSP.
19 "Flu Danger May Stir Research, Says Salk," *San Diego Union*, September 10, 1976.
20 Salk KPBS interview by Dr. Jeff Kirsch, August 24, 1976, JSP.
21 "Sabin, Salk Split over Flu Shot Plan," *Washington Post*, June 29, 1976.
22 "Swine Flu False Alarm," *New York Times*, June 28, 1976.
23 "Right on Swine Flu," *New York Times*, July 20, 1976.
24 "The Swine Flu Snafu," *Newsweek*, July 12, 1976.
25 Lawrence Altman, "In Philadelphia 30 Years Ago, an Eruption of Illness and Fear," *New York Times*, August 1, 2006; Harold Schmeck, Jr., "Legionnaire's Disease: 5 Years Later the Mystery is all But," *New York Times*, January 19, 1982.
26 Lawrence Altman, "20 Flu-like Deaths in Pennsylvania, 115 Ill, a Mystery," *New York Times*, August 4, 1976.
27 Lori Heller, "Six Days, 25 Deaths, and Still No Answer," *Tribune-Review*, August 5, 1976.
28 Neustadt and Fineberg, *Swine Flu Affair*, 139.
29 On Guillain-Barré: Boffey, "Guillain-Barre: Rare Disease Paralyzes Swine Flu Campaign"; Kolata, *Flu*; Schonberger et al., "Guillain-Barre Syndrome Following Vaccination in the National Influenza Immunization Program, United States, 1976–1977."
30 Schonberger et al., "Guillain-Barre Syndrome," 120.
31 Boffey, "Guillain-Barre," 155.
32 Osborn, *History, Science, and Politics*, 49.
33 Samuel Katz interview.
34 Testimony before US Senate Committee on Labor and Public Welfare, March 31, 1977, JSP.
35 "Flu Danger May Stir Research, Says Salk," *San Diego Union*, September 10, 1976.

CHAPTER 28

1 "Vaccine Made Life Hell in Slow Motion," *Washington Star*, February 12, 1981.
2 Boffey, "Polio: Salk Challenges Safety of Sabin's Live-Virus Vaccine."

3 "Justices Refuse Appeal of Alert to Polio Vaccine," *New York Law Journal*, December 24, 1974; Curran, "Public Warnings of the Risk in Oral Polio Vaccine."

4 Salk, "Poliomyelitis: Reflections after Twenty Years," *San Diego Union*, March 28, 1973.

5 "Polio: The Cure for the New Controversy," *New York Times*, May 26, 1973.

6 JES to Maloney, November 15, 1974, JSP.

7 "News Plus Comment," *AAP News* 25, no. 16, 1974.

8 Katz to JES, January 10, 1975, JSP.

9 Lynch to JES, February 5, 1975, JSP; JES to Lynch, February 19, 1975, JSP.

10 Katz to JES, January 10, 1975, JSP.

11 Brian Henderson interview.

12 Gabe Stickle interview of JES, September 8, 1984, MOD.

13 "Polio Victim Wins Lawsuit," *San Diego Union*, June 6, 1975, JSP.

14 J. Salk and D. Salk, "Control of Influenza and Poliomyelitis with Killed Virus Vaccines"; D. Salk and J. Salk, "Vaccinology of Poliomyelitis."

15 Kevin Kimberlin interview.

16 Text of the oath can be found on the website Greek Medicine—The Hippocratic Oath, http://nlm.nih.gov/hmd/greek/greek_oath.html.

17 Samuel Katz interview.

18 Katz to JES, April 24, 1975, JSP.

19 JES to Meyer, August 4, 1976, JSP.

20 *Polio Immunization Program, 1976: Hearing before the Subcommittee on Health of the Committee on Labor and Public Welfare, United States Senate* (Washington, DC: US Government Printing Office, 1976), 8.

21 *NBC Nightly News*, September 23, 1976.

22 "In Polio Epidemic Vaccine Shortage Predicted," *San Diego Union*, February 10, 1976.

23 JES to Troan, October 6, 1976, JSP.

24 Chasan, "The Polio Paradox," 38.

25 Bodian to JES, June 23, 1976, JSP.

26 JES to Yau, October 1, 1976, JSP.

27 Night notes, August 5, 1977, JSP.

28 Salk presentation before the National Immunization Conference, NIH, November 12–14, 1976, JSP.

29 Fred Westall interview.

30 Ettinger to JES, October 7, 1977, JSP.

31 "Polio Fatal to Man Suing for Damages," *Arizona Daily Star*, September 23, 1977.

32 Karl Schindler v. the United States, March 1977, JSP; Katkowsky to JES, March 8, 1977, JSP.

33 Katkowsky to JES, January 10, 1985, JSP.

34 Chasan, "Polio Paradox," 39.

35 *Medical World News*, May 2, 1977, JSP.

36 Presidential Medal of Freedom, July 4, 1977, JSP.

37 JES to Carter, October 7, 1977, JSP.

38 Samuel Katz interview; Debbe Sabin interview.

39 Debbe Sabin interview.

40   Samuel Katz interview.

41   "A Long and Bitter Quarrel about Which Vaccine to Use," *New York Daily News*, December 20, 1976, JSP.

42   *Chicago Reader*, May 29, 1987.

43   Neal Nathanson interview.

44   Debbe Sabin interview.

45   Ezra Bowen, "Albert Sabin," *People*, July 2, 1984.

46   Neal Nathanson interview.

47   Faith Fitzgerald interview.

48   "Jonas Salk: Optimism Still Motivates Him," *San Diego Union*, April 10, 1983.

49   Floyd Bloom interview.

50   "The Polio Pioneers Are Still Busy," *Newsweek*, May 19, 1980.

51   Arnold Mandell interview.

52   BOC to ABS, July 12, 1955, ASA.

53   Debbe Sabin interview.

54   Peter Salk interview.

55   Author conversation with Darrell Salk.

56   Author conversation with Darrell Salk.

57   Chasan, "Polio Paradox," 39.

58   Ben MacNitt, "Vaccine Alternative Available When Man Died," *Tucson Daily Citizen*, July 11, 1981.

59   Carol Mooney and Howard Fisher, "Salk Says Sabin Vaccine Caused Death," *Arizona Daily Star*, July 11, 1981.

60   John Troan, "How Many More Must We Cripple?" *Pittsburgh Press*, September 30, 1979.

61   Salk, "The Virus of Poliomyelitis: From Discovery to Extinction," 810.

62   Ronald Moss interview.

63   Seytre and Shaffer, *The Death of a Disease: A History of the Eradication of Poliomyelitis*.

64   Charles Merieux to Ito, December 22, 1980, JSP.

65   Seytre and Shaffer, *Death of a Disease*, 93.

66   National Foundation grant, January 25, 1978, JSP.

67   Charles Merieux to JES, April 11, 1983, JSP.

68   JES to Stoeckel, May 5, 1977, JSP.

69   Charles Merieux to Ito, December 22, 1980, JSP.

70   JES to Stoeckel, January 6, 1981, JSP.

71   Salk, "Virus of Poliomyelitis," 810.

72   Bendiner, "Salk: Adulation, Animosity, and Achievement," 194.

73   M. Cimons, "Polio Heroes Still at Odds over Vaccine," *Los Angeles Times*, March 12, 1983.

74   Ezra Bowen, "Albert Sabin," *People*, July 2, 1984; "Dr. Albert Sabin, Developer of Oral Polio Vaccine, Dies," *Los Angeles Times*, March 4, 1993; Debbe Sabin interview.

75   Ezra Bowen, "Albert Sabin," *People*, July 2, 1984.

76   Debbe Sabin interview.

77   Debbe Sabin interview.

CHAPTER 29

1 Board of Trustees meeting, January 15, 1980, JSP.

2 Floyd Bloom interview.

3 Executive Committee meeting, May 27, 1980, JSP.

4 Paul Berg interview.

5 Joan Abrahamson interview.

6 Board of Trustees meeting, January 15, 1980, JSP.

7 Board of Trustees meeting, January 19, 1982, JSP.

8 Floyd Bloom interview.

9 Maureen Dulbecco interview.

10 Floyd Bloom interview.

11 Joan Abrahamson interview.

12 Night notes, July 27, 1984, JSP.

13 Kathleen Murray interview.

14 Delbert Glanz interview.

15 Night notes, July 27, 1984, JSP.

16 Wiseman, *Louis I. Kahn, Beyond Time and Style: a Life in Architecture*, 106–7.

17 Floyd Bloom interview.

18 Draft Aide-mémoire on the Possible Arrangements with Dr. Salk on Reaching the Age of Seventy, August 3, 1983, JSP.

19 JES to de Hoffmann, December 8, 1983, JSP.

20 Draft Aide-mémoire on the Possible Arrangements with Dr. Salk on Reaching the Age of Seventy, August 3, 1983, JSP.

21 Joan Abrahamson interview.

22 JES to de Hoffmann, December 8, 1983, JSP.

23 Remarks by the Founding Director to the Board of Trustees, January 2, 1984, JSP.

24 Remarks by the Founding Director to the Board of Trustees, January 2, 1984, JSP.

25 Transcribed minutes from the Board of Trustees meeting, January 25, 1984, JSP.

26 Dulbecco to de Hoffman, January 23, 1984, JSP.

27 Transcribed minutes from the Board of Trustees meeting, January 25, 1984, JSP.

28 Transcribed minutes from the Board of Trustees meeting, January 25, 1984, JSP.

29 Transcribed minutes from the Board of Trustees meeting, January 25, 1984, JSP.

30 Roget Guillemin interview.

31 Peter Salk interview.

32 Barbara Robinson interview.

33 Gerald Edelman interview.

34 Maureen Dulbecco interview.

35 Night notes, July 27, 1984, JSP.

36 Agreement, October 28, 1984, JSP.

37 Joan Abrahamson interview.

38 Fred Westall interview.

39 Jack MacAllister interview.

40 Joan Abrahamson interview.

41 Arnold Mandell interview.

CHAPTER 30

1 Lowan to JES, January 9, 1986, JSP.
2 Acceptance Address, Jawaharlal Nehru Award for International Understanding, January 10, 1977, JSP.
3 Goodfield, *The Planned Miracle*, 64.
4 JES to Juan, May 29, 1986, JSP.
5 J. Salk and J. Salk, *World Population and Human Values: A New Reality*.
6 Draft preface for *World Population and Human Values: A New Reality*, JSP.
7 "Jonas Salk & Son: A New Reality," *North County Express*, December 15, 1981.
8 "Jonas Salk & Son: A New Reality," *North County Express*, December 15, 1981.
9 Wheeler to JES, includes clip of review by Robert Rosen in *Journal of Social and Biological Structures*, May 5, 1982.
10 Salk, *Anatomy of Reality: Merging of Intuition and Reason*.
11 Jonathan Salk interview.
12 JES to Harman, April 16, 1980, JSP.
13 Paul Goldberger, "Louis I. Kahn Dies; Architect Was 73," *New York Times*, March 20, 1974.
14 Antonio Damasio interview.
15 Ted Mohns interview.
16 Ted Mohns interview.
17 Barbara Robinson interview.
18 Kathleen Murray interview.
19 Kathleen Murray interview.
20 Lorraine Friedman interview.
21 Fred Westall interview.
22 Hubbard to JES, June 11, 1981, JSP.
23 Eva Seilitz Horney, in honor of Jonas Salk's birthday, October 28, 1994, in private collection of Eva Seilitz Horney.
24 Eva Seilitz Horney interview.
25 JES to Horney, October 30, 1974, JSP.
26 Eva Seilitz Horney interview.
27 Eva Seilitz Horney interview.
28 Horney, personal communication, August 16, 2012.
29 Horney to JES, March 1, 1993, JSP.
30 Joan Abrahamson interview.
31 "In Perfect Balance," *Los Angeles Times*, November 3, 1985.
32 Joan Abrahamson interview.
33 JES to Abrahamson, April 1, 1985, JSP.
34 Joan Abrahamson interview.
35 Barbara Robinson interview.
36 Jon Cohen interview.
37 Heather Wood Ion interview.
38 Heather Wood Ion interview.

39 Ion to JES, May 11, 1992, JSP.
40 Ion to JES, July 26, 1992, JSP.
41 Barbara Robinson interview.
42 Lisa Longworth interview.
43 Lisa Longworth interview.
44 Lisa Longworth interview.
45 Lisa Longworth interview.
46 Information from Lisa Longworth's website, http://lisalongworth.com.
47 Carol Anne Bundy interview.
48 Carol Anne Bundy interview.
49 Carol Anne Bundy interview.
50 Bundy, personal communication, October 2, 2013.
51 Joan Abrahamson interview.
52 Kathleen Murray interview.
53 Joan Abrahamson interview.
54 Joan Abrahamson interview.
55 Horney, personal communication, April 15, 2012.
56 Eva Seilitz Horney interview.
57 Jack MacAllister interview.
58 Jon Cohen interview.
59 Steven Brostoff interview.
60 Brill to JES, September 25, 1987, JSP.
61 Brill to JES, October 1, 1990, JSP.
62 Kathleen Murray interview.
63 Arnold Mandell interview.
64 Lisa Longworth interview.
65 Eva Seilitz Horney interview.
66 Françoise Gilot interview.
67 Marsha Kaye, "Gilot (I'm Famous Myself) Is Still Painted into a Corner by Picasso," *Chicago Tribune*, December 3, 1981, JSP.
68 Ted Mohns interview.
69 "An Hour with French Painter Françoise Gilot," *Charlie Rose*, PBS, February 13, 1998.
70 Lisa Longworth interview.
71 Lisa Longworth interview.
72 Arnold Mandell interview.
73 Jonathan Salk interview.
74 Heather Wood Ion interview.
75 Barbara Beretich interview.

CHAPTER 31

1 J. Cohen, *Shots in the Dark: The Wayward Search for an AIDS Vaccine*; Shilts, *And the Band Played On: Politics, People, and the AIDS Epidemic*.

2 "Twentieth Century Miracle Worker," *Modern Maturity*, December 1984.

3 Gottlieb et al., "*Pneumocystis carinii* Pneumonia and Mucosal Candidiasis in Previously Healthy Homosexual Men: Evidence of a New Acquired Cellular Immunodeficiency."

4 Centers for Disease Control, "Kaposi's Sarcoma and *Pneumocystis* Pneumonia among Homosexual men—New York and California."

5 HIV/AIDS Surveillance Report, Centers for Disease Control, available online at http://www.cdc.gov/hiv/library/reports/surveillance/.

6 Fauci and Land, "Human Immunodeficiency Virus Disease: AIDS and Related Disorders."

7 Centers for Disease Control, "*Pneumocystis carinii* Pneumonia among Persons with Hemophilia A."

8 Centers for Disease Control, "Possible Transfusion-Associated Acquired Immune Deficiency Syndrome (AIDS)—California."

9 Centers for Disease Control, "Immunodeficiency among Female Sexual Partners of Males with Acquired Immune Deficiency Syndrome (AIDS)—New York."

10 Gallo and Montagnier, "AIDS in 1988"; Hellman, *Great Feuds in Medicine*; "The Chronology of AIDS Research."

11 Barre-Sinoussi et al., "Isolation of a T-Lymphocyte Retrovirus from a Patient at Risk for Acquired Immune Deficiency Syndrome (AIDS)."

12 Gallo et al., "Isolation of Human T-cell Leukemia Virus in Acquired Immune Deficiency Syndrome (AIDS)"; Gelmann et al., "Proviral DNA of a Retrovirus, Human T-cell Leukemia Virus in Two Patients with AIDS."

13 Fauci and Land, "Human Immunodeficiency Virus Disease."

14 HIV/AIDS Surveillance Report, Centers for Disease Control, available online at http://www.cdc.gov/hiv/library/reports/surveillance/.

15 Joan Abrahamson interview.

16 Robert Gallo interview.

17 Robert Gallo interview.

18 Lawrence Lasky interview.

19 Murray Gardner interview.

20 Lawrence Lasky interview.

21 Salk, "Prospects for the Control of AIDS by Immunizing Seropositive Individuals."

22 Notes from conference call among JES, Paul Luciw, Murray Gardner, September 19, 1986, JSP.

23 Notes dictated at 2:30–3:55 a.m. in AIDS Journal, March 14, 15, 1987, JSP.

24 Murray Gardner interview.

25 Faith Fitzgerald interview.

26 Kevin Kimberlin interview.

27 Kevin Kimberlin interview.

28 Kevin Kimberlin interview.

29 James Glavin interview.

30 Kevin Kimberlin interview.

31 Draft of "A business plan pertaining to developing, testing, licensing and marketing products related to the control of AIDS," October 7, 1987, JSP.

32 Kevin Kimberlin interview.

33 AIDS Journal, March 18, 1987, JSP.

34 Robert Gallo interview; Hellman, *Great Feuds in Medicine.*

35 J. Cohen, *Shots in the Dark*, 45.

36 "Chronology of AIDS Research."

37 Steven Brostoff interview.

38 Carol Anne Bundy interview.

39 Ronald Moss interview.

40 Dennis Carlo interview.

41 Steven Richieri interview.

42 Dennis Carlo interview.

43 Salk, "Prospects for the Control of AIDS."

44 Sana Siwolop, "A Tough Old Soldier Joins the Fight against AIDS," *Business Week*, July 27, 1987, 69.

45 Lawrence Altman, "New, Unorthodox Strategy on AIDS Proposed by Salk," *New York Times*, June 11, 1987.

46 "Ethics and an AIDS Vaccine," *Chicago Tribune*, July 24, 1991.

47 Katherine Bishop, "California Acts to Speed AIDS Drug Testing," *New York Times*, September 30, 1987.

48 Notice of Claimed Investigational Exemption for a New Drug, Salk AIDS Immunotherapeutic, submitted to Dr. Ray Wilson, California Department of Health Services, Food and Drug Branch, September 30, 1987, JSP.

49 Murray Gardner interview.

50 Alexandra Levine interview.

51 Alexandra Levine interview.

52 Dennis Carlo interview.

53 Copy of Alexandra Levine talk at a gathering of friends invited by the Salk family, July 9, 1995, private collection of Jonathan Salk.

54 Murray Gardner interview.

55 Sheryl Stolberg, "Hero With Something to Prove," *Los Angeles Times*, March 7, 1993.

56 Levine and Henderson to Human Subjects, January 14, 1988, JSP.

57 Alexandra Levine interview.

58 M. Glover, "UCD Drops Plan to Test Salk's AIDS Vaccine," *Sacramento Bee*, July 10, 1988.

59 E. Robinson-Haynes, "A New Setback for 95 Hoping to Beat AIDS," *Sacramento Bee*, July 13, 1988.

60 JES to Williams, July 12, 1988, JSP.

61 Salk, "Studies on HIV Immunotherapy," draft, January 17, 1990, JSP.

62 Gibbs et al., "Observations after Human Immunodeficiency Virus Seropositive and Seronegative Chimpanzees."

63 Lawrence Altman, "Salk Says Tests of Vaccine Show Halt of AIDS Infection in Chimps," *New York Times*, June 9, 1989, JSP.

64 Jon Van, "Hopes Rise for AIDS Vaccine," *Chicago Tribune*, June 9, 1989.

65 James Glavin interview.

66 Delbert Glanz, Roger Guillemin interviews; W. K. Stevens, "Frederic de Hoffmann, 65, Dies; Physicist and Salk Institute Chief," *New York Times*, October 7, 1989.

67 Delbert Glanz interview.
68 Levine et al., "Immunization of HIV-Infected Individuals with Inactivated HIV Immunogen: Significance of HIV-Specific Cell-Mediated Immune Response."
69 Salk, "Perspectives on an AIDS Vaccine," Sixth International Conference on AIDS, San Francisco, JSP.
70 Daniel Hoth interview.
71 J. Cohen, *Shots in the Dark*, 219.
72 J. Cohen, *Shots in the Dark*, 121.
73 "Ninth International Conference Draws 15000 to Berlin," *Global AIDSnews* 3:3–5, 1993.
74 Carlo, draft press release, 9th International AIDS Conference, 1993, JSP.
75 Trauger et al., "Effect of Immunization with Inactivated gp120-Depleted Human Immunodeficiency Virus Type 1 (HIV-1) Immunogen on HIV-1 Immunity, Viral DNA and Percentage of CD4 Cells."
76 Sheryl Stolberg, "Salk Report on AIDS Vaccine Meets Skepticism at Convention," *Los Angeles Times*, June 10, 1993.
77 Kevin Kimberlin interview.
78 Sheryl Stolberg, "Salk Report on AIDS Vaccine Meets Skepticism at Convention," *Los Angeles Times*, June 10, 1993.
79 Lawrence Altman, "Hopes Are Dashed on AIDS Therapy," *New York Times*, June 10, 1993.
80 J. Cohen, "Immune Response Corp.—Take Two."
81 Dennis Carlo interview.

CHAPTER 32

1 Ronald Moss interview.
2 Irene Lacher, "A Place of Her Own," *Los Angeles Times*, March 6, 1991
3 *Cleveland Plain Dealer*, May 10, 1984.
4 Mary Jane Salk interview.
5 Ronald Moss interview.
6 Joan Abrahamson interview.
7 "Avian Influenza Vaccines," http://www.uptodate.com/contents/avian-influenza-vaccines.
8 Lambert and Fauci, "Influenza Vaccines for the Future."
9 Transcription of recorded conversations, Jonas Salk and Bruce J. West, July 19, 1984, JSP.
10 *Arizona Republic*, April 13, 1985, JSP.
11 Debbe Sabin interview.
12 Joan Abrahamson interview.
13 Charles Massey interview.
14 Lawrence Lasky interview.
15 "The Thirty Million Dollar Temple of Thought," *Detroit News*, March 20, 1966.
16 Night notes, June 8, 1995, in private collection of Eva Seilitz Horney.

17 Carol Anne Bundy interview.

18 Robert Gallo interview.

19 Jonathan Salk interview.

20 Irene Lacher, "A Place of Her Own," *Los Angeles Times*, March 6, 1991.

21 Night notes, June 15, 1995, in private collection of Eva Seilitz Horney.

22 Eva Seilitz Horney interview.

23 Salk, "In Memory of a Meaningful Life," March 1, 1992, in private collection of Eva Seilitz Horney.

24 Salk, "The Meaning of Meaningful Life—A tribute to Lee Salk," n.d., JSP.

25 Heather Wood Ion interview.

26 Joan Abrahamson interview.

27 Kevin Kimberlin interview.

28 Night notes, June 9, 1995, in private collection of Eva Seilitz Horney.

29 Patrick Whelan interview; Silver and Wilson, *Polio Voices: An Oral History from the American Polio Epidemics and Worldwide Eradication Efforts*.

30 Patrick Whelan interview.

31 Silver and Wilson, *Polio Voices*, 145.

32 Ronald Moss interview.

33 Jonathan Salk interview.

34 Carol Anne Bundy interview.

35 Silver and Wilson, *Polio Voices*, 146.

36 "An Hour with French Painter Francoise Gilot," *Charlie Rose*, PBS, February 13, 1998.

37 Jonathan Salk interview.

38 Patrick Whelan interview.

39 Grace Glueck, "Salk Studies Man's Future," *New York Times*, April 8, 1980.

40 Heather Wood Ion interview.

41 Lorraine Friedman interview.

42 Christine Forrester interview.

43 Jane Krieger, "What Price Fame—to Dr. Salk," *New York Times Magazine*, July 17, 1955.

44 Charles Massey interview.

45 "The Price of Fame," *News Front*, July 1967.

46 Jonathan Salk interview.

47 George Johnson, "Once Again a Man with a Mission," *New York Times*, November 25, 1990.

48 Dulbecco, "Obituary: Jonas Salk (1914–95)."

49 Lawrence Lasky interview.

50 Arnold Mandell interview.

51 Robert Gallo interview.

52 "Stages and Phases of My Life"; "Chapters and Episodes of My Life," autobiographical material, 1985, JSP.

53 "Closing in on Polio," *Time*, March 29, 1954, 64.

Bibliography

MANUSCRIPT COLLECTIONS

Albert B. Sabin Archives (ASA), Henry R. Winkler Center for the History of the Health
Professions, University of Cincinnati Libraries, Cincinnati, OH

Archives, Frederick L. Ehrman Medical Library, New York University School of
Medicine, New York, NY

Archives and Special Collections, the City College of the City University of New York,
New York, NY

Jon Cohen AIDS Research Collection, University of Michigan, Ann Arbor

Jonas Salk Papers (JSP), Mandeville Special Collections Library, University of California,
San Diego, La Jolla, CA

March of Dimes Archives (MOD), March of Dimes Foundation, White Plains, NY

Salk Institute for Biological Studies, La Jolla, CA

Townsend Harris High School Archives, Flushing, NY

BOOKS AND JOURNAL ARTICLES

Aimone, F. The 1918 Influenza Epidemic in New York City: A Review of the Public
Health Response. *Public Health Reports.* 2010;125:71–79.

Alvord, E. C., C. M. Shaw, S. Hruby, and K. W. Kies. Encephalitogen-Induced Inhibition
of Experimental Allergic Encephalomyelitis: Prevention, Suppression and Therapy.
Ann NY Acad Sci. 1965;122:333–45.

Announcements. *Science.* 1962;136:769.

Antin, Mary. *From Plotzk to Boston.* Boston: W. B. Clarke, 1899.

Ayres, Alex, ed. *The Wit and Wisdom of Abraham Lincoln: An A–Z Compendium of Quotes from the Most Eloquent of American Presidents*. New York: Penguin, 1995.

Bainbridge, William S. *Across the Secular Abyss: From Faith to Wisdom*. Lanham, MD: Lexington, 2007.

Barre-Sinoussi, F., J. C. Chermann, F. Rey, M. T. Nugeyre, et al. Isolation of a T-Lymphocyte Retrovirus from a Patient at Risk for Acquired Immune Deficiency Syndrome (AIDS). *Science*. 1983;220:868–71.

Bendiner, E. Salk: Adulation, Animosity, and Achievement. *Hospital Practice*. 1983;18: 194–96, 200–201, 204–5, 208–11, 214-15, 218.

Benison, Saul. *Tom Rivers: Reflections on a Life in Medicine and Science*. Cambridge, MA: MIT Press, 1967.

Beveridge, W. I. B. *Influenza: The Last Great Plague*. New York: Prodist, 1977.

Bodian, D. Poliomyelitis Immunization. *Science*. 1961;134:819–22.

Bodian, D., T. Francis, Jr., C. Larson, et al. Interim Report, Public Health Service Technical Committee on Poliomyelitis Vaccine. *JAMA*. 1955;159:1444–47.

Boffey, P. M. Anatomy of a Decision: How the Nation Declared War on Swine Flu. *Science*. 1976;192:636–41.

Boffey, P. M. Guillain-Barre: Rare Disease Paralyzes Swine Flu Campaign. *Science*. 1977;195:155–59.

Boffey, P. M. National Academy of Sciences: How the Elite Choose Their Peers. *Science*. 1977;196:738–41.

Boffey, P. M. Polio: Salk Challenges Safety of Sabin's Live-Virus Vaccine. *Science*. 1977;196:35–36.

Bornstein, M. B. A Tissue Culture Approach to Demyelinative Disorders. *Natl Cancer Inst Monogr*. 1963;11:197–214.

Bourgeois, Suzanne. *Genesis of the Salk Institute: The Epic of Its Founders*. Berkeley: University of California Press, 2013.

Bronowski, R. "Bruno: A Personal View." *Leonardo*. 1985;18:223.

Brownlee, David B., and David G. De Long. *Louis I. Kahn: In the Realm of Architecture*. New York: Rizzoli International, 1991.

Campbell, B., P. J. Vogel, E. Fisher, and R. Lorenz. Myelin Basic Protein Administration in Multiple Sclerosis. *Arch Neurol*. 1973;29:10–15.

Carter, Richard. *Breakthrough: The Saga of Jonas Salk*. New York: Trident, 1966.

Caverly, Charles. "Anterior Poliomyelitis in Vermont in the Year 1910." In *Infantile Paralysis in Vermont, 1894–1922: A Memorial to Charles S. Caverly, MD*, 39–55. Brattleboro VT: State Department of Public Health, 1924.

Caverly, Charles. "Epidemic Poliomyelitis: A Review of the Epidemics of 1914 and 1915." In *Infantile Paralysis in Vermont, 1894–1922: A Memorial to Charles S. Caverly, MD*, 97–143. Brattleboro VT: State Department of Public Health, 1924.

Caverly, Charles. "Notes of an Epidemic of Acute Anterior Poliomyelitis." In *Infantile Paralysis in Vermont, 1894–1922: A Memorial to Charles S. Caverly, MD*, 21–38. Brattleboro VT: State Department of Public Health, 1924.

Caverly, Charles. "Preliminary Report of an Epidemic of Paralytic Disease, Occurring in Vermont, in the Summer of 1894." In *Infantile Paralysis in Vermont, 1894–1922: A Memorial to Charles S. Caverly, MD*, 15–20. Brattleboro VT: State Department of Public Health, 1924.

Centers for Disease Control. Immunodeficiency among Female Sexual Partners of Males with Acquired Immune Deficiency Syndrome (AIDS)—New York. *MMWR* 1983;31:697–98.

Centers for Disease Control. Kaposi's Sarcoma and *Pneumocystis* Pneumonia among Homosexual Men—New York and California. *MMWR* 1981;30:305–7.

Centers for Disease Control. *Pneumocystis carinii* Pneumonia among Persons with Hemophilia A. *MMWR* 1982;31:365–67.

Centers for Disease Control. Possible Transfusion-Associated Acquired Immune Deficiency Syndrome (AIDS)—California. *MMWR* 1982;31:652–54.

Chasan, D. J. The Polio Paradox. *Science.* 1986; 7(3): 37–39.

Chronology of AIDS Research. *Nature.* 1987;326:435–36.

Cohen, G. N. The Early Influence of the Institut Pasteur on the Emergence of Molecular Biology. *J Biol Chem.* 2002;277:50215–18.

Cohen, J. Immune Response Corp.—Take Two. *Science.* 1994;264:1402.

Cohen, Jon. *Shots in the Dark: The Wayward Search for an AIDS Vaccine.* New York: W. W. Norton, 2001.

Cohn, Victor. *Four Billion Dimes.* Minneapolis: Minneapolis Star & Tribune, 1955.

Correspondent. International Conferences: Poliomyelitis. *The Lancet.* 1954;264:650–51.

Cowen, Tyler. *What Price Fame.* Cambridge, MA: Harvard University Press, 2000.

Crosby, Alfred W. *America's Forgotten Pandemic.* Cambridge, UK: Cambridge University Press, 1989.

Cruse, Julius M., and R. E. Lewis. *Historical Atlas of Immunology.* London: Taylor & Francis, 2005.

Curphey, T. J. Fatal Allergic Reaction Due to Influenza Vaccine. *JAMA.* 1947;133:1062–64.

Curran, W. J. Public Warnings of the Risk in Oral Polio Vaccine. *Am J Public Health.* 1975;65:501–2.

Curson, Marjorie. *Jonas Salk.* Englewood Cliffs, NJ: Silver Burdett, 1990.

Debre, R., and S. Thieffry. Symptomatology and Diagnosis of Poliomyelitis. *Monogr Ser World Health Organ.* 1955;26:109–36.

Ducas, D. Unto the Least of These. *Sigma Phi Epsilon Journal.* February 1941;6.

Dulbecco, R. Obituary: Jonas Salk (1914–95). *Nature.* 1995;376:216.

Editorial. "Narrow is the Way." *N Engl J Med* 1955;252:1096–97.

Evans, Andrew, and Glenn D. Wilson. *Fame: The Psychology of Stardom.* London: Vision, 1999.

Eylar, E. H., J. Salk, G. C. Beveridge, and L. V. Brown. Experimental Allergic Encephalomyelitis. *Arch Biochem Biophys.* 1969;132:34–48.

Fauci, A. S., and H. C. Land. "Chapter 189. Human Immunodeficiency Virus Disease: AIDS and Related Disorders." In *Harrison's Principles of Internal Medicine,* edited by D. L. Longo, A. S. Fauci, D. L. Kapser, S. L. Nauser, J. L. Jameson, and J. Localzo, 1506–87. 18th ed. New York: McGraw-Hill, 2012.

Flexner, Simon, and James Thomas Flexner. *William Henry Welch and the Heroic Age of American Medicine.* New York: Viking, 1941.

Francis, T., Jr. Influenza: Methods of Study and Control. *Bull NY Acad Med.* 1945;21: 337–55.

Francis, T., Jr. A New Type of Virus from Epidemic Influenza. *Science.* 1940;92:405–8.

Francis, T., Jr. Transmission of Influenza by a Filterable Virus. *Science.* 1934;80:457–59.

Francis, T., Jr., and T. P. Magill. Immunological Studies with the Virus of Influenza. *J Exp Med.* 1935;62:505–16.

Francis, T., Jr., and J. E. Salk. A Simplified Procedure for the Concentration and Purification of Influenza Virus. *Science.* 1942;96:499–500.

Francis, T, Jr., J. E. Salk, J. E. Pearson, and P. N. Brown. Protective Effect of Vaccination against Induced Influenza A. *J Clin Invest.* 1945;24:536–46.

Francis, Thomas, Jr., John A. Napier, Robert B. Voight, Fay M. Hemphill, Herbert A. Wenner, Robert F. Korns, Morton Boisen, Eva Tolchinsky, and Earl L. Diamond. *Evaluation of the 1954 Field Trial for Poliomyelitis Vaccine: Final Report.* Ann Arbor, MI: Edwards Brothers, 1957.

Freud, Sigmund. *The Future of an Illusion.* Edited by James Starchey. New York: W. W. Norton, 1961.

Fuller, R. Buckminster. *I Seem To Be a Verb.* New York: Bantam, 1970.

Gallagher, Hugh Gregory. *FDR'S Splendid Deception.* New York: Dodd, Mead, 1985.

Gallo, R. C., and L. Montagnier. AIDS in 1988. *Sci Am.* 1988;259:41–48.

Gallo, R. C., P. S. Sarin, E. P. Gelmann, et al. Isolation of Human T-cell Leukemia Virus in Acquired Immune Deficiency Syndrome (AIDS). *Science.* 1983;220:865–67.

Gaydos, J. C., R. A. Hodder, F. H. Top, Jr., R. G. Allen, V. J. Soden, T. Nowosiwsky, and P. K. Russell. Swine Influenza A at Fort Dix, New Jersey (January–February 1976): II. Transmission and Morbidity in Units with Cases. *J Infect Dis.* 1977;136:S363–68.

Gaydos, J. C., R. A. Hodder, F. H. Top, Jr., V. J. Soden, R. G. Allen, J. D. Bartley, J. Zabkar, T. Nowosiwsky, and P. K. Russell. Swine Influenza A at Fort Dix, New Jersey (January–February 1976). I. Case Finding and Clinical Study of Cases. *J Infect Dis.* 1977;136:S365–62.

Gaydos, J. C., F. H. Top, Jr., R. A. Hodder, and P. K. Russell. Swine Influenza A Outbreak, Fort Dix, New Jersey, 1976. *Emerg Infect Dis.* 2006;12:23–28.

Gelmann, E., M. Popovic, D. Blayney, H. Masur, G. Sidhu, R. E. Stahl, and R. C. Gallo. Proviral DNA of a Retrovirus, Human T-Cell Leukemia Virus in Two Patients with AIDS. *Science.* 1983;220:862–65.

Gibbons, A. The Salk Institute at a Crossroads. *Science.* 1990;249:360–62.

Gibbs, C. J., Jr., R. Peters, M. Gravell, et al. Observations after Human Immunodeficiency Virus Immunization and Challenge of Human Immunodeficiency Virus Seropositive and Seronegative Chimpanzees. *Proc Natl Acad Sci.* 1991;88:3348–52.

Gilot, Françoise. *Françoise Gilot: An Artist's Journey / Un Voyage Pictural.* New York: The Atlantic Monthly Press, 1987.

Gilot, Françoise, and Carlton Lake. *Life with Picasso.* New York: McGraw-Hill, 1964; Anchor/Doubleday, 1989.

Gomery, D. Two Documents: "Your Priceless Gift" and "The 1946 Film Daily Yearbook." *Historical Journal of Film, Radio and Television.* 1995;15:125–35.

Gonsette, R. E., P. Delmotte, and L. Demonty. Failure of Basic Protein Therapy for Multiple Sclerosis. *J Neurol.* 1977;216:27–31.

Goodfield, June. *The Planned Miracle.* London: Scribners, 1991.

Gottlieb, M. S., R. Schroff, H. M. Schanker, et al. *Pneumocystis carinii* Pneumonia and Mucosal Candidiasis in Previously Healthy Homosexual Men: Evidence of a New Acquired Cellular Immunodeficiency. *N Engl J Med.* 1981;305:1425–31.

Gould, Tony. *A Summer Plague: Polio and its Survivors.* New Haven, CT: Yale University Press, 1995.

Greenberg, Louis. *The Jews in Russia: The Struggle for Emancipation.* New York: Schocken, 1976.

Griffin, H. E., and Thomas Francis, Jr. Epidemiologist to the Military. *Arch Environ Health.* 1970;21:252–55.

Hammon W. M., L. L. Coriell, and J. Stokes, Jr. Evaluation of Red Cross Gamma Globulin as a Prophylactic Agent for Poliomyelitis: 1. Plan of Controlled Field Tests and Results of 1951 Pilot Study in Utah. *JAMA.* 1952;150:739–49.

Hammon, W. M., et al. Evaluation of Red Cross Gamma Globulin as a Prophylactic Agent for Poliomyelitis: 3. Preliminary Report of Results Based on Clinical Diagnoses. *JAMA.* 1952;150:757–60.

Heaton, C. E., and A. E. Dumont. *The First One Hundred Twenty-Five Years of the New York University School of Medicine.* New York: New York University, 1966.

Hellman, Hal. *Great Feuds in Medicine.* New York: John Wiley & Sons, 2001.

Hirst, G. K. The Quantitative Determination of Influenza Virus and Antibodies by Means of Red Cell Agglutination. *J Exp Med.* 1942;75:49–64.

Howe, H. A. Antibody Response of Chimpanzees and Human Beings to Formalin-Inactivated Trivalent Poliomyelitis Vaccine. *Am J Hyg.* 1952;56:265–86.

Howe, Irving. *World of Our Fathers.* New York: Harcourt Brace Jovanovich, 1976.

Hubbard, Barbara Marx. *The Hunger of Eve.* Eastsound, WA: Island Pacific Northwest, 1989.

Ibbotson, Patricia. *Eloise: Poorhouse, Farm, Asylum and Hospital, 1839–1984.* Charleston, SC: Arcadia, 2012.

Iezzoni, Lynette. *Influenza 1918.* New York: TV Books, 1999.

Kane, F. F. The Second International Poliomyelitis Conference. *Med J Aust.* 1951; 2:790–92.

Katz, S. L. From Culture to Vaccine: Salk and Sabin. *N Engl J Med.* 2004;351:1485–87.

Keller, Werner. *Diaspora: The Post-Biblical History of the Jews.* New York: Harcourt, Brace, & World, 1966.

Klein, Aaron E. *Trial by Fury: The Polio Vaccine Controversy.* New York: Charles Scribner's Sons, 1972.

Kipling, Rudyard. *Rewards and Fairies.* London: Macmillan, 1910.

Kluger, Jeffrey. *Splendid Solution: Jonas Salk and the Conquest of Polio.* New York: J. P. Putnam's Sons, 2004.

Kolata, Gina. *Flu: The Story of the Great Influenza Pandemic of 1918 and the Search for the Virus that Caused It.* New York: Farrar, Straus & Giroux, 1999.

Kroeger, Otto, and Janet M Thuesen. *Type Talk.* New York: Dell, 1988.

Lambert, L. C., and A. S. Fauci. Influenza Vaccines for the Future. *N Engl J Med.* 2010;363:2036–44.

Lanouette, William, with Bela Szilard. *Genius in the Shadows: A Biography of Leo Szilard, the Man behind the Bomb.* New York: C. Scribner's Sons, 1992.

Larson, Kent. *Louis I. Kahn: Unbuilt Masterworks.* New York: Monacelli, 2000.

Lebow, Eileen F. *The Bright Boys: A History of Townsend Harris High School.* Westport CT: Greenwood, 2000.

Leonell C. Strong. *CA Cancer J Clin*. 1979;29:54–56.

Leslie, S. W. A Different Kind of Beauty: Scientific and Architectural Style in I. M. Pei's Mesa Laboratory and Louis Kahn's Salk Institute. *Historical Studies in the Natural Sciences*. 2008;38:173–221.

Levine A., B. E. Henderson, S. Groshen, and J. Salk. Immunization of HIV-Infected Individuals with Inactivated HIV Immunogen: Significance of HIV-Specific Cell-Mediated Immune Response [Abst. ThA337]. Sixth International Conference on AIDS. 1990:204.

McCarter, Robert. *Louis I Kahn*. New York: Phaidon, 2005.

McPherson, Stephanie Sammartino. *Jonas Salk: Conquering Polio*. Minneapolis: Lerner, 2002.

Members of the Commission on Influenza, Board for the Investigation and Control of Influenza and Other Epidemic Diseases in the Army, Preventive Medicine Service, Office of the Surgeon General, United States Army. A Clinical Evaluation of Vaccination against Influenza. *JAMA*. 1944;124:982–85.

Milton, John. *Paradise Lost*. New York: A. S. Barnes, 1867.

Nathanson, N., and A. D. Langmuir. The Cutter Incident: Poliomyelitis Following Formaldehyde-Inactivated Poliovirus Vaccination in the United States during the Spring of 1955. I. Background. *Amer Jour Hyg*. 1963;78:16–28.

Nathanson, N., and A. D. Langmuir. The Cutter Incident: Poliomyelitis Following Formaldehyde-Inactivated Poliovirus Vaccination in the United States during the Spring of 1955. II. Relationship of Poliomyelitis to Cutter Vaccine. *Amer Jour Hyg*. 1963;78:29–60.

Neustadt, Richard E., and Harvey V. Fineberg. *The Swine Flu Affair: Decision Making on a Slippery Disease*. US Department of Health, Education, and Welfare, 1978; repr., Honolulu: University Press of the Pacific, 2005.

Norrby, Erling. *Nobel Prizes and Life Sciences*. Singapore: World Scientific Publishing, 2010.

Offit, Paul A. *The Cutter Incident*. New Haven, CT: Yale University Press, 2005.

Osborn, June E. *History, Science, and Politics: Influenza in America, 1918–1976*. New York: Prodist, 1977.

Oshinsky, David M. *Polio: An American Story*. New York: Oxford University Press, 2005.

Paul, J. R. Epidemiology of Poliomyelitis. *Monogr Ser World Health Organ*. 1955;26:9–57.

Paul, John R. *A History of Poliomyelitis*. New Haven, CT: Yale University Press, 1971.

Paul, J. R. "Thomas Francis, Jr., 1900–1969." In *Biographical Memoirs*, vol. 44, 58–113. Washington, DC: National Academy of Sciences, 1974.

Paull, Barbara I. *A Century of Medical Excellence*. Pittsburgh: University of Pittsburgh, Medical Alumni Association, 1986.

Philbrook, F. R., and T. H. Ingalls. Poliomyelitis Vaccination in Southeast Massachusetts in 1955. *N Engl J Med*. 1956;255:385–87.

Plotkin, Stanley A., and Edward A. Mortimer, Jr. *Vaccines*. Philadelphia: W. B. Saunders, 1988.

Poskanzer, D. C., and D. A. Raymond. "Multiple Sclerosis and Other Demyelinating Diseases." In *Principles of Internal Medicine*, edited by K. J. Isselbacher, R. D. Adams, E. Braunwald, R. G. Petersdorf, and J. D. Wilson, 1971–77. 9th ed. New York: McGraw-Hill, 1980.

Rischin, Moses. *The Promised City*. Cambridge, MA: Harvard University Press, 1977.

Rivers, T., D. H. Sprunt, and G. P. Berry. Observations on Attempts to Produce Acute Disseminated Encephalomyelitis in Monkeys. *J Exp Med*. 1933;58:39–53.

Romine, J. S., J. Salk, W. C. Wiederholt, F. C. Westall, and C. K. Jablecki. Preliminary Phase Studies of Myelin Basic Protein in Multiple Sclerosis: II. Clinical Observations. *Neurology*. 1979;29:572.

Romine, J. S., J. Salk, W. C. Wiederholt, F. C. Westall, and C. K. Jablecki. "Studies on Myelin Basic Protein Administration in Multiple Sclerosis Patients: 2. Preliminary Report of Clinical Observations." In *Progress in Multiple Sclerosis Research*, edited by H. Bauer, S. Poser, and G. Ritter, 428–33. New York: Springer-Verlag, 1980.

Rose, David W. *Images of America: March of Dimes*. Charleston, SC: Arcadia, 2003.

Rudy, S. Willis. *The College of the City of New York: A History, 1847–1947*. New York: City College Press, 1949.

Ruskin, A. P., H. Rosner, B. Marshall, and J. B. Rogoff. Poliomyelitis Following Sabin Type III Vaccine: Report of a Case Stressing Importance of Electro-Diagnostic Studies. *Arch Phys Med Rehabil*. 1964;451:93–96.

Sabin, A. B. Vaccine-Associated Poliomyelitis Cases. *Bull World Health Organ*. 1969;40: 947–49.

Sachar, Howard M. *The Course of Modern Jewish History*. Cleveland: World Publishing, 1958.

Salk Institute Goes Public. *Nature*. 1970; 225:788.

Salk, D., and J. Salk. Vaccinology of Poliomyelitis. *Vaccine*. 1984;2(1):59–74.

Salk, Jonas. *Anatomy of Reality: Merging of Intuition and Reason*. New York: Columbia University Press, 1983.

Salk, J. E. Biological Basis of Disease and Behavior. *Perspectives in Biology and Medicine*. 1962;5:198–206.

Salk, J. E. Biology in the Future. *Perspectives in Biology and Medicine*. 1962;5:423–31.

Salk, J. Immunological Paradoxes: Theoretical Considerations in the Rejection or Retention of Grafts, Tumors, and Normal Tissue. *Ann NY Acad Sci*. 1969;164:365–80.

Salk, J. E. An Interpretation of the Significance of Influenza Virus Variation for the Development of an Effective Vaccine. *Bull NY Acad Med*. 1952;28:748–65.

Salk, Jonas. *Man Unfolding*. New York: Harper & Row, 1972.

Salk, J. E. Method for Separation of Micro-organisms from Large Quantities of Broth Culture. *Proc Soc Exp Biol Med*. 1938;38:228–30.

Salk, J. The Next Evolutionary Step in the Ascent of Man in the Cosmos. *Leonardo*. 1985;18:237–42.

Salk, J. E. Poliomyelitis Vaccine in the Fall of 1955. *Am J Public Health Nations Health*. 1956;46:1–14.

Salk, J. Prospects for the Control of AIDS by Immunizing Seropositive Individuals. *Nature*. 1987;327:473–76.

Salk, J. E. Reactions to Influenza Virus Vaccines. *JAMA*. 1947;134:393.

Salk, J. The Restless Spirit of Thomas Francis, Jr., Still Lives. *Arch Environ Health*. 1970;21:273–75.

Salk, J. E. Studies in Human Subjects on Active Immunization against Poliomyelitis. *JAMA*. 1953;151:1081–98.

Salk, Jonas. *The Survival of the Wisest.* New York: Harper & Row, 1973.

Salk, J. E. Vaccination against Paralytic Poliomyelitis Performance and Prospects. *Am J Public Health Nations Health.* 1955;45:575–96.

Salk, J. The Virus of Poliomyelitis: From Discovery to Extinction. *JAMA.* 1983;250:808–10.

Salk, J. E., and T. Francis, Jr. Immunization against Influenza. *Ann Int Med.* 1946;25:443–52.

Salk, J. E., and J. B. Gori. A Review of Theoretical, Experimental, and Practical Considerations in the Use of Formaldehyde for the Inactivation of Poliovirus. *Ann NY Acad Sci.* 1960;83:609–37.

Salk, J. E., U. Krech, J. S. Youngner, M. B. Bennett, L. J. Lewis, and P. L. Bazeley. Formaldehyde Treatment and Safety Testing of Experimental Poliomyelitis Vaccines. *Am J Public Health Nations Health.* 1954;44:563–70.

Salk, J. E., L. J. Lewis, J. S. Youngner, and B. L. Bennett. The Use of Adjuvants to Facilitate Studies on the Immunologic Classification of Poliomyelitis Viruses. *Amer J Hyg* 1951;54:157–73.

Salk, J. E., W. J. Menke, and T. Francis, Jr. A Clinical, Epidemiological and Immunological Evaluation of Vaccination against Epidemic Influenza. *Am J Hyg.* 1945;42:57–93.

Salk, J. E., H. E. Pearson, P. N. Brown, and T. Francis, Jr. Protective Effect of Vaccination against Induced Influenza B. *J Clin Invest.* 1945;24:547–53.

Salk, J., and D. Salk. Control of Influenza and Poliomyelitis with Killed Virus Vaccines. *Science.* 1977;195:834–47.

Salk, Jonas, and Jonathan Salk. *World Population and Human Values: A New Reality.* New York: Harper & Row, 1981.

Salk, J. E., and P. C. Suriano. Importance of Antigenic Composition of Influenza Virus Vaccine in Protecting against the Natural Disease. *Am J Public Health Nations Health.* 1949;39:345–55.

Salk, J., and E. N. Ward. Some Characteristics of a Continuously Propagating Cell Derived from Monkey Heart Tissue. *Science.* 1957;126:1338–39.

Salk, J. E., J. M. Wilbur, and T. Francis, Jr. Identification of Influenza Virus Type A in Current Outbreak of Respiratory Disease. *JAMA.* 1944;124:93.

Salk, J. E., J. S. Youngner, and E. N. Ward. Use of Color Change of Phenol Red as the Indicator in Titrating Poliomyelitis Virus or Its Antibody in a Tissue-Culture System. *Amer J Hyg.* 1954;60(2):214–30.

Salk, Lee. *My Father, My Son.* New York: G. P. Putnam's Sons, 1982.

Schlesinger, R. W., I. M. Morgan, and P. K. Olitsky. Transmission to Rodents of Lansing Type Poliomyelitis Virus in the Middle East. *Science* 1943;98:452–54.

Schonberger, L. B, D. J. Bregman, J. Z. Sullivan-Bolyal, et al. Gulllain-Barre Syndrome Following Vaccination in the National Influenza Immunization Program, United States, 1976–1977. *Am J Epidemiol.* 1979;110:105–23.

Seavey, Nina Gilden, Jane S. Smith, and Paul Wagner. *A Paralyzing Fear: The Triumph over Polio in America.* New York: TV Books, 1998.

Seytre, Bernard, and Mary Shaffer. *The Death of a Disease: A History of the Eradication of Poliomyelitis.* New Brunswick, NJ: Rutgers University Press, 2005.

Shapiro, C. S. Jacob Bronowski: A Retrospective. *Leonardo* 1985;18:215–22.

Shilts, Randy. *And the Band Played On: Politics, People, and the AIDS Epidemic.* New York: St. Martin's, 1987.

Shimkin, M. B. Leonell C. Strong, 1894–1982. *Cancer Res.* 1984;44:2740.

Shorter, Edward. *The Health Century.* New York: Doubleday, 1987.

Sills, David L. *The Volunteers.* Glencoe, IL: Free Press, 1957.

Silver, Julie, and Daniel Wilson. *Polio Voices: An Oral History from the American Polio Epidemics and Worldwide Eradication Efforts.* Westport, CT: Praeger, 2007.

Smith, Jane S. *Patenting the Sun.* New York: William Morrow, 1990.

Smith, W., C. H. Andrewes, and P. P. Laidlaw. A Virus Obtained from Influenza Patients. *Lancet.* 1933;222:66–68.

Stoller, Ezra. *The Salk Institute.* New York: Princeton Architectural Press, 1999.

Thomas, Gwyn. *A Few Selected Exits.* Boston: Little, Brown, 1968.

Timiras, P. S. Remembrance: Elizabeth Roboz Einstein (1904–1995). *Neurochemical Research.* 1995;20:885.

Trauger. R. J., F. Ferre, A. E. Daigle, et al. Effect of Immunization with Inactivated gp120-Depleted Human Immunodeficiency Virus Type 1 (HIV-1) Immunogen on HIV-1 Immunity, Viral DNA and Percentage of CD4 Cells. *JID.* 1994;169: 1256–64.

Troan, John. *Passport to Adventure.* Pittsburgh, PA: Neworks Press, 2000.

Vaughan, Victor C. *A Doctor's Memories.* Indianapolis: Bobbs-Merrill, 1926.

Wade, N. Salk Institute: Elitist Pursuit of Biology with a Conscience. *Science.* 1972;178:846–49.

Walsh, J. Two Cultures. *Science.* 1959;130:652–54.

Watson, James D. *The Double Helix.* New York: Atheneum, 1968.

Weller, Thomas H. *Growing Pathogens in Tissue Cultures.* Canton, MA: Science History Publications, 2004.

Williams, Greer. *Virus Hunters.* New York: Alfred A. Knopf, 1959.

Wilson, John Rowan. *Margin of Safety.* Garden City, NY: Doubleday, 1963.

Wiseman, Carter. *Louis I. Kahn, Beyond Time and Style: A Life in Architecture.* New York: W. W. Norton, 2007.

Woolley, P. G. The Epidemic of Influenza at Camp Devens, Mass. *J Lab Clin Med.* 1919;4:330–43.

Youngner, J. S., E. N. Ward, and J. E. Salk. Studies on Poliomyelitis Viruses in Cultures of Monkey Testicular Tissue: I. Propagation of Viruses in Roller Tubes. *Amer J Hyg.* 1952;55(2):291–300.

AUTHOR'S INTERVIEWS

Abrahamson, Joan

Altman, Lawrence

Bailen-Rose, Frances

Bailey, Ethel

Baltimore, David

Bencken, Betsy

Beretich, Barbara

Berg, Paul

Bernstein, Isidor

Bloom, Floyd
Brostoff, Steven
Brown, Harriet Press
Bundy, Carol Anne
Carlos, Dennis
Cohen, Jon
Damasio, Antonio
Damin, Anita
DeHoff, John
Dribbon, Robert
Dribbon, Stanley
Drosd, Rudy
Dulbecco, Maureen
Dulbecco, Renato
Eckhart, Walter
Edelman, Gerald
Elkes, Joel
Fisher, Barnard
Fitzgerald, Faith
Flower, Michael
Forester, Christine
Francis, Mary Jane
Franken, Jessica
Friedman, Lorraine
Gallo, Robert
Gardner, Murray
Gildred, Theodore
Gilot, Françoise
Gitenstein, Seymour
Glanz, Delbert
Glavin, James
Glusman, Murray
Goldstein, Harold
Guillemin, Roger
Hamburg, David
Henderson, Brian
Hollingsworth, Rogers
Horney, Eva Seilitz
Hoth, Daniel
Hubbard, Barbara Marx
Ion, Heather Wood
Kahn, James
Katz, Samuel
Kees, Walter
Kessler, Eileen

Kimberlin, Kevin
Korr, David
Kraemer, Mortimer
Lasky, Lawrence
Lennox, Edwin
Levine, Alexandra
Longworth, Lisa
Luciw, Paul
MacAllister, Jack
Mack, June
Mack, Walter
Mandell, Arnold
Massey, Charles
Mohns, Theodore
Moses, Campbell
Moss, Ronald
Murray, Kathleen
Nathan, Murray
Nathanson, Neal
Norwick, Sydney
Paley, Ethel Schneider
Richieri, Steven
Robinson, Barbara
Rose, David
Rosenfeld, Albert
Sabin, Debbe
Salk, Darrell (brief conversation)
Salk, Jonathan
Salk, Mary Jane
Salk, Peter
Salk, Sylvia
Sechzer, Philip
Seil, Frederick
Seligmann, Arthur
Selikov, Anne
Selnik, Ann
Shearer, Gene
Stimpert, Audrey
Strumpf, Paul
Terzo, Frederick
Wegemer, Donald
Westall, Fred
Whelan, Patrick
Zuckerman, Herman

Index

O'Connor, Daniel Basil (*continued*)
and Sabin, 194–95, 224, 334, 390
and Salk Institute board of
trustees, 244
and Salk Institute concept, 232–33
and Salk Institute design and
construction, 237, 252, 256,
257, 260
and Salk Institute fellows, 241–42
and Salk Institute funding, 246–47,
249, 264, 330–31
and Salk Institute's funding withdrawn,
331–32
and Salk Institute's name, 246–47,
257, 334
and Salk's depression, 229, 334
and Salk's divorce and remarriage,
307, 335
and Salk's lifestyle, 278
Salk's productive/close relationship
with, 91–93, 127, 142, 172, 211, 334,
340, 409
Salk's strained relationship with, 266,
267, 269, 273, 294, 298, 332–35
and scientific community, 211
and Slater's leadership, 326, 328–29
on success of organization, 179
and Vaccine Advisory Committee,
154–55
and volunteers of polio vaccine field
trials, 146
and Weaver, 74–75, 123–24
wife's death, 195
See also National Foundation (NF);
National Foundation for Infantile
Paralysis (NFIP)
O'Connor, Elvira, 195
O'Connor, Hazel Royall, 207, 235
O'Connor, Sheelagh, 334–35
Olitsky, Peter, 77
"Operational Memoranda," 146
oral poliovirus vaccine (OPV)
advantages of, 382
advocates for, 219–20
Bodian's position on, 385

and cases of polio infection, 221–22,
223, 226–27, 372, 378–79, 381, 382,
383, 386–87, 394, 447
field trials for, 220–22
and herd immunity, 382, 383
immunity provided by, 219
lawsuits following infections from, 372,
379–80, 382, 386–87
and lifetime immunity question, 212,
225, 382
oral administration of, 219
and policy-making groups, 384,
385–87, 391–92
revaccinations with, 225, 226, 227
and reversion to virulence concerns,
220, 221, 224, 383
and "Sabin Oral Sunday" campaign,
223, 226
Salk's concerns about safety of, 381,
383, 385, 391
in subtropical regions, 394
wide-spread acceptance of, 373, 446
Order of the Quetzal, Guatemala, 175
Orgel, Leslie, 263, 268, 347, 357
Oshinsky, David, 209, 213
Ousley, H., 353

Paley, Karl, 22
Paradise Lost (Milton), 281
Parenting, 455
Parents Magazine, 50
Park, William, 99
Parke, Davis and Company
conspiracy and price-fixing charges
against, 216
contaminated vaccine batches from,
138–39
and Cutter affair, 189
and influenza vaccine, 47, 60, 61, 62
initial distribution of polio vaccine, 180
and polio vaccine production, 132–33,
138, 144
Salk's relationship with, 49
and swine flu vaccine, 368, 372
and tuberculosis results, 137

women in Salk's life
  extramarital relationships, 279, 280,
    282–86, 410–21 (*see also* Hubbard,
    Barbara Marx)
  wives (*see* Gilot, Françoise; Salk, Donna)
  See also Friedman, Lorraine
Woodward-Baltimore, Sandra, 267–68
work ethic of Salk, 15, 45, 57, 93–94,
    133–34, 434
Workman, William
  and Ann Arbor symposium, 166, 167
  and Cutter affair, 183
  and field trial for polio vaccine, 138
  and licensure of polio vaccine, 137,
    167, 196
  and Merthiolate mandate, 153–54
  retirement of, 196
World Health Organization (WHO)
  immunization goals of, 407
  and Sabin's Russian trial, 222
  and Salk's concerns about live virus
    vaccine, 391
  Stockholm conference, 198–99
World Health Organization's Expert
    Committee on Influenza, 60
*World Population and Human Values:
    A New Reality* (Salk), 407–8
World Telegram, 135
Wright, Jessie, 107, 165
writings and publications of Salk
  on AIDS vaccine research, 434
  Anatomy of Reality, 408
  Man Unfolding, 317–18, 320, 408
  The Millennium of the Mind, 416
  papers, 23, 50, 51, 84, 89–90,
    150–52, 313

"Polio: The Cure for the New
    Controversy", 380
The Survival of the Wisest, 319–20, 321,
    362, 408
"The Use of Adjuvants to Facilitate
    Studies on the Immunologic
    Classification of Poliomyelitis
    Virus", 84
*World Population and Human Values:
    A New Reality* , 407–8
writing style of Salk, 119, 407–8, 457
  See also correspondence of Salk;
    night-notes
Wyeth Laboratories, 368, 379, 384

Yale Medical Journal, 65
Yang, Chen Ning "Frank," 402–3
yellow fever, 24, 39, 46, 65, 141
Youmans, John, 225
Young, Robert, 71
Youngner, Julius
  and Ann Arbor symposium, 209
  criticisms of Salk, 133, 209–10,
    457–58
  and *JAMA* article, 119
  laboratory work of, 83
  and publishing results of research, 90
  relationship with Salk, 81
  resignation of, 210
  and Salk's crediting of team, 210
  and vaccine development, 102–3
Ypsilanti State Hospital, 43–44, 46
Yurochko, Francis, 81

Zagury, Dan, 435
Zhdanov, Viktor, 225